Fourth Edition

MEDICAL ASSISTANT
CARDIOPULMONARY & ELECTROCARDIOGRAPHY—MODULE D

Material selected from:

Essentials of Medical Assisting: Administrative and Clinical Competencies
by Bonnie F. Fremgen

Medical Terminology with Human Anatomy, Fourth Edition
by Jane Rice

Structure & Function of the Human Body
by Frederic H. Martini and Edwin F. Bartholomew

Workbook
by Bonnie F. Fremgen and Kathleen Wallington
for *Essentials of Medical Assisting: Administrative and Clinical Competencies*
by Bonnie F. Fremgen

Medical Assistant Test Review Programmed Learner
by Bonnie F. Fremgen, Kathleen Wallington, and Mary King

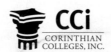

CCi
CORINTHIAN
COLLEGES, INC.

Learning Solutions

New York   Boston   San Francisco
London   Toronto   Sydney   Tokyo   Singapore   Madrid
Mexico City   Munich   Paris   Cape Town   Hong Kong   Montreal

Cover Art: Courtesy of Getty Images, Inc.

Excerpts taken from:

Essentials of Medical Assisting: Administrative and Clinical Competencies
by Bonnie F. Fremgen
Copyright © 1998 by Pearson Education, Inc.
Published by Prentice Hall
Upper Saddle River, New Jersey 07458

Medical Terminology with Human Anatomy, Fourth Edition
by Jane Rice
Copyright © 1999, 1995, 1991 by Appleton & Lange
Published by Prentice Hall

Structure & Function of the Human Body
by Frederic H. Martini and Edwin F. Bartholomew
Copyright © 1999 by Frederic H. Martini, Inc.
Published by Prentice Hall

Workbook
by Bonnie F. Fremgen and Kathleen Wallington
for *Essentials of Medical Assisting: Administrative and Clinical Competencies*
by Bonnie F. Fremgen
Copyright © 1998 by Pearson Education, Inc.
Published by Prentice Hall

Medical Assistant Test Review Programmed Learner
by Bonnie F. Fremgen, Kathleen Wallington, and Mary King
Copyright © 1999 by Pearson Education, Inc.
Published by Prentice Hall

Pearson Learning Solutions, 501 Boylston Street, Suite 900, Boston, MA 02116
A Pearson Education Company
www.pearsoned.com

Printed in the United States of America

3 4 5 6 7 8 9 10 V011 14 13 12 11 10

2009380079

KW/SB

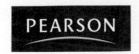

ISBN 10: 0-558-58509-4
ISBN 13: 978-0-558-58509-9

Credits and Acknowledgments

CCi Medical Assistant Program Series (Modules A-G)

Publisher

Pearson Learning Solutions in cooperation with Corinthian Colleges, Inc.

Editors and Project Managers

Alicia Mata, BSBM, CMA, Allied Health Program Manager, CCi

Kathy Case, MSN, RN, Program Manager Health Sciences

Donna Patterson, AA, CMA, Program Coordinator

Authors

Cheryl Niblett, CMA, BSC, Medical Assistant Program Chair

Kellie Stock, CMA, Medical Assistant Instructor

Ted Volkmann, BS, Mathematics

Shaun Holland, CMA, Lead Medical Assistant Instructor

Tanya Mercer, Medical Assistant Instructor

Irma Blanco, BS, Director of Education

Blanca Zepeda, AA, CMA, Medical Assistant Program Chair

Vince Dick, Medical Assistant Instructor

Claudia Chaparro, AA, CMA, Medical Assistant Instructor

Sally Stegmeier, CMA, Medical Assistant Instructor

Berta Williams, NRCMA, Director of Education

Brad Johnson, Medical Assistant Program Chair

Jennifer Montoya, Medical Assistant Instructor

Steve Dovalina, CMA, Medical Assistant Instructor

Gwen Schrader, Medical Assistant Program Chair

Christine Cusano, AA, CMA, Medical Assistant & Medical Administrative Assistant Instructor

Maria Leal, Allied Health Instructor

Rachael Washington, Placement Representative

Amanda Gaugler, BS, Director of Education

Niki Good, BA Education, School President

Jacqueline Ferguson, BA, Academic Dean

Joan Jeong, BA, AA, CMA, Medical Program Director

John Etheridge, Medical Assistant Program Chair

Judith Enlow, CMA, Medical Assistant Instructor and Program Chair

Marchelle (Mickey) Weaver, BSBA, Director of Education

Kathryn Cremeans, Medical Assistant Program Chair

Sandra Shepherd, Medical Assistant Instructor

Dorit Soltanovich, MD, Medical Program Director

Dottie Fields, RMA, Education Chair, Medical Assistant and Medical Administrative Assistant Programs

Ron Mendez, Program Chair Medical Assisting Instructor, B.S. Medical Technology, NCMA, CPT1

Doris R. Owens, Medical Assisting Instructor, AA, CMA, CCTC, CAHA, NRPT

Donna McCord, Medical Assisting Instructor, CMA, CPT 1

Shirley Marie Crews, Medical Assisting & Coding/Billing Instructor, CCMA A-C, NCPT, X-ray Technician

Dora Perez, Medical Program Chair, BS, CMA

CONTENTS

3. MEDICAL TERMINOLOGY OF THE RESPIRATORY SYSTEM 81

Material selected from: *Medical Terminology with Human Anatomy*, Fourth Edition
by Jane Rice

Section One
MEDICAL TERMINOLOGY AND ANATOMY AND PHYSIOLOGY

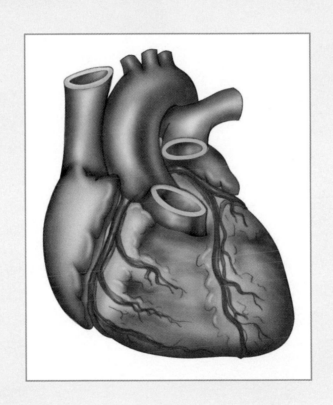

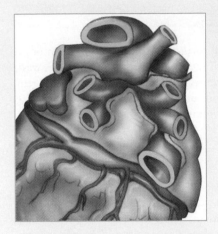

1

MEDICAL TERMINOLOGY OF THE CARDIOVASCULAR SYSTEM

- Anatomy and Physiology Overview
- The Heart
- The Flow of Blood
- Arteries
- Blood Pressure
- Veins
- Capillaries
- Life Span Considerations
- Terminology With Surgical Procedures & Pathology
- Vocabulary Words
- Abbreviations
- Drug Highlights
- Diagnostic and Laboratory Tests
- Communication Enrichment
- Study and Review Section
    Learning Exercises
    Word Parts Study Sheet
    Review Questions
    Critical Thinking Activity

OBJECTIVES

On completion of this chapter, you should be able to:

- Describe the cardiovascular system.

- Describe and state the functions of arteries, veins, and capillaries.

- Describe cardiovascular differences of the child and the older adult.

- Identify the commonly used pulse checkpoints of the body.

- Describe blood pressure.

- Analyze, build, spell, and pronounce medical words that relate to surgical procedures and pathology.

- Identify and give the meaning of selected vocabulary words.

- Identify and define selected abbreviations.

- Review Drug Highlights presented in this chapter.

- Provide the description of diagnostic and laboratory tests related to the cardiovascular system.

- Successfully complete the study and review section.

▶ ANATOMY AND PHYSIOLOGY OVERVIEW

Through the cardiovascular system, blood is circulated to all parts of the body by the action of the heart. This process provides the body's cells with oxygen and nutritive elements and removes waste materials and carbon dioxide. The *heart,* a muscular pump, is the central organ of the system, which also includes *arteries, veins,* and *capillaries.* The various organs and components of the cardiovascular system are described in this chapter, along with some of their functions.

▶ THE HEART

The *heart* is a four-chambered, hollow muscular pump that circulates blood throughout the cardiovascular system. The heart is the center of the cardiovascular system from which the various blood vessels originate and later return. It is slightly larger than a man's fist and weighs approximately 300 g in the average adult male. It lies slightly to the left of the midline of the body and is shaped like an inverted cone with its apex downward. The heart has three layers or linings:

Endocardium. The inner lining of the heart
Myocardium. The muscular, middle layer of the heart
Pericardium. The outer, membranous sac surrounding the heart

CHAMBERS OF THE HEART

The human heart acts as a double pump and is divided into the right and left heart by a partition called the *septum.* Each side contains an upper and lower chamber. The *atria* or upper chambers are separated by the interatrial septum. The *ventricles* or lower chambers are separated by the interventricular septum. The atria receive blood from the various parts of the body, whereas the ventricles pump blood to body parts. A description of the heart's four chambers and some of their functions is given below.

The Right Atrium

The right upper portion of the heart is called the *right atrium.* It is a thin-walled space that receives blood from all body parts except the lungs. Two large veins bring the blood into the right atrium and are known as the superior and inferior vena cavae.

THE CARDIOVASCULAR SYSTEM

ORGAN/STRUCTURE	PRIMARY FUNCTIONS
Heart	Hollow muscular pump that circulates blood throughout the cardiovascular system
Arteries	Branching system of vessels that transports blood from the right and left ventricles of the heart to all body parts
Veins	Vessels that transport blood from peripheral tissues to the heart
Capillaries	Microscopic blood vessels that connect arterioles with venules; facilitate passage of life-sustaining fluids containing oxygen and nutrients to cell bodies and the removal of accumulated waste and carbon dioxide

The Right Ventricle

The right lower portion of the heart is called the *right ventricle*. It receives blood from the right atrium through the atrioventricular valve and pumps it through a semilunar valve to the lungs.

The Left Atrium

The left upper portion of the heart is called the *left atrium*. It receives blood rich in oxygen as it returns from the lungs via the left and right pulmonary veins.

The Left Ventricle

The left lower portion of the heart is called the *left ventricle*. It receives blood from the left atrium through an atrioventricular valve and pumps it through a semilunar valve to a large artery known as the aorta and from there to all parts of the body except the lungs.

HEART VALVES

The *valves* of the heart are located at the entrance and exit of each ventricle. The functions of each of the four heart valves are described below.

The Tricuspid Valve

The *right atrioventricular* or *tricuspid valve* guards the opening between the atrium and the right ventricle. The tricuspid valve allows the flow of blood into the ventricle and prevents its return to the right atrium.

The Pulmonary Semilunar Valve

The exit point for blood leaving the right ventricle is called the *pulmonary semilunar valve*. Located between the right ventricle and the pulmonary artery, it allows blood to flow from the right ventricle through the pulmonary artery to the lungs.

The Bicuspid or Mitral Valve

The left atrioventricular valve between the left atrium and ventricle is called the *bicuspid* or *mitral valve*. It allows blood to flow to the left ventricle and closes to prevent its return to the left atrium.

The Aortic Semilunar Valve

Blood exits from the left ventricle through the *aortic semilunar valve*. Located between the left ventricle and the aorta, it allows blood to flow into the aorta and prevents its return to the ventricle.

VASCULAR SYSTEM OF THE HEART

Due to the membranous lining of the heart *(endocardium)* and the thickness of the myocardium, it is essential that the heart have its own vascular system. The coronary arteries supply the heart with blood, and the cardiac veins, draining into the coronary sinus, collect the blood and return it to the right atrium (Fig. 1–1).

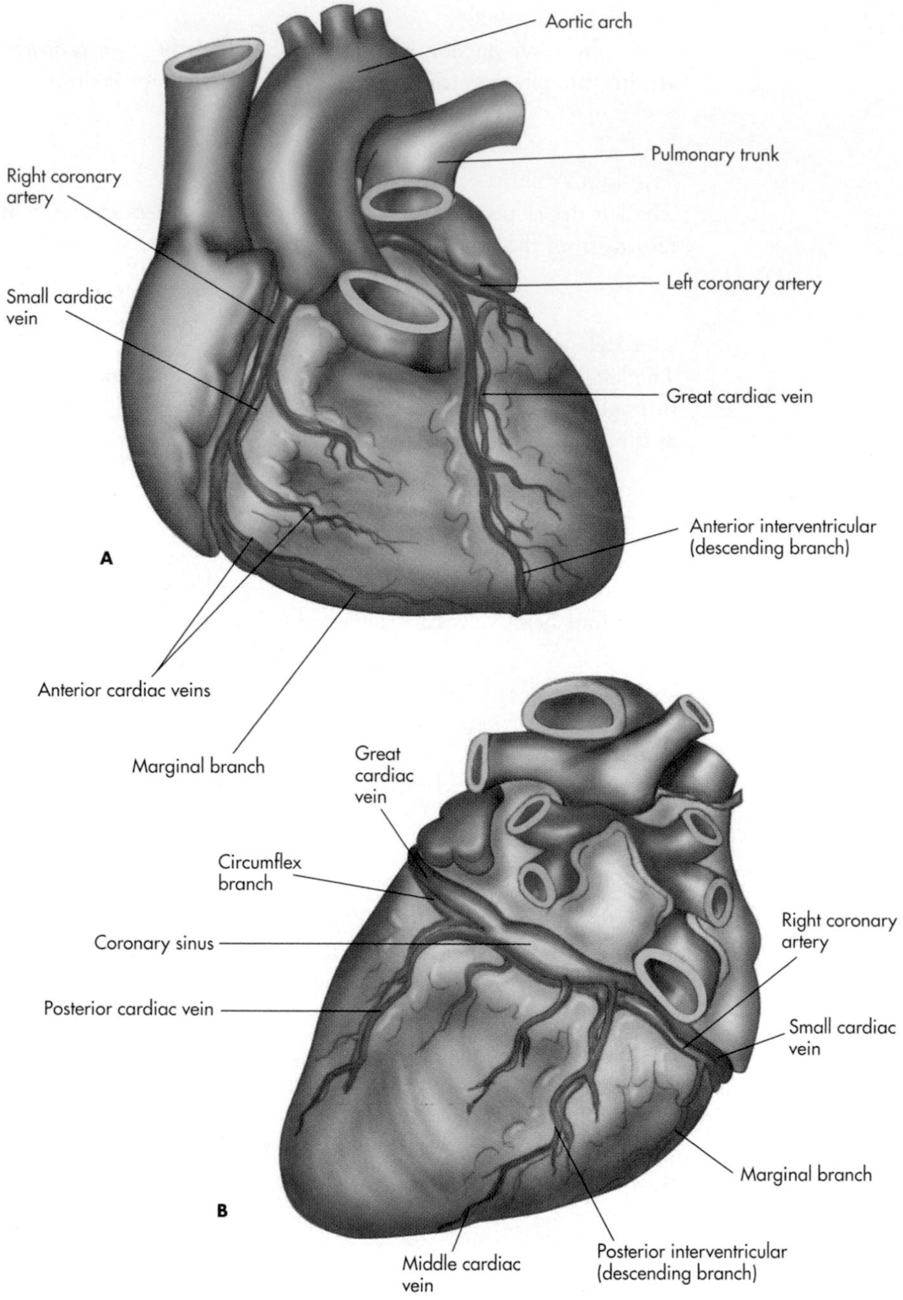

FIGURE 1–1

Coronary circulation. **(A)** Coronary vessels portraying the complexity and extent of the coronary circulation. **(B)** Coronary vessels that supply the anterior surface of the heart.

► THE FLOW OF BLOOD

Blood flows through the heart, to the lungs, back to the heart, and on to the various body parts as indicated in Figure 1–2. Blood from the superior and inferior vena cavae enters the right atrium and subsequently passes through the tricuspid valve and into the right ventricle, which pumps it through the pulmonary semilunar valve into the left and right pulmonary arteries, which carry it to the lungs. In the lungs, the blood gives up wastes and takes on oxygen as it passes through cap-

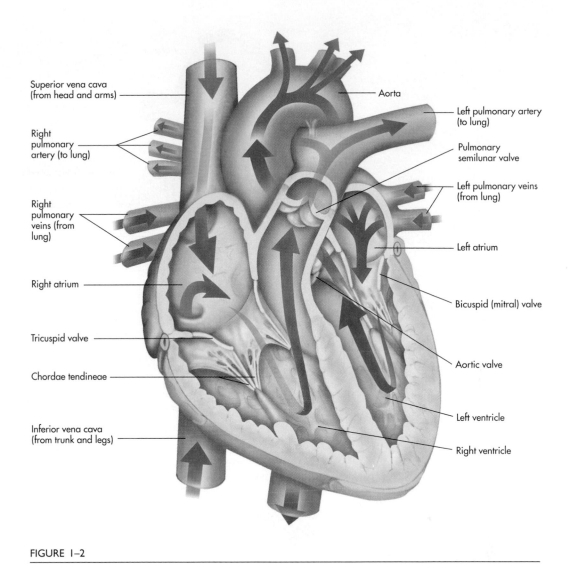

Superior vena cava
(from head and arms)

Aorta

Left pulmonary artery
(to lung)

Right
pulmonary
artery (to lung)

Pulmonary
semilunar valve

Left pulmonary veins
(from lung)

Right
pulmonary
veins (from
lung)

Left atrium

Right atrium

Bicuspid (mitral) valve

Tricuspid valve

Aortic valve

Chordae tendineae

Left ventricle

Inferior vena cava
(from trunk and legs)

Right ventricle

FIGURE 1–2

The flow of blood through the heart.

illaries into veins. Blood leaves the lungs through the left and right pulmonary veins, which carry it to the heart's left atrium. The oxygenated blood then passes through the bicuspid or mitral valve into the left ventricle, which pumps it out through the aortic valve and into the *aorta*. This large artery supplies a branching system of smaller arteries that connect to tiny capillaries throughout the body.

Capillaries are microscopic blood vessels with thin walls that allow the passage of oxygen and nutrients to the body and let the blood pick up waste and carbon dioxide. Veins lead away from the capillaries as tiny vessels and increase in size until they join the superior and inferior vena cavae as they return to the heart.

THE HEARTBEAT

The *heartbeat* is controlled by the autonomic nervous system. It is normally generated by specialized neuromuscular tissue of the heart that is capable of causing cardiac muscle to contract rhythmically. The neuromuscular tissue of the heart comprises the *sinoatrial node,* the *atrioventricular node,* and the *atrioventricular bundle* (Fig. 1–3).

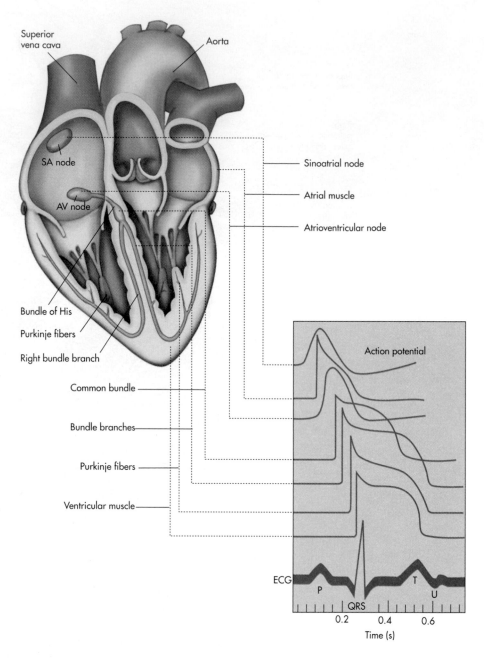

FIGURE 1–3

The conduction system of the heart. Action potentials for the SA and AV nodes, other parts of the conduction system, and the atrial and ventricular muscles are shown along with the correlation to recorded electrical activity (electrocardiogram ECG [EKG]).

Sinoatrial Node (SA Node)

Often called the *pacemaker of the heart*, the *SA node* is located in the upper wall of the right atrium, just below the opening of the superior vena cava. It consists of a dense network of *Purkinje fibers (atypical muscle fibers)* considered to be the source of impulses initiating the heartbeat. Electrical impulses discharged by the SA node are distributed to the right and left atria and cause them to contract.

Atrioventricular Node (AV Node)

Located beneath the endocardium of the right atrium, the *AV node* transmits electrical impulses to the *bundle of His (atrioventricular bundle)*.

Atrioventricular Bundle (Bundle of His)

The *bundle of His* forms a part of the conducting system of the heart. It extends from the AV node into the intraventricular septum, where it divides into two branches within the two ventricles. The *Purkinje system* includes the bundle of His and the peripheral fibers. These fibers end in the ventricular muscles, where the excitation of muscle is initiated, causing contraction. The average heartbeat *(pulse)* is between 60 and 100 beats per minute for the average adult. The rate of heartbeat may be affected by emotions, smoking, disease, body size, age, stress, the environment, and many other factors.

ELECTROCARDIOGRAM

An *electrocardiogram* (ECG, EKG) records the electrical activity of the heart. A standard electrocardiogram consists of 12 different leads. With electrodes placed on the patient's arms, legs, and six positions on the chest, a 12-lead ECG can be recorded. The leads that are recorded on an electrocardiograph are I, II, III, aVR, aVL, aVF, and six chest leads V_1, V_2, V_3, V_4, V_5, and V_6. The standard limb leads, leads I, II, and III, each record the differences in potential between two limbs. Augmented limb leads, aVR, aVL, and aVF, record between one limb and the other two limbs. There are six unipolar chest leads that record electrical activity of different parts of the heart. An ECG provides valuable information in the diagnosing of cardiac abnormalities, such as myocardial damage and arrhythmias (Fig. 1–4).

▶ ARTERIES

The *arteries* constitute a branching system of vessels that transports blood from the right and left ventricles of the heart to all body parts (Table 1–1, and Fig. 1–5). In a normal state, arteries are elastic tubes that recoil and carry blood in pulsating waves. All arteries have a pulse, reflecting the rhythmical beating of the heart; however, certain points are commonly used to check the rate, rhythm, and condition of the arterial wall. These checkpoints are listed below and shown in Figure 1–6.

Radial. Located on the radial *(thumb side)* of the wrist. This is the most common site for taking a pulse

Brachial. Located in the antecubital space of the elbow. This is the most common site used to check blood pressure

Carotid. Located in the neck. In an emergency *(cardiac arrest),* this site is the most readily accessible

Temporal. Located at the temple

Femoral. Located in the groin

Popliteal. Located behind the knee

Dorsalis pedis. Located on the upper surface of the foot

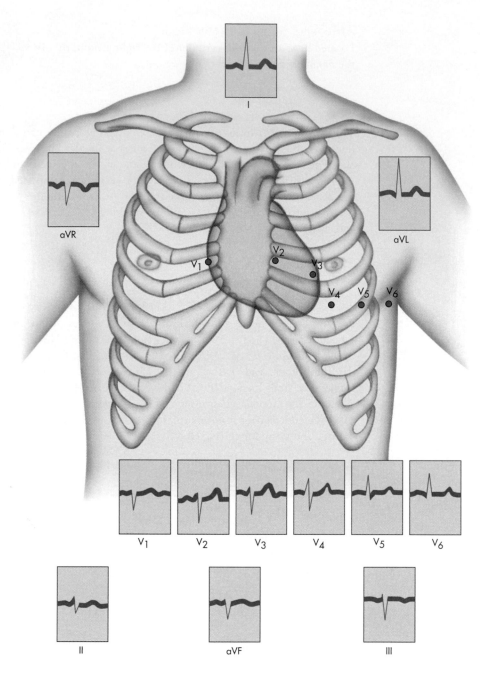

FIGURE 1–4

A normal electrocardiogram (ECG [EKG]).

▶ BLOOD PRESSURE

Blood pressure, generally speaking, is the pressure exerted by the blood on the walls of the vessels. The term most commonly refers to the pressure exerted in large arteries at the peak of the pulse wave. This pressure is measured with a *sphygmomanometer* used in concert with a *stethoscope*. Pressure is reported in millimeters of mercury as observed on a graduated column. With the use of a pressure cuff, circulation is interrupted in the brachial artery just above the elbow. Pressure from the cuff is shown on the graduated column of the sphygmomanometer, and as the pressure is released,

TABLE 1–1   Selected Arteries

Artery	Tissue Supplied
Right common carotid	Right side of the head and neck
Left common carotid	Left side of the head and neck
Left subclavian	Left upper extremity
Brachiocephalic	Head and arm
Aortic arch	Branches to head, neck, and upper extremities
Celiac	Stomach, spleen, and liver
Renal	Kidneys
Superior mesenteric	Lower half of large intestine
Inferior mesenteric	Small intestines and first half of the large intestine
Axillary	Axilla
Brachial	Arm
Radial	Lateral side of the hand
Ulnar	Medial side of the hand
Internal iliac	Pelvic viscera and rectum
External iliac	Genitalia and lower trunk muscles
Deep femoral	Deep thigh muscles
Femoral	Thigh
Popliteal	Leg and foot
Anterior tibial	Leg
Dorsalis pedis	Foot

blood again flows past the cuff. At this point, using a stethoscope, one hears a heartbeat and records the systolic pressure. Continued release of pressure results in a change in the heartbeat sound from loud to soft, at which point one records the diastolic pressure. This method results in a ratio of systolic over diastolic readings expressed in millimeters of mercury (mm Hg). In the average adult, the systolic pressure usually ranges from 100 to 140 mm Hg and the diastolic from 60 to 90 mm Hg. A typical blood pressure showing systolic over diastolic readings might be expressed as 120/80. Two types of sphygmomanometers are shown in Figure 1–7.

PULSE PRESSURE

The *pulse pressure* is the difference between the systolic and diastolic readings. This reading is an indication of the tone of the arterial walls. The normal pulse pressure is found when the systolic pressure is about 40 points higher than the diastolic reading. For example, if the blood pressure is 120/80, the pulse pressure would be 40.

▶ VEINS

The vessels that transport blood from peripheral tissues to the heart are the *veins* (see Table 1–2, and Fig. 1–8). In a normal state, veins have thin walls and valves that prevent the backflow of blood. Veins are the vessels used when blood is removed for analysis. The process of removing blood from a vein is called *venipuncture*.

▶ CAPILLARIES

The *capillaries* are microscopic blood vessels with single-celled walls that connect *arterioles* (small arteries) with *venules* (small veins). Blood, passing through capillaries, gives up the oxygen and nutrients carried to this point by the arteries and picks up waste and carbon dioxide as it enters veins. The extremely thin walls of capillaries facilitate passage of life-sustaining fluids containing oxygen and nutrients to cell bodies and the removal of accumulated waste and carbon dioxide.

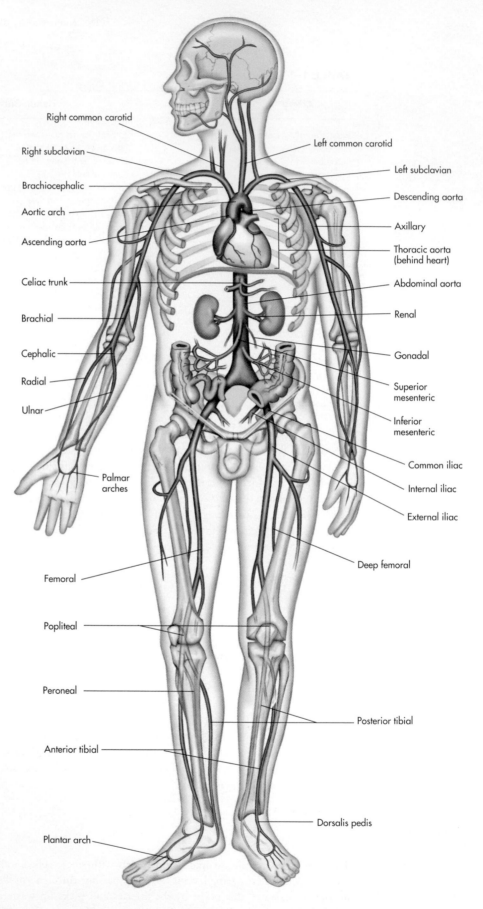

Right common carotid

Right subclavian

Brachiocephalic

Aortic arch

Ascending aorta

Celiac trunk

Brachial

Cephalic

Radial

Ulnar

Palmar arches

Femoral

Popliteal

Peroneal

Anterior tibial

Plantar arch

Left common carotid

Left subclavian

Descending aorta

Axillary

Thoracic aorta (behind heart)

Abdominal aorta

Renal

Gonadal

Superior mesenteric

Inferior mesenteric

Common iliac

Internal iliac

External iliac

Deep femoral

Posterior tibial

Dorsalis pedis

FIGURE 1–5

An overview of the arterial system.

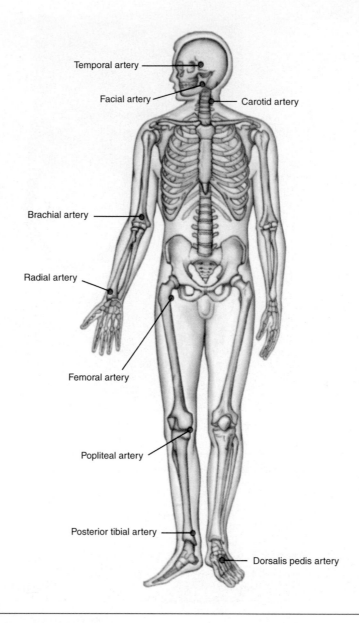

Temporal artery

Facial artery

Carotid artery

Brachial artery

Radial artery

Femoral artery

Popliteal artery

Posterior tibial artery

Dorsalis pedis artery

FIGURE 1–6

The primary pulse points of the body.

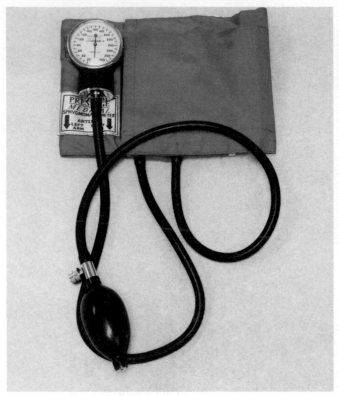
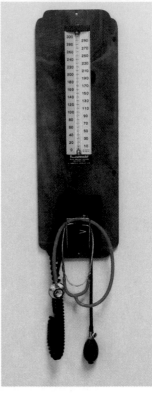

A   B

FIGURE 1–7

Sphygmomanometers: **(A)** aneroid type, **(B)** mercury type.

TABLE 1–2   Selected Veins

Vein	Tissue Drained
External jugular	Superficial tissues of the head and neck
Internal jugular	Sinuses of the brain
Subclavian	Upper extremities
Superior vena cava	Head, neck, and upper extremities
Inferior vena cava	Lower body
Hepatic	Liver
Hepatic portal	Liver and gallbladder
Superior mesenteric	Small intestine and most of the colon
Inferior mesenteric	Descending colon and rectum
Cephalic	Lateral arm
Axillary	Axilla and arm
Basilic	Medial arm
External iliac	Lower limb
Internal iliac	Pelvic viscera
Femoral	Thigh
Great saphenous	Leg
Popliteal	Lower leg
Peroneal	Foot
Anterior tibial	Deep anterior leg and dorsal foot

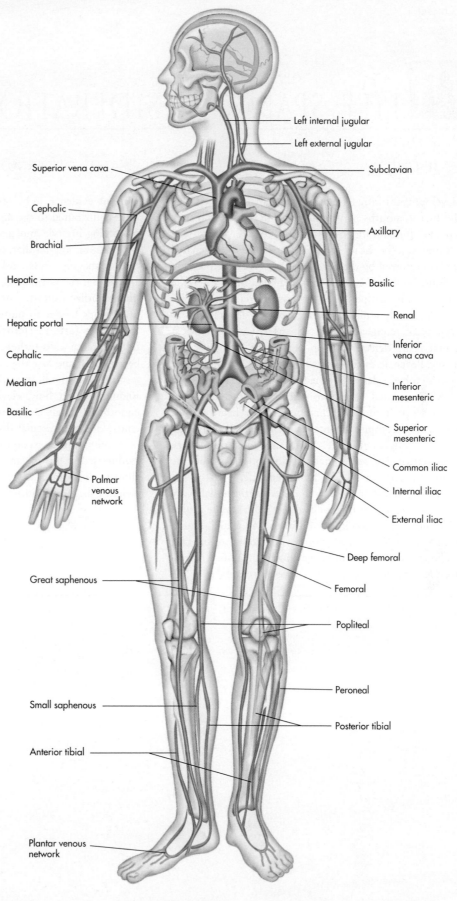

Left internal jugular

Left external jugular

Superior vena cava

Subclavian

Cephalic

Axillary

Brachial

Hepatic

Basilic

Hepatic portal

Renal

Cephalic

Inferior vena cava

Median

Inferior mesenteric

Basilic

Superior mesenteric

Palmar venous network

Common iliac

Internal iliac

External iliac

Deep femoral

Great saphenous

Femoral

Popliteal

Peroneal

Small saphenous

Posterior tibial

Anterior tibial

Plantar venous network

FIGURE 1–8

An overview of the venous system.

LIFE SPAN CONSIDERATIONS

► THE CHILD

The development of the fetal heart is usually completed during the first 2 months of intrauterine life. It is completely formed and functioning by 10 weeks. At 16 weeks fetal heart tones can be heard with a **fetoscope.** Oxygenated blood is transported by the umbilical vein from the placenta to the fetus. Fetal circulation is terminated at birth when the umbilical cord is clamped. The newborn's circulation begins to function shortly after birth and if proper adaptations do not take place, congenital heart disease may occur. Most congenital heart defects develop before the 10th week of pregnancy. Pediatric cardiologists have recognized more than 50 congenital heart defects. If the left side of the heart is not completely separated from the right side, various septal defects develop. If the four chambers of the heart do not occur normally, complex anomalies form, such as tetralogy of Fallot, a congenital heart defect involving pulmonary stenosis, ventricular septal defect, dextroposition of the aorta, and hypertrophy of the right ventricle.

The **pulse, blood pressure,** and **respirations** will vary according to the age of the child. A newborn's pulse rate is irregular and rapid, varying from 120 to 140 beats/minute. Blood pressure is low and may vary with the size of the cuff used. The average blood pressure at birth is 80/46. The respirations are approximately 35 to 50 per minute.

► THE OLDER ADULT

Current evidence indicates that cardiac changes that were once contributed to the aging process may be minimized by modifying lifestyle and personal habits, such as following a low-sodium, low-fat diet, not smoking, drinking in moderation, managing stress, and exercising regularly. Studies have shown that the normal aging heart is able to provide an adequate cardiac output. But in some older adults, the heart must work harder to pump blood because of hardening of the arteries **(arteriosclerosis)** and a buildup of fatty plaques in the arterial walls **(atherosclerosis).** Arteries may gradually become stiff and lose their elastic recoil. The aorta and arteries supplying the heart and brain are generally affected first. Reduced blood flow, elevated blood lipids, and defective endothelial repair that can be seen in aging accelerate the course of cardiovascular disease.

Some common symptoms seen in the older adult with cardiovascular disease are confusion, syncope, palpitations, shortness of breath, dry, hacking cough, fatigue, chest pain, weight gain, and fluid retention, especially in the legs.

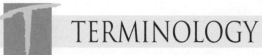

TERMINOLOGY

WITH SURGICAL PROCEDURES & PATHOLOGY

TERM	WORD PARTS			DEFINITION
anginal (ăn′ jĭ-năl)	angin al	R S	to choke, quinsy pertaining to	Pertaining to attacks of choking or suffocation
angioblast (ăn′ jĭ-ō-blăst)	angio blast	CF S	vessel immature cell, germ cell	The germ cell from which blood vessels develop
angiocardiog- raphy (ăn″ jĭ-ō-kăr″ dĭ-ŏg′ ră-fē)	angio cardio graphy	CF CF S	vessel heart recording	The process of recording the heart and vessels after an intravenous injection of a radiopaque solution
angiocarditis (ăn″ jĭ-ō-kăr-dī′ tĭs)	angio card itis	CF R S	vessel heart inflammation	Inflammation of the heart and its great vessels
angioma (ăn″ jĭ-ō′ mă)	angi oma	CF S	vessel tumor	A tumor of a blood vessel. See Figure 1–9.
angionecrosis (ăn″ jĭ-ō-nēc-rō′ sĭs)	angio necr osis	CF R S	vessel death condition of	A condition of the death of blood vessels
angiopathy (ăn″ jĭ-ŏp′ ă-thē)	angio pathy	CF S	vessel disease	Disease of blood vessels
angioplasty (ăn′ jĭ-ō-plăs″ tē)	angio plasty	CF S	vessel surgical repair	Surgical repair of a blood vessel or vessels
angiorrhaphy (ăn″ jĭ-or′ ă-fē)	angio rrhaphy	CF S	vessel suture	Suture of a blood vessel or vessels
angiospasm (ăn′ jĭ-ō-spăzm)	angio spasm	CF S	vessel contraction, spasm	Contraction or spasm of a blood vessel
angiostenosis (ăn″ jĭ-ō-stĕ-nō′ sĭs)	angio sten osis	CF R S	vessel narrowing condition of	A condition of narrowing of a blood vessel
aortitis (ā″ ōr-tī′ tĭs)	aort itis	R S	aorta inflammation	Inflammation of the aorta

continued

Terminology - continued

TERM	WORD PARTS			DEFINITION
aortomalacia (ā-ōr″ tō-mă-lā′ shĭ-ă)	aorto malacia	CF S	aorta softening	Softening of the walls of the aorta
arrhythmia (ă-rĭth′ mĭ-ă)	a rrhythm ia	P R S	lack of rhythm condition	A condition in which there is a lack of rhythm of the heartbeat
arterectomy (ăr″ tĕ-rĕk′ tō-mē)	arter ectomy	R S	artery excision	Surgical excision of an artery
arterial (ăr-tē′ rĭ-ăl)	arteri al	CF S	artery pertaining to	Pertaining to an artery
arteriolith (ăr-tĕ′ rĭ-ō-lĭth)	arterio lith	CF S	artery stone	An arterial stone
arteriosclerosis (ăr-tē″ rĭ-ō-sklĕ-rō′ sĭs)	arterio scler osis	CF R S	artery hardening condition of	A condition of hardening of an artery
arteriotome (ăr-tē′ rĭ-ō-tōm)	arterio tome	CF S	artery instrument to cut	An instrument used to cut an artery
arteriotomy (ăr″ tē-rĭ-ŏt′ ō-mē)	arterio tomy	CF S	artery incision	Incision into an artery
arteritis (ăr″ tĕ-rī′ tĭs)	arter itis	R S	artery inflammation	Inflammation of an artery. See Figure 1–10.
atheroma (ăth″ ĕr-ō′ mă)	ather oma	R S	fatty substance, porridge tumor	Tumor of an artery containing a fatty substance
atherosclerosis (ăth″ ĕr-ō-sklĕ-rō′ sĭs)	athero scler osis	CF R S	fatty substance, porridge hardening condition of	A condition of the arteries characterized by the buildup of fatty substances and hardening of the walls
atrioventricular (ăt″ rĭ-ō-vĕn-trĭk′ ū-lăr)	atrio ventricul ar	CF R S	atrium ventricle pertaining to	Pertaining to the atrium and the ventricle
bicuspid (bī-kŭs′ pĭd)	bi cuspid	P S	two point	Having two points or cusps; pertaining to the mitral valve

Terminology - continued

TERM	WORD PARTS			DEFINITION
bradycardia (brăd″ ĭ-kăr′ dĭ-ă)	brady card ia	P R S	slow heart condition	A condition of slow heartbeat
cardiac (kăr′ dĭ-ăk)	cardi ac	CF S	heart pertaining to	Pertaining to the heart
cardiocentesis (kăr″ dĭ-ō-sĕn-tē′ sĭs)	cardio centesis	CF S	heart surgical puncture	Surgical puncture of the heart
cardiodynia (kăr″ dĭ-ō-dĭn′ ĭ-ă)	cardio dynia	CF S	heart pain	Pain in the heart
cardiokinetic (kăr″ dĭ-ō-kĭ-nĕt′ ĭk)	cardio kinet ic	CF R S	heart motion pertaining to	Pertaining to heart motion
cardiologist (kăr-dē-ŏl′ ō-jĭst)	cardio log ist	CF R S	heart study of one who specializes	One who specializes in the study of the heart
cardiology (kăr″ dĭ-ōl′ ō-jē)	cardio logy	CF S	heart study of	The study of the heart
cardiomegaly (kăr″ dĭ-ō-mĕg′ ă-lē)	cardio megaly	CF S	heart enlargement, large	Enlargement of the heart
cardiometer (kăr″ dĭ-ōm′ ĕ-tĕr)	cardio meter	CF S	heart instrument to measure	An instrument used to measure the action of the heart
cardiopathy (kăr″ dĭ-ŏp′ ă-thē)	cardio pathy	CF S	heart disease	Heart disease
cardioplegia (kăr″ dĭ-ŏ-plē′ jĭ-ă)	cardio plegia	CF S	heart stroke, paralysis	Paralysis of the heart
cardioptosis (kăr″ dĭ-ō-tō′ sĭs)	cardio ptosis	CF S	heart prolapse, drooping	Prolapse of the heart; a downward displacement
cardiopulmonary (kăr″ dĭ-ō-pŭl′ mō-nĕr-ē)	cardio pulmonar y	CF R S	heart lung pertaining to	Pertaining to the heart and lungs

continued

Terminology - continued

TERM	WORD PARTS			DEFINITION
cardioscope (kăr′ dĭ-ō-skōp″)	cardio scope	CF S	heart instrument	An instrument used to examine the interior of the heart
cardiotonic (kăr″ dĭ-ō-tŏn′ ĭk)	cardio ton ic	CF R S	heart tone pertaining to	Pertaining to increasing the tone of the heart; a type of medication
cardiovascular (kăr″ dĭ-ō-văs′ kū-lar)	cardio vascul ar	CF R S	heart small vessel pertaining to	Pertaining to the heart and small blood vessels
carditis (kăr-dī′ tĭs)	card itis	R S	heart inflammation	Inflammation of the heart
constriction (kən-strĭk′ shən)	con strict ion	P R S	together, with to draw, to bind process	The process of drawing together as in the narrowing of a vessel
cyanosis (sī-ăn-ō′ sĭs	cyan osis	R S	dark blue condition of	A dark blue condition of the skin and mucus membranes caused by oxygen deficiency
dextrocardia (děks″ trō-kăr′ dĭ-ă)	dextro card ia	CF R S	to the right heart condition	The condition of the heart being on the right side of the body
electrocardio-graph (ē-lěk″ trō-kăr′ dĭ-ō-grăf)	electro cardio graph	CF CF S	electricity heart to write, record	A device used for recording the electrical impulses of the heart muscle
electrocardio-phonograph (ē-lěk″ trō-kăr″ dĭ-ō-fō′ nō-grăf)	electro cardio phono graph	CF CF CF S	electricity heart sound to write, record	A device used to record heart sounds
embolism (ěm′ bō-lĭzm)	embol ism	R S	a throwing in condition of	A condition in which a blood clot obstructs a blood vessel; *a moving blood clot*
endarterectomy (ěn″ dăr-těr-ěk′ tō-mē)	end arter ectomy	P R S	within artery excision	Surgical excision of the inner portion of an artery
endocarditis (ěn″ dō-kăr-dī′ tĭs)	endo card itis	P R S	within heart inflammation	Inflammation of the endocardium

Terminology - continued

TERM	WORD PARTS			DEFINITION
endocardium (ĕn″ dō-kăr′ dē-ŭm)	endo cardi um	P CF S	within heart tissue	The inner lining of the heart
extrasystole (ĕks″ tră-sĭs′ tō-lē)	extra systole	P S	outside contraction	A cardiac contraction caused by an impulse arising outside the sinoatrial node
hemangiectasis (hē″ măn-jĭ-ĕk′ tă-sĭs)	hem angi ectasis	R CF S	blood vessel dilatation	Dilatation of a blood vessel
hemangioma (hē-măn″ jĭ-ō′ mă)	hem angi oma	R CF S	blood vessel tumor	A benign tumor of a blood vessel. See Figures 1–11 and 1–12.
hypertension (hī″ pĕr-tĕn′ shŭn)	hyper tens ion	P R S	excessive, above pressure process	High blood pressure; a disease of the arteries caused by such pressure

 TERMINOLOGY SPOTLIGHT

Hypertension is a medical term that is used to describe a blood pressure higher than normal: a systolic reading above 140 millimeter (mm) of mercury (Hg) and a diastolic reading above 90 mm Hg. With hypertension (HBP), the blood vessels can become tight and constricted. See Figure 1–13. These changes can cause the blood to press on the vessel walls with extra force. When this force exceeds a certain level and remains there, one has high blood pressure. Hypertension often has no symptoms and is frequently called "the silent killer," because if left untreated it can lead to kidney failure, stroke, heart attack, peripheral artery disease, and eye damage. See Figure 1–14. There are various factors that can contribute to developing hypertension (see Table 1–3).

Hypertension can be controlled by a variety of methods, such as taking blood pressure medicine as prescribed, seeing a physician on a regular basis, establishing healthy eating habits, exercising, avoiding stress, and making lifestyle changes.

TABLE 1–3   Contributing Factors to Hypertension

Those That One Can Control:

Smoking	Avoid the use of tobacco products
Overweight	Maintain a proper weight for age and body size
Lack of Exercise	Exercise regularly
Stress	Learn to manage stress
Alcohol	Limit intake of alcohol

Other Contributing Factors:

Heredity	Family history of high blood pressure, heart attack, stroke, or diabetes
Race	There is a greater incidence of hypertension among African-Americans
Sex	Males have a greater chance of developing hypertension
Age	The likelihood of hypertension increases with age

continued

Terminology - continued

TERM	WORD PARTS			DEFINITION
hypotension (hī″ pō-těn′ shŭn)	hypo	P	deficient, below	Low blood pressure
	tens	R	pressure	
	ion	S	process	
ischemia (ĭs-kē′ mĭ-ă)	isch	R	to hold back	A condition in which there is a lack of blood supply to a part caused by constriction or obstruction of a blood vessel
	emia	S	blood condition	
mitral stenosis (mī′ trăl stě-nō′ sĭs)	mitr	R	mitral valve	A condition of narrowing of the mitral valve
	al	S	pertaining to	
	sten	R	narrowing	
	osis	S	condition of	
myocardial (mī″ ō-kăr′ dĭ-ăl)	myo	CF	muscle	Pertaining to the heart muscle
	cardi	CF	heart	
	al	S	pertaining to	
myocarditis (mī″ ō-kăr-dī′ tĭs)	myo	CF	muscle	Inflammation of the heart muscle
	card	R	heart	
	itis	S	inflammation	
oxygen (ŏk′ sĭ-jěn)	oxy	R	sour, sharp, acid	A colorless, odorless, tasteless gas essential in the respiration of animals
	gen	S	formation, produce	
pericardial (pěr″ ĭ-kăr′ dĭ-ăl)	peri	P	around	Pertaining to the pericardium, the sac surrounding the heart
	cardi	CF	heart	
	al	S	pertaining to	
pericardio-rrhaphy (pěr″ ĭ-kăr″ dĭ-ōr′ ă-fē)	peri	P	around	Suture of the pericardium
	cardio	CF	heart	
	rrhaphy	S	to suture	
pericarditis (pěr″ ĭ-kăr-dī′ tĭs)	peri	P	around	Inflammation of the pericardium
	card	R	heart	
	itis	S	inflammation	
phlebitis (flě-bī′ tĭs)	phleb	R	vein	Inflammation of a vein
	itis	S	inflammation	
phlebolith (flěb′ ō-lĭth)	phlebo	CF	vein	A stone within a vein
	lith	S	stone	
phlebotomy (flě-bŏt′ ō-mē)	phlebo	CF	vein	Incision into a vein
	tomy	S	incision	

Terminology - continued

TERM	WORD PARTS		DEFINITION
presystolic (prē″ sĭs-tōl′ ĭk)	pre systol ic	P R S	before contraction pertaining to	Pertaining to before the systole (regular contraction) of the heart
semilunar (sĕm″ ĭ-lū′ năr)	semi lun ar	P R S	half moon pertaining to	Valves of the aorta and pulmonary artery
sinoatrial (sīn″ ō-ā′ trĭ-ăl)	sino atri al	CF R S	a curve atrium pertaining to	Pertaining to the sinus venosus and the atrium
sphygmomano- meter (sfĭg″ mō-măn-ōm ĕt-ĕr)	sphygmo mano meter	CF CF S	pulse thin instrument to measure	An instrument used to measure the arterial blood pressure
stethoscope (stĕth′ ō-skōp)	stetho scope	CF S	chest instrument	An instrument used to listen to the sounds of the heart, lungs, and other internal organs
tachycardia (tăk″ ĭ-kăr′ dĭ-ă)	tachy card ia	P R S	fast heart condition	A fast heartbeat
thrombosis (thrŏm-bō′ sĭs)	thromb osis	R S	clot of blood condition of	A condition in which there is a blood clot within the vascular system; *a stationary blood clot*
tricuspid (trī-kŭs′ pĭd)	tri cuspid	P S	three a point	Having three points; pertaining to the tricuspid valve
triglyceride (trī-glĭs′ ĕr-īd)	tri glyc er ide	P R S S	three sweet, sugar relating to having a particular quality	Pertaining to a compound consisting of three molecules of fatty acids
vasoconstrictive (văs″ ō-kŏn-strĭk′ tĭv)	vaso con strict ive	CF P R S	vessel together to draw, to bind nature of, quality of	The drawing together, as in the narrowing of a blood vessel

continued

Terminology - continued

TERM	WORD PARTS			DEFINITION
vasodilator (văs″ ō-dĭ-lā′ tor)	vaso dilat or	CF R S	vessel to widen one who, a doer	A nerve or agent that causes dilation of blood vessels
vasospasm (văs′ ō-spăzm)	vaso spasm	CF S	vessel contraction, spasm	Contraction of a blood vessel
vasotonic (văs″ ō-tŏn′ ĭk)	vaso ton ic	CF R S	vessel tone pertaining to	Pertaining to the tone of a blood vessel
vasotripsy (văs′ ō-trĭp″ sē)	vaso tripsy	CF S	vessel crushing	The crushing of a blood vessel to arrest hemorrhaging
vectorcardiogram (vĕk″ tor-kăr′ dĭ-ō-grăm)	vector cardio gram	R CF S	a carrier heart a mark, record	A record of the direction and magnitude of the electromotive forces of the heart during one complete cycle
venipuncture (vĕn′ ĭ-pŭnk″ chūr)	veni puncture	CF S	vein to pierce	To pierce a vein
venoclysis (vē-nŏk′ lĭ-sĭs)	veno clysis	CF S	vein injection	The injection of medicine or nutritional fluid via a vein
venotomy (vē-nŏt′ ō-mē)	veno tomy	CF S	vein incision	Incision into a vein
ventricular (vĕn-trĭk′ ū-lăr)	ventricul ar	R S	ventricle pertaining to	Pertaining to a ventricle

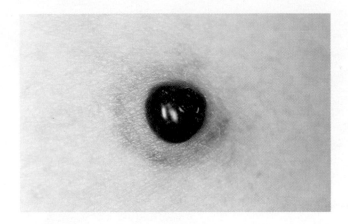

FIGURE 1–9

Infarction angioma. *(Courtesy of Jason L. Smith, MD.)*

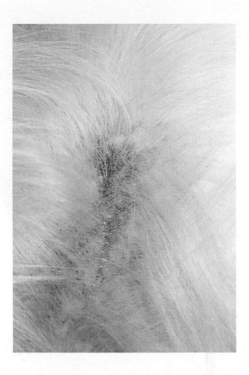

FIGURE 1–10

Temporal arteritis. *(Courtesy of Jason L. Smith, MD.)*

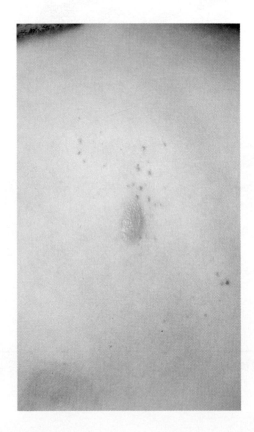

FIGURE 1–11

Hemangioma. *(Courtesy of Jason L. Smith, MD.)*

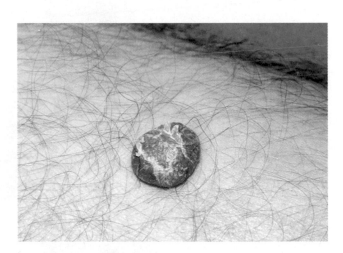

FIGURE 1–12

Sclerosing hemangioma. *(Courtesy of Jason L. Smith, MD.)*

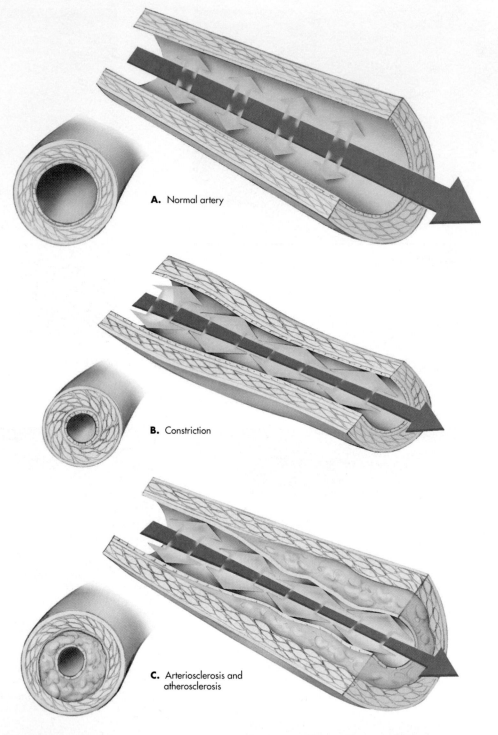

A. Normal artery

B. Constriction

C. Arteriosclerosis and atherosclerosis

FIGURE 1–13

Blood vessels: **(A)** normal artery, **(B)** constriction, **(C)** arteriosclerosis and atherosclerosis.

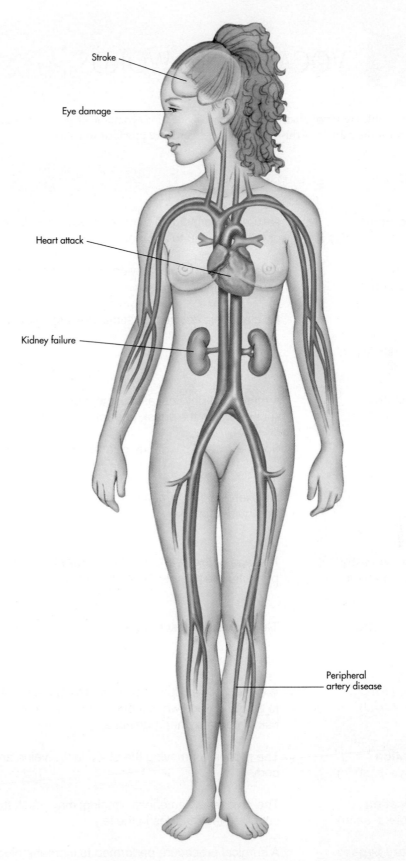

Stroke

Eye damage

Heart attack

Kidney failure

Peripheral
artery disease

FIGURE 1–14

Uncontrolled hypertension can lead to kidney failure, stroke, heart attack, peripheral artery disease, and eye damage.

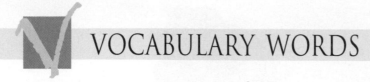

VOCABULARY WORDS

Vocabulary words are terms that have not been divided into component parts. They are common words or specialized terms associated with the subject of this chapter. These words are provided to enhance your medical vocabulary.

WORD	DEFINITION
anastomosis (ă-năs″ tō-mō′ sĭs)	A surgical connection between blood vessels or the joining of one hollow or tubular organ to another
aneurysm (ăn′ ū-rĭ′zm)	A sac formed by a local widening of the wall of an artery or a vein; usually caused by injury or disease
artificial pacemaker (ăr″ tĭ-fĭsh′ ăl pās′ māk-ĕr)	An electronic device that stimulates impulse initiation within the heart
auscultation (ŏs″ kool-tā′ shŭn)	A method of physical assessment using a stethoscope to listen to sounds within the chest, abdomen, and other parts of the body
bruit (br$\overline{oo}$t)	Noise, a sound of venous or arterial origin heard on auscultation
cardiocybernetics (kăr″ dē-ō-sī″ bĕr-nĕt′ ĭks)	An exercise program that combines a daily workout with relaxation therapy and guided imagery
cardiomyopathy (kăr″ dē-ō-mī-ŏp′ ă-thē)	Disease of the heart muscle that may be caused by a viral infection, a parasitic infection, or overconsumption of alcohol
catheterization (kăth″ ĕ-tĕr-ĭ-zā′ shŭn)	The process of inserting a catheter into the heart or the urinary bladder
cholesterol (kō-lĕs′ tĕr-ŏl)	A waxy, fat-like substance in the bloodstream of all animals. It is believed to be dangerous when it builds up on arterial walls and contributes to the risk of coronary heart disease.
circulation (sər″-kyə lā′ shən)	The process of moving the blood in the veins and arteries throughout the body
claudication (klaw-dĭ-kā′ shŭn)	The process of lameness, limping; may result from inadequate blood supply to the muscles in the leg
coronary bypass (kŏr′ ō-nă-rē bī′ păs)	A surgical procedure performed to increase blood flow to the myocardium by using a section of a saphenous vein or internal mammary artery to bypass the obstructed or occluded coronary artery

Vocabulary - continued

WORD	DEFINITION
diastole (dī-ăs′ tō-lē)	The relaxation phase of the heart cycle during which the heart muscle relaxes and the heart chambers fill with blood
dysrhythmia (dĭs-rĭth′ mē-ă)	An abnormal, difficult, or bad rhythm
echocardiography (ĕk″ ō-kăr″ dē-ŏg′ rah-fē)	A noninvasive ultrasound method for evaluating the heart for valvular or structural defects and coronary artery disease
extracorporeal circulation (ĕks-tră-kòr-pōr′ ē-ăl sər″-kyə lā′ shən)	Pertaining to the circulation of the blood outside the body via a heart–lung machine or hemodialyzer
fibrillation (fĭ″ brĭl-ā′ shŭn)	Quivering of muscle fiber; may be atrial or ventricular
flutter (flŭt′ ər)	A condition of the heartbeat in which the contractions become extremely rapid
harvest (hăr′ vĭst)	To gather an organ and make it ready for transplantation
heart–lung transplant (hart-lŭng trăns′ plănt)	The surgical process of transferring the heart and lungs from a donor to a patient
heart transplant (hart trăns′ plănt)	The surgical process of transferring the heart from a donor to a patient
hemodynamic (hē″ mō-dī-năm′ ĭk)	Pertaining to the study of the heart's ability to function as a pump; the movement of the blood and its pressure
infarction (ĭn-fărk′ shŭn)	Process of development of an infarct, which is necrosis of tissue resulting from obstruction of blood flow
Korotkoff sounds (kor′ ŏt-kŏf sowndz)	Tapping sounds heard during auscultation of blood pressure
laser angioplasty (lā′ zĕr ăn′ jĭ-ō-plăs″ tē)	The use of light beams to clear a path through a blocked artery. Once the blockage is located, a laser probe is inserted into the blood vessel and advanced to the clogged area. The laser is activated by a qualified physician and, in an instant, the blockage is vaporized and blood flow is restored in the artery.

continued

WORD	DEFINITION
lipoproteins (lĭp-ō-prō′ tēns)	*Fat (lipid)* and *protein molecules* that are bound together. They are classified as: **VLDL**—very-low-density lipoproteins; **LDL**—low-density lipoproteins; and **HDL**—high-density lipoproteins. High levels of VLDL and LDL are associated with cholesterol and triglyceride deposits in arteries, which could lead to coronary heart disease, hypertension, and atherosclerosis. One's total cholesterol level should be below 200 mg/dL and HDL (good cholesterol) above 35 mg/dL. Elevated levels of LDL (bad cholesterol) is a risk factor associated with developing **coronary heart disease** *(CHD)* or **coronary artery disease** *(CAD)*. The more risk factors that one has, the greater the possibility of developing coronary artery disease, a major cause of heart attacks. See Table 1–4 for associated coronary heart disease risk factors.
lubb-dupp (lŭb-dŭp)	The two separate heart sounds that can be heard with the use of a stethoscope
murmur (mər′ mər)	A soft blowing or rasping sound heard by auscultation of various parts of the body, especially in the region of the heart
occlusion (ŏ-kloo′ zhŭn)	The process or state of being closed
palpitation (păl-pĭ-tā′ shŭn)	Rapid throbbing or fluttering of the heart
percutaneous transluminal coronary angioplasty (pĕr″ kū-tā′ nē-ŭs trăns-lū′ mĭ-năl kȯr′ ō-nă-rē ăn′ jĭ-ō-plăs″ tē)	The use of a balloon-tipped catheter to compress fatty plaques against an artery wall. When successful, the plaques remain compressed, and this permits more blood to flow through the artery, thereby relieving the symptoms of heart disease.
Raynaud's phenomenon (rā-nōz fĕ-nŏm′ ĕ-nŏn)	A disorder that generally affects the blood vessels in the fingers and toes; it is characterized by intermittent attacks that cause the blood vessels in the digits to narrow. The attack is usually due to exposure to cold or occurs during emotional stress. Once the attack begins, the patient may experience pallor, cyanosis, and/or rubor in the affected part. See Figure 1–15.
rheumatic heart disease (roo-măt′ĭk hart dĭ-zēz′)	Endocarditis or valvular heart disease as a result of complications of acute rheumatic fever
septum (sĕp′ tŭm)	A wall or partition that divides or separates a body space or cavity

Vocabulary - continued

WORD	DEFINITION
shock (shŏk)	A state of disruption of oxygen supply to the tissues and a return of blood to the heart
spider veins (spī′dĕr vāns)	Hemangioma in which numerous telangiectatic vessels radiate from a central point. See Figure 1–16.
stroke (strōk)	A sudden severe attack such as a blockage or rupture of a blood vessel within the brain
systole (sĭs′ tō-lē)	The contractive phase of the heart cycle during which blood is forced into the aorta and the pulmonary artery
telangiectasis (tĕl-ăn″jĕ-ĕk-tă′sĭs)	A vascular lesion formed by dilatation of a group of small blood vessels; it may appear as a birthmark or be caused by long-term exposure to the sun. See Figure 1–17.
thrombophlebitis (thrŏm″bō-flē-bī′tĭs)	Inflammation of a vein associated with the formation of a thrombus. See Figure 1–18.
tissue plasminogen activator (tĭsh′ ū plăz-mĭn′ ŏ-jĕn ăk′ tĭ-vā″ tor)	A drug that is used within the first 6 hours of a myocardial infarction to dissolve fibrin clots. It reduces the chance of dying after a myocardial infarction by 50%. Examples are *Kabikinase (streptokinase)* and *Activase (alteplase recombinant).*

TABLE 1–4   Risk Factors Associated With Developing Coronary Heart Disease

Male age 45 or older	Diabetes mellitus
Female age 55 or older	High-density lipoprotein (HDL) below
Female under age 55 with premature	35 mg/dL
menopause and not on estrogen	Family history of early heart disease
replacement therapy	(parent or sibling; male less than 55,
Smoker	female less than 65)
Hypertension	Obesity

Note: To help lower cholesterol one should limit intake of foods that are high in saturated fat:

Wholemilk	Bacon
Dairy cream	Ribs
Cheese	Ground red meat
Butter	Cold cuts
Red meat, heavily marbled with fat	Poultry skin
Prime cuts	Coconut or palm oil
Sausage	Hydrogenated vegetable oil

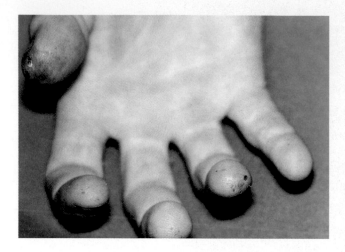

FIGURE 1–15

Raynaud's phenomenon. *(Courtesy of Jason L. Smith, MD.)*

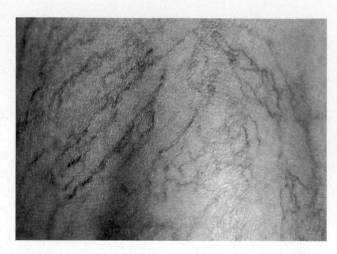

FIGURE 1–16

Spider veins. *(Courtesy of Jason L. Smith, MD.)*

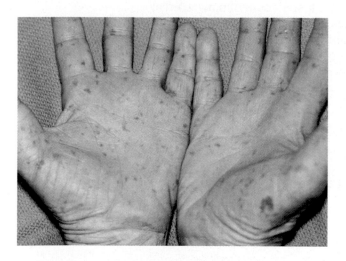

FIGURE 1–17

Telangiectasis. *(Courtesy of Jason L. Smith, MD.)*

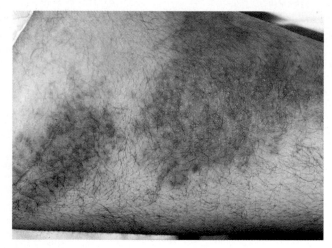

FIGURE 1–18

Thrombophlebitis. *(Courtesy of Jason L. Smith, MD.)*

ABBREVIATIONS

ACG	angiocardiography		IHSS	idiopathic hypertrophic subaortic stenosis
AI	aortic insufficiency		LA	left atrium
AMI	acute myocardial infarction		LBBB	left bundle branch block
AS	aortic stenosis		LD	lactic dehydrogenase
ASD	atrial septal defect		LDL	low-density lipoproteins
ASH	asymmetrical septal hypertrophy		LV	left ventricle
ASHD	arteriosclerotic heart disease		MI	myocardial infarction
AST	aspartate aminotransferase		MS	mitral stenosis
A-V, AV	atrioventricular		MVP	mitral valve prolapse
BBB	bundle branch block		OHS	open heart surgery
BP	blood pressure		PAT	paroxysmal atrial tachycardia
CAD	coronary artery disease		PMI	point of maximum impulse
CC	cardiac catheterization			
CCU	coronary care unit		PTCA	percutaneous transluminal coronary angioplasty
CHD	coronary heart disease			
CHF	congestive heart failure			
CK	creatine kinase			
CO	cardiac output		PVCs	premature ventricular contractions
CPR	cardiopulmonary resuscitation			
CVP	central venous pressure		RA	right atrium
DVTs	deep vein thromboses		RV	right ventricle
ECC	extracorporeal circulation		S-A, SA	sinoatrial
ECG	electrocardiogram		SCD	sudden cardiac death
EKG	electrocardiogram		TEE	transesophageal echocardiography
FHS	fetal heart sound			
HDL	high-density lipoproteins		tPA	tissue plasminogen activator
H&L	heart and lungs		VLDL	very-low-density lipoproteins
			VSD	ventricular septal defect

DRUG HIGHLIGHTS

Drugs that are generally used for cardiovascular diseases and disorders include digitalis preparations, antiarrhythmic agents, vasopressors, vasodilators, antihypertensive agents, and antilipemic agents.

Digitalis Drugs   Strengthen the heart muscle, increase the force and velocity of myocardial systolic contraction, slow the heart rate, and decrease conduction velocity through the atrioventricular (AV) node. These drugs are used in the treatment of congestive heart failure, atrial fibrillation, atrial flutter, and paroxysmal atrial tachycardia. With the administration of digitalis, toxicity may occur. The

most common early symptoms of digitalis toxicity are anorexia, nausea, vomiting, and arrhythmias.
Examples: Crystodigin (digitoxin), Lanoxin (digoxin), and Cedilanid-D (deslanoside).

Antiarrhythmic Agents

Used in the treatment of cardiac arrhythmias.
Examples: Tambocor (flecainide acetate), Tonocard (tocainide HCl), Inderal (propranolol HCl), and Calan (verapamil).

Vasopressors

Cause contraction of the muscles associated with capillaries and arteries, thereby narrowing the space through which the blood circulates. This narrowing results in an elevation of blood pressure. Vasopressors are useful in the treatment of patients suffering from shock.
Examples: Intropin (dopamine HCl), Aramine (metaraminol bitartrate), and Levophed Bitartrate (norepinephrine).

Vasodilators

Cause relaxation of blood vessels and lower blood pressure. Coronary vasodilators are used for the treatment of angina pectoris.
Examples: Sorbitrate (isosorbide dinitrate), nitroglycerin, amyl nitrate, and Cardilate (erythrityl tetranitrate).

Antihypertensive Agents

Used in the treatment of hypertension.
Examples: Catapres (clonidine HCl), Aldomet (methyldopa), Lopressor (metoprolol tartrate), and Capoten (captopril).

Antilipemic Agents

Used to lower abnormally high blood levels of fatty substances (lipids) when other treatment regimens fail.
Examples: Nicolar or Nicobid (niacin), Mevacor (lovastatin), Lopid (gemfibrozil), Atromid-S (clofibrate), and Questran (cholestyramine).

DIAGNOSTIC AND LABORATORY TESTS

Test	Description
angiogram (ăn′ jē-ō-grăm)	A test used to determine the size and shape of arteries and veins of organs and tissues. A radiopaque substance is injected into the blood vessel, and x-rays are taken.
angiography (ăn″ jē-ŏg′ ră-fē)	The x-ray recording of a blood vessel after the injection of a radiopaque substance. Used to determine the condition of the blood vessels, organ, or tissue being studied. Types: aortic, cardiac, cerebral, coronary, digital subtraction (use of a computer technique), peripheral, pulmonary, selective, and vertebral.
cardiac catheterization (kăr′dĭ-ăk kăth″ ĕ-tĕr-ĭ-zā′ shŭn)	A test used in diagnosis of heart disorders. A tiny catheter is inserted into an artery in the groin area of the patient and is fed through this artery to the heart. Dye is then pumped through the catheter, enabling the physician to locate by x-ray any blockages in the arteries supplying the heart.

Test	Description
cardiac enzymes (kar′ dĭ-ăk ĕn′- zīmz)	Blood tests performed to determine cardiac damage in an acute myocardial infarction.
alanine aminotransferase (ALT)	Levels begin to rise 6 to 10 hours after an MI and peak at 24 to 48 hours.
aspartate aminotransferase (AST)	Levels begin to rise 6 to 10 hours after an MI and peak at 24 to 48 hours.
creatine phosphokinase (CPK)	Used to detect area of damage.
creatine kinase (CK)	Level may be 5 to 8 times normal.
creatine kinase isoenzymes	Used to indicate area of damage; CK-MB heart muscle, CK-MM skeletal muscle, and CK-BB brain.
cholesterol (kōl-lĕs′ tĕr-ŏl)	A blood test to determine the level of cholesterol in the serum. Elevated levels may indicate an increased risk of coronary heart disease. Any level greater than 200 mg/dL is considered too high for good heart health.
electrophysiology (ē-lĕk″ trō-fĭz″ ĭ-ŏl′ ō-jē)	A cardiac procedure that maps the electrical activity of the heart from within the heart itself.
Holter monitor (hōlt′ ər mŏn′ ĭ-tər)	A method of recording a patient's ECG for 24 hours. The device is portable and small enough to be worn by the patient during normal activity.
lactic dehydrogenase (LDH) (lăk′ tĭk dē-hī-drŏj′ ĕ-nās)	Increased 6 to 12 hours after cardiac injury.
stress test (strĕs test)	A method of evaluating cardiovascular fitness. The ECG is monitored while the patient is subjected to increasing levels of work. A treadmill or ergometer is used for this test.
triglycerides (trī-glĭs′ ĕr-īds)	A blood test to determine the level of triglycerides in the serum. Elevated levels (greater than 200 mg/dL) may indicate an increased risk of coronary heart disease and diabetes mellitus.
ultrasonography (ŭl-tră-sŏn-ŏg′ ră-fē)	A test used to visualize an organ or tissue by using high-frequency sound waves. It may be used as a screening test or as a diagnostic tool to determine abnormalities of the aorta, arteries and veins, and the heart.

COMMUNICATION ENRICHMENT

This segment is provided for those who wish to enhance their ability to communicate in either English or Spanish.

RELATED TERMS

English	Spanish	English	Spanish
blood pressure	presión sanguinea (*p rě*-sĭ-ōn săn-gĭ-ně-ă)	artery	arteria (ăr-*tě*-rĭ-ă)
cholesterol	colesterol (*kō*-lĕs-tĕ-rōl)	capillary	capilar (*că*-pĭ-lăr)
clot	coagulo (kō-*ă*-gŭ-lō)	vessel	vaso (*vă*-sō)
heart	corazón (*kō*-ră-zōn)	choke, suffocate	sofocar (sō-*fō*-kăr)
heart disease	enfermedad del corazón (ĕn-fĕr-*mě*-dăd dĕl *kō*-ră-zōn)	injection	inyeccion (*ĭn*-jĕc-sĭ-ōn)
		record	registro (*rě*-hĭs-trō)
high blood pressure	presion alta (*p rě*-sĭ-ōn ăl-tă)	motion	mocíon (*mō*-sĭ-ōn)
murmur	murmullo (*mūr*-mū-jō)	inflammation	inflamación (ĭn-*flă*-mă-sĭ-ōn)
palpitations	palpitaciónes (*păl*-pĭ-tă-sĭ-ō-nĕs)	spasm	espasmo (ĕs-*păs*-mō)
pulse	pulso (*pūl*-sō)	oxygen	oxigeno (ōx-sĭ-*hě*-nō)
system	sistema (sĭs-*tě*-mă)	narrowing	estrecho (ĕs-*trě*-chō)
varicose veins	venas varicosas (*vě*-năs vă-rĭ-*kō*-săs)	puncture	pinchazo (pĭn-*chă*-sō)
veins	venas (*vě*-năs)	soften	ablandar (*ă*-blăn-dăr)
heartbeat	latidos del corazón (*lă*-tĭ-dōs dĕl kō-*ră*-zōn)	rhythm	ritmo (*rĭt*-mō)

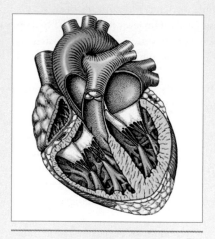

2

ANATOMY AND PHYSIOLOGY OF THE HEART AND CIRCULATION

OBJECTIVES

On completion of this chapter, you should be able to:

• Describe the location and general features of the heart.

• Trace the flow of blood through the heart, identifying the major blood vessels, chambers, and heart valves.

• Identify the layers of the heart wall.

• Describe the events of a typical heartbeat, or cardiac cycle.

• Describe the components and functions of the conducting system of the heart.

• Describe the structure and function of arteries, capillaries, and veins.

• Describe how tissues and various organ systems interact to regulate blood flow and pressure in tissues.

• Distinguish among the types of blood vessels on the basis of their structure and function.

• Identify the major arteries and veins and the areas they serve.

• Describe the age-related changes that occur in the cardiovascular system.

All the cells of the human body require a supply of oxygen and nutrients and a means of waste disposal. As we saw in the last chapter, blood meets both of these needs. However, blood must be kept moving. If blood remains stationary, its oxygen and nutrient supplies are quickly exhausted, its capacity to absorb wastes is soon reached, and neither hormones nor white blood cells can reach their intended targets.

All these vital activities thus depend on the pumping action of the heart. This muscular organ beats approximately 100,000 times each day, pumping roughly 8000 L of blood—enough to fill forty 55-gal drums.

The blood pumped by the heart is carried within tubes of varying diameter (the blood vessels) to all parts of the body. Blood vessels carrying blood away from the heart, the *arteries*, gradually decrease in size; the vessels carrying blood back to the heart, the *veins*, gradually increase in size. The smallest of all blood vessels, the *capillaries*, connect the smallest arteries with the smallest veins. It is through the thin walls of the capillaries that gases, nutrients, and wastes are exchanged between the blood and the body's cells.

What makes the heart such a powerful organ? How are the blood vessels specialized for transporting blood? This chapter focuses on the cardiovascular structures involved in the pumping and transportation of blood. It also describes the major blood vessels of the body.

▶ THE HEART AND THE CIRCULATORY SYSTEM

Blood is pumped by the heart through a closed network of blood vessels that extend between the heart and all the tissues of the body. There are two general networks of blood vessels that make up the circulatory system. In the **pulmonary circulation** the blood completes a round-trip from the heart to the exchange surfaces of the lungs. In the **systemic circulation** the blood completes a round-trip from the heart to all portions of body *except* the exchange surfaces of the lungs. Each circuit begins and ends at the heart. **Arteries** carry blood away from the heart; **veins** return blood to the heart. **Capillaries** are small, thin-walled vessels that connect the smallest arteries to the smallest veins.

As indicated in Figure 2-1, blood travels through the two circuits in sequence. For example, blood returning to the heart in the systemic veins must first go to the lungs and return to the heart before it can reenter the systemic arteries. The heart contains four muscular chambers. The **right atrium** (Ā-trē-um; hall) receives blood from the systemic circulation, and the **right ventricle** (VEN-tri-k'l) discharges it into the pulmonary circulation. The **left atrium** collects blood from the pulmonary circulation, and the **left ventricle** pushes it into the systemic circulation. When the heart beats, the two ventricles contract at the same time and eject equal volumes of blood. The heart, then, is really a double pump, with a ventricle and an atrium associated with each circuit.

▶ STRUCTURE OF THE HEART

The heart is a small, cone-shaped organ roughly the size of a clenched fist. It lies near the anterior chest wall, directly behind the sternum, and sits at an angle with its blunt tip pointed downward and to the left side of the body. It is surrounded by the **pericardial** (per-i-KAR-dē-al) **cavity**. This cavity is lined by a serous membrane called the **pericardium**.

The pericardium is subdivided into a **visceral pericardium**, or **epicardium**, that covers the outer surface of the heart, and a **parietal pericardium** that lines the opposing inner surface of the fibrous sac surrounding the heart. The space between these surfaces contains a small amount of pericardial fluid that acts as a lubricant, reducing friction as the heart beats.

The great veins and arteries of the circulatory system are connected to the heart at the **base** (see Figure 2-2). The pointed tip formed by the two ventricles is the **apex** (Ā-peks) of the heart. A typical heart measures approximately 12.5 cm (5 in.) from the attached base to the apex.

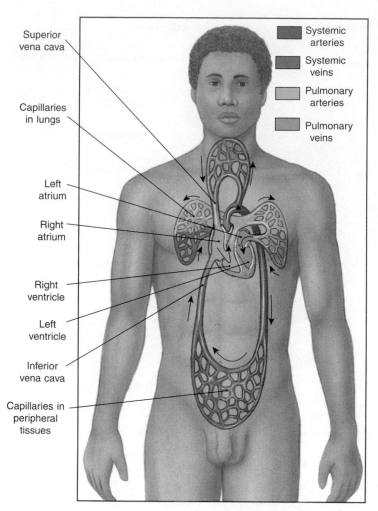

Superior
vena cava

Capillaries
in lungs

Left
atrium

Right
atrium

Right
ventricle

Left
ventricle

Inferior
vena cava

Capillaries in
peripheral
tissues

Systemic
arteries

Systemic
veins

Pulmonary
arteries

Pulmonary
veins

FIGURE 2-1

An Overview of Blood Flow.

Blood flows through separate pulmonary and systemic circulations, driven by the pumping of the heart. Each pathway begins and ends at the heart and contains arteries, capillaries, and veins.

INTERNAL ANATOMY OF THE HEART

inter, between + *atrium,* room; or *ventriculus,* a little belly
septum, a wall
interatrial septum, interventricular septum: muscular walls that separate the two atria and the two ventricles, respectively

Figure 2-3 shows the internal appearance and structure of the four chambers of the heart. Muscular walls, or *septa*, separate the right atrium from the left atrium, and the right ventricle from the left ventricle. These dividing walls are called the **interatrial septum** and **interventricular septum**. The septa ensure that no mixing of blood occurs between the left and right chambers of the heart. On each side of the heart, blood flows from the atrium into the ventricle through an **atrioventricular (AV) valve**. The structure of this valve ensures that blood flows in one direction only, from the atrium into the ventricle.

Note that Figure 2-3 also shows the path of blood flow through both sides of the heart. The right atrium receives blood from the systemic circulation through two large veins, the **superior vena cava** (VĒ-na KĀ-va) and the **inferior vena cava**. The superior vena cava delivers blood from the head, neck, upper limbs, and chest. The inferior vena cava carries blood returning from the rest of the trunk, organs in the abdominopelvic cavity, and the lower limbs.

Blood travels from the right atrium into the right ventricle through a broad opening bounded by three flaps of fibrous tissue. These flaps, called *cusps*, are part of the **right atrioventricular (AV) valve**, also known as the **tricuspid** (trī-KUS-pid; *tri*, three) **valve**. Each cusp is braced by strong fibers, the *chordae tendineae* (KOR-dē TEN-di-nē-ē), that are connected to small muscles that project from the inner surface of the right ventricle.

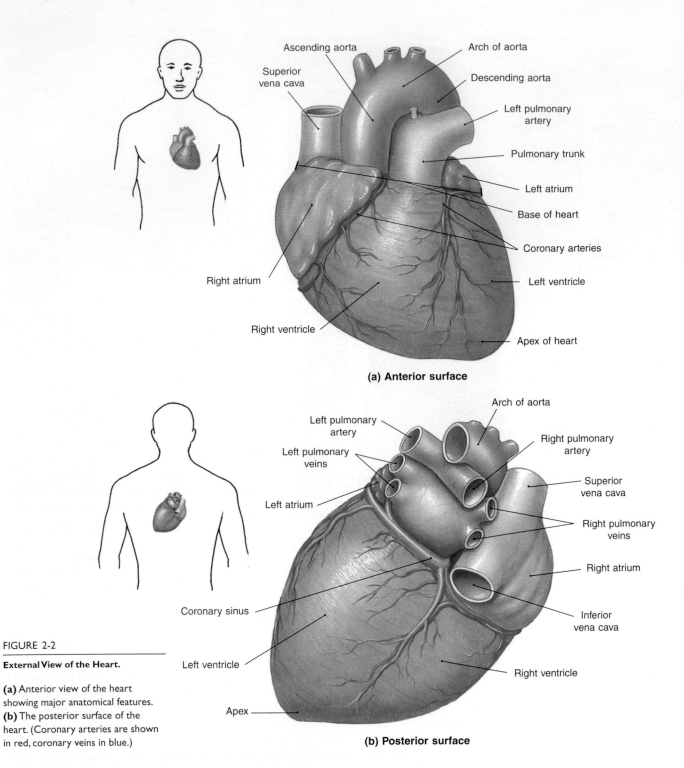

Ascending aorta

Arch of aorta

Superior
vena cava

Descending aorta

Left pulmonary
artery

Pulmonary trunk

Left atrium

Base of heart

Coronary arteries

Left ventricle

Right atrium

Right ventricle

Apex of heart

(a) Anterior surface

Arch of aorta

Left pulmonary
artery

Left pulmonary
veins

Right pulmonary
artery

Left atrium

Superior
vena cava

Right pulmonary
veins

Right atrium

Coronary sinus

Inferior
vena cava

Left ventricle

Right ventricle

Apex

(b) Posterior surface

FIGURE 2-2

External View of the Heart.

(a) Anterior view of the heart
showing major anatomical features.
(b) The posterior surface of the
heart. (Coronary arteries are shown
in red, coronary veins in blue.)

Blood leaving the right ventricle flows into the large **pulmonary trunk** through the **pulmonary semilunar** (half-moon) **valve**. Once within the pulmonary trunk, blood flows into the **left** and **right pulmonary arteries**. These vessels branch repeatedly within the lungs, supplying the capillaries where gas exchange occurs. As blood leaves these respiratory capillaries it then passes through the **left** and **right pulmonary veins** before entering the left atrium.

As in the right atrium, the opening between the left atrium and the left ventricle has a valve—the **left atrioventricular (AV) valve**, or **bicuspid** (bī-KUS-pid; *bi*, two) **valve**—which prevents

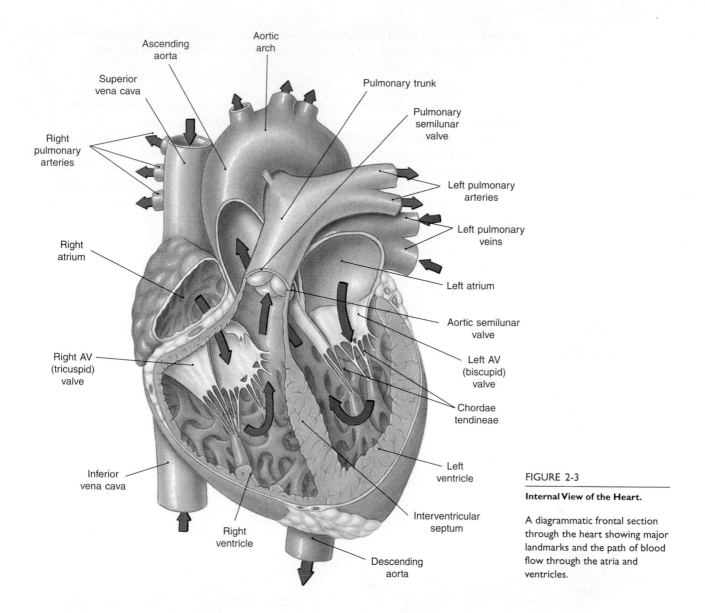

Ascending
aorta

Aortic
arch

Superior
vena cava

Pulmonary trunk

Pulmonary
semilunar
valve

Right
pulmonary
arteries

Left pulmonary
arteries

Left pulmonary
veins

Right
atrium

Left atrium

Aortic semilunar
valve

Right AV
(tricuspid)
valve

Left AV
(biscupid)
valve

Chordae
tendineae

Left
ventricle

Inferior
vena cava

Interventricular
septum

Right
ventricle

Descending
aorta

FIGURE 2-3

Internal View of the Heart.

A diagrammatic frontal section
through the heart showing major
landmarks and the path of blood
flow through the atria and
ventricles.

backflow from the ventricle into the atrium. As the name *bicuspid* implies, the left AV valve contains a pair of cusps rather than three. Because its shape resembles a bishop's hat, or *mitre*, this valve is also known as the **mitral** (MĪ-tral) **valve.**

Internally, the left ventricle resembles the right ventricle. Blood leaving the left ventricle passes through the **aortic semilunar valve** and into the systemic circuit by way of the *ascending aorta*.

The Ventricles

The close relationship between structure and function are clearly evident in the heart. For example, the function of an atrium is to collect blood returning to the heart and deliver it to the attached ventricle. Because the workloads placed on the right and left atria are very similar, the two chambers look almost identical. However, the demands placed on the right and left ventricles are very different, and there are structural differences between the two.

The lungs are close to the heart, and the pulmonary arteries and veins are relatively short and wide. As a result, the right ventricle normally does not need to push very hard to propel blood through the pulmonary circulation. As you can see in Figure 2-3, the wall of the right ventricle is relatively thin compared with that of the left ventricle. Because the systemic circulation has a more extensive network of blood vessels, the left ventricle must exert much more force than the right ventricle. As might be expected, the left ventricle has an extremely thick muscular wall.

The Heart Valves

The atrioventricular valves prevent backflow of blood from the ventricles into the atria. When a ventricle is relaxed and filling with blood, the AV valve offers no resistance to the flow of blood from atrium to ventricle (Figure 2-4a). When the ventricle begins to contract, blood moving back toward the atrium swings the cusps together, closing the valve (Figure 2-4b). The chordae tendineae attached to the cusps prevent their ballooning back into the atrium and allowing the backflow of blood into the atrium when the ventricle contracts. However, a small amount of backflow often occurs, even in normal individuals. The swirling action creates a soft but distinctive sound, called a *heart murmur*.

The pulmonary and aortic semilunar valves prevent backflow of blood from the pulmonary trunk and aorta into the right and left ventricles. When these valves close, the three symmetrical cusps support one another like the legs of a tripod (Figure 2-4a).

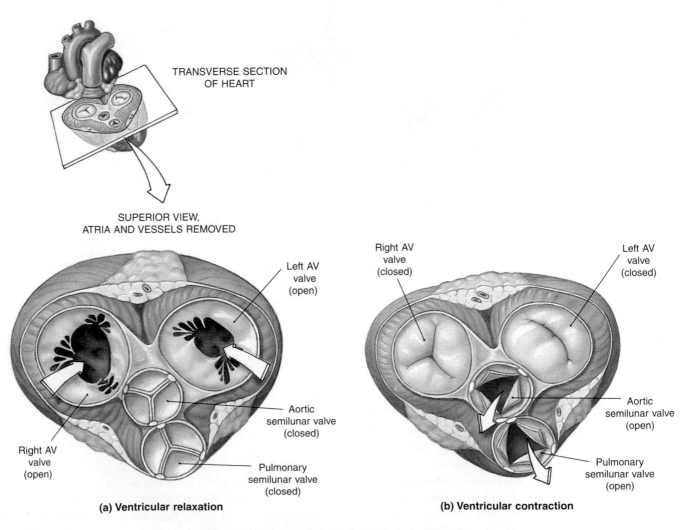

FIGURE 2-4

Valves of the Heart.

(a) Valve position during ventricular relaxation, when the AV valves are open and the semilunar valves are closed. **(b)** The appearance of the cardiac valves during ventricular contraction, when the AV valves are closed and the semilunar valves are open.

THE HEART WALL

The wall of the heart is made up of three distinct layers (Figure 2-5). The **epicardium**, which covers the outer surface of the heart, is a serous membrane that consists of an exposed epithelium and an underlying layer of loose connective tissue. The **myocardium**, or muscular wall of the heart, contains cardiac muscle tissue and associated connective tissues, blood vessels, and nerves. The inner surfaces of the heart, including the valves, are covered by the **endocardium** (en-dō-KAR-dē-um), whose squamous epithelium is continuous with the epithelium, or *endothelium*, that lines the attached blood vessels.

Cardiac Muscle Cells

Cardiac muscle cells within the myocardium interconnect at specialized sites known as **intercalated** (in-TER-ka-lā-ted) **discs**. Specialized connections and tiny pores at these sites strengthen and stabilize the cells and provide for the movement of ions, small molecules, and electrical impulses. In addition, the myofibrils of adjacent cells are attached to the disc. This increases the efficiency of the cells, as they can "pull together" whenever the heart contracts.

BLOOD SUPPLY TO THE HEART

The heart works continuously, and cardiac muscle cells require reliable supplies of oxygen and nutrients. During maximum exertion the oxygen demand rises considerably, and the blood flow to the heart may increase to nine times that of resting levels. Although the heart is filled with blood, the surrounding heart muscle relies on its own network of blood vessels. The vessels that supply blood to cells of the heart form the **coronary circulation**.

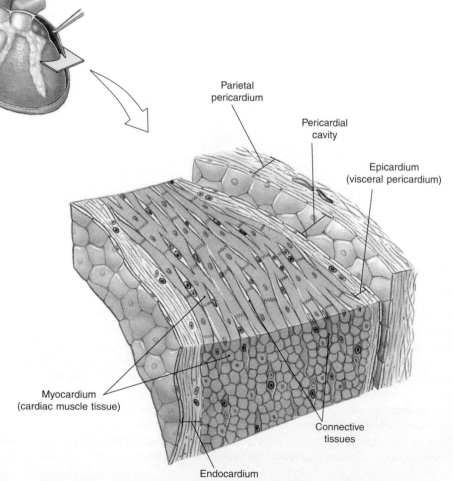

Parietal
pericardium

Pericardial
cavity

Epicardium
(visceral pericardium)

Myocardium
(cardiac muscle tissue)

Connective
tissues

Endocardium

FIGURE 2-5

Layers of the Heart Wall.

A diagram of a section through the heart wall showing the epicardium, myocardium, and endocardium. The cardiac muscle cells of the myocardium branch and interconnect at sites called intercalated discs.

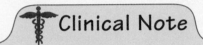

Clinical Note

Coronary Circulation and Heart Attacks

Cardiac muscle cells need a constant supply of oxygen and nutrients, and any reduction in coronary circulation reduces the heart's performance. A reduction in the coronary blood supply, a process called a **coronary ischemia** (is-KĒ-mē-a), usually results from a partial or complete blockage of one or more coronary arteries. The usual cause is the formation of a fatty deposit, or *plaque*, in the wall of a coronary blood vessel.

A general term for these degenerative changes in the coronary circulation is **coronary artery disease (CAD)**. One of the first symptoms of CAD is **angina pectoris** (an-JĪ-na PEK-tō-ris) which means "a pain spasm in the chest." In the most common form of angina, pain radiates from the sternal area to the arms, back, and neck when the individual exerts himself or is under emotional stress. Angina develops with exertion because the partially blocked coronary vessels cannot meet the increased demand for oxygen and nutrients.

In a heart attack, or **myocardial** (mī-ō-KAR-dē-al) **infarction (MI)**, a portion of the coronary circulation becomes blocked and the cardiac muscle cells die from lack of oxygen. The affected tissue then degenerates, creating a nonfunctional area known as an *infarct*. Heart attacks most often result from severe coronary heart disease. The consequences of a heart attack depend on the site and duration of the circulatory blockage.

There are roughly 1.3 million MIs in the United States each year, and half of the victims die within a year of the incident. Factors that increase the risk of a heart attack include smoking, high blood pressure, high blood cholesterol levels, diabetes, male gender (below 70 years old), severe emotional stress, and obesity. Eliminating as many risk factors as possible will improve one's chances of preventing or surviving a heart attack.

Concept Questions

✔ Damage to the semilunar valves on the right side of the heart would interfere with blood flow to what vessel?

✔ What prevents the AV valves from opening back into the atria?

✔ Why is the left ventricle more muscular than the right ventricle?

The coronary circulation begins with the left and right **coronary arteries**, which originate at the base of the ascending aorta (see Figure 2-2a). Blood pressure here is the highest found anywhere in the systemic circulation, and this pressure ensures a continuous flow of blood to meet the demands of active cardiac muscle tissue. Each coronary artery splits in two, and smaller branches form a maze of interconnections called **anastomoses** (a-nas-to-MŌ-ses). Because the arteries are interconnected in this way, the blood supply to the cardiac muscle remains relatively constant, regardless of pressure changes within the left and right coronary arteries. Two main **cardiac veins** carry blood away from the coronary capillaries. These veins drain into the **coronary sinus**, a large, thin-walled vein (see Figure 2-2b). Blood from the coronary sinus flows into the right atrium near the base of the inferior vena cava.

▶ THE HEARTBEAT

The average heart beats about 100,000 times per day, or about 70 to 80 beats per minute. During 1 minute, the heart can pump 4 to 6 L (about 1 to 1.5 gal) of blood, that is, the entire volume of blood in the body. During strenuous activity, some five to seven times this volume of blood could be pumped in the same amount of time.

CARDIAC CYCLE

What happens during one heartbeat? One complete heartbeat makes up a single **cardiac cycle** and takes about 0.8 seconds to complete. During each cardiac cycle any one chamber undergoes alternating periods of contraction and relaxation. During contraction, or **systole** (SIS-to-lē), the chamber pushes blood into an adjacent chamber or into an arterial trunk (see Figure 2-6). Systole is followed by the second phase, one of relaxation, or **diastole** (dī-AS-to-lē), during which the chamber fills with blood and prepares for the next heartbeat.

During the cardiac cycle, the pressure within each chamber rises in systole and falls in diastole. Because fluids will move from an area of high pressure to one of lower pressure, an increase in pressure in one chamber will cause the blood to flow to another chamber of lesser pressure. One-way valves between adjacent chambers help to ensure that blood flows in the desired direction.

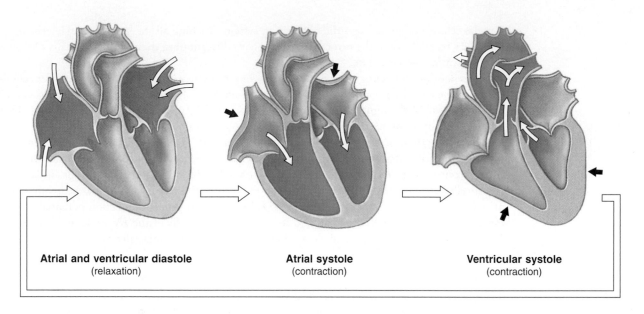

| **Atrial and ventricular diastole** (relaxation) | **Atrial systole** (contraction) | **Ventricular systole** (contraction) |

FIGURE 2-6

The Cardiac Cycle.

The atria and ventricles go through repeated cycles of systole and diastole. A cardiac cycle is made up of one period of systole and diastole.

The amount of blood ejected by a ventricle during a single heartbeat is known as the **stroke volume**. The amount of blood pumped by a ventricle in 1 minute is called the **cardiac output**. The cardiac output of an adult is about equal to the total volume of blood in the body.

Heart Sounds

When you listen to your own heart with a stethoscope, you hear the familiar "lubb-dupp" that accompanies each heartbeat. These sounds accompany the action of the heart valves. The first heart sound ("lubb") marks the start of ventricular systole, and the sound is produced as the AV valves close and the semilunar valves open. The second heart sound, "dupp," occurs at the beginning of ventricular diastole, when the semilunar valves close.

CONDUCTING SYSTEM OF THE HEART

The correct pressure relationships that occur in a normal heartbeat depend on the careful timing of contractions. In the normal pattern of blood flow, the atria contract first and then the ventricles. Each time the heart beats, the contractions of individual cardiac muscle cells are coordinated and harnessed to ensure that blood flows in the right direction at the proper time. Unlike skeletal muscle fibers, cardiac muscle cells can contract on their own without stimulation from hormones or nerves. This is a property called *automaticity*, or *autorhythmicity*. Normally, however, cardiac muscle cells do not contract independently of one another; this would disrupt the cardiac cycle. Instead, the cardiac muscle cells wait for the arrival of a signal generated and distributed by smaller, specialized muscle cells that make up the *conducting system* of the heart. The conducting system includes **nodal cells** that establish the heartbeat rate and **conducting cells** that distribute the stimulus for contraction throughout the myocardium.

Nodal Cells

Nodal cells are unusual because they can generate electrical impulses, or *action potentials*, at regular intervals. Nodal cells are electrically connected to one another and to conducting cells, which are in turn connected to normal cardiac muscle cells. As a result, when an electrical impulse appears in a nodal cell, it sweeps through the conducting system, reaching all the cardiac muscle cells in less than 0.25 second. When the myocardial cells receive this stimulus, they contract. In this way nodal cells determine the heart rate.

There are two different groups of nodal cells, or **pacemaker cells**. The main pacemaker cells are found in the **cardiac pacemaker**, or **sinoatrial** (sī-nō-Ā-trē-al) **node** (**SA node**), which is embedded in the wall of the right atrium near the entrance of the superior vena cava (Figure 2-7). These pacemaker cells spontaneously generate 70 to 80 electrical impulses per minute.

The other group of nodal cells is located at the junction between the atria and the ventricles. They make up the **atrioventricular** (ā-trē-ō-ven-TRIK-ū-lar) **node** (**AV node**). These cells are electrically connected to the SA nodal cells through conducting cells in the atrial walls. Isolated AV nodal cells generate only 40 to 60 electrical impulses per minutes. In the normal heart, these cells are stimulated by impulses from the SA node before they can produce an action potential on their own. If the SA nodal cells are unable to function, then the cells of the AV node will become the new pacemakers of the heart, and the resting heart rate becomes unusually low.

Conducting Cells

The stimulus for a contraction must be distributed so that (1) the atria contract together, before the ventricles, and (2) the ventricles contract together, in a wave that begins at the apex and spreads toward the base. When the ventricles contract in this way, blood is pushed toward the base of the heart, into the aortic and pulmonary trunks.

The conducting network of the heart is shown in Figure 2-7. The cells of the SA node are electrically connected to those of the AV node by conducting cells. After electrical impulses reach the AV node from the SA node, they travel to the **AV bundle**, also known as the *bundle of His* (hiss). This bundle of conducting cells travels along the interventricular septum before dividing into **left** and **right bundle branches** that radiate across the inner surfaces of the left and right ventricles. At this point specialized **Purkinje** (pur-KIN-jē) **cells** (*Purkinje fibers*) carry the impulses to the contractile cells of the ventricles. This entire process takes place in slightly less than one-quarter of a second!

Normal pacemaker activity results in an average heart rate of 70 to 75 beats per minute (bpm). A number of clinical problems result from abnormal pacemaker activity. **Bradycardia** (brā-di-KAR-dē-a) means "slow heart" and is the term used to indicate a resting heart rate that is slower than normal (less than 60 bpm), whereas **tachycardia** (tak-i-KAR-dē-a), meaning "swift heart," indicates a faster than normal resting heart rate (100 or more bpm).

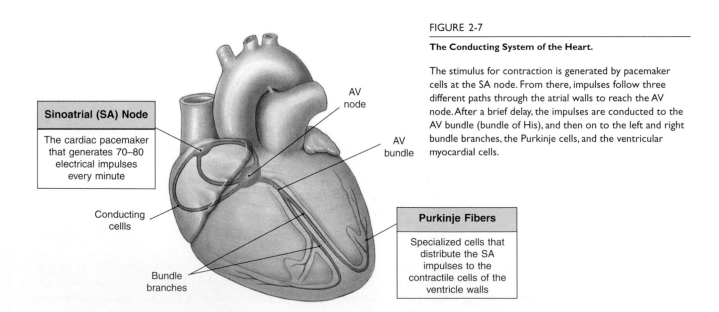

FIGURE 2-7

The Conducting System of the Heart.

The stimulus for contraction is generated by pacemaker cells at the SA node. From there, impulses follow three different paths through the atrial walls to reach the AV node. After a brief delay, the impulses are conducted to the AV bundle (bundle of His), and then on to the left and right bundle branches, the Purkinje cells, and the ventricular myocardial cells.

AV node

AV bundle

Sinoatrial (SA) Node

The cardiac pacemaker that generates 70–80 electrical impulses every minute

Conducting cells

Bundle branches

Purkinje Fibers

Specialized cells that distribute the SA impulses to the contractile cells of the ventricle walls

THE ELECTROCARDIOGRAM

The electrical impulses occurring in the heart can be detected by electrodes attached to the body surface. A recording of these electrical activities constitutes an **electrocardiogram** (ē-lek-trō-KAR-dē-ō-gram), also called an **ECG** or **EKG** (Figure 2-8). Each time the heart beats, an electrical impulse radiates through the atria, reaches the AV node, travels down the interventricular septum, turns at the apex, and spreads through the muscle tissue of the ventricles toward the base.

Figure 2-8 shows the important features of a standard electrocardiogram. The small **P wave** accompanies the electrical impulse generated by the SA node. The atria begin contracting shortly after the start of the P wave. The **QRS complex** appears as the electrical impulse passes into the walls of the ventricles. This is a relatively strong electrical signal because the amount of ventricular muscle is much larger than that of the atria. The ventricles begin contracting shortly after the peak of the R wave. The smaller **T wave** indicates the return of the unstimulated condition in the ventricles as they prepare for another contraction. By this time, the atria have recovered and are preparing for their next contraction.

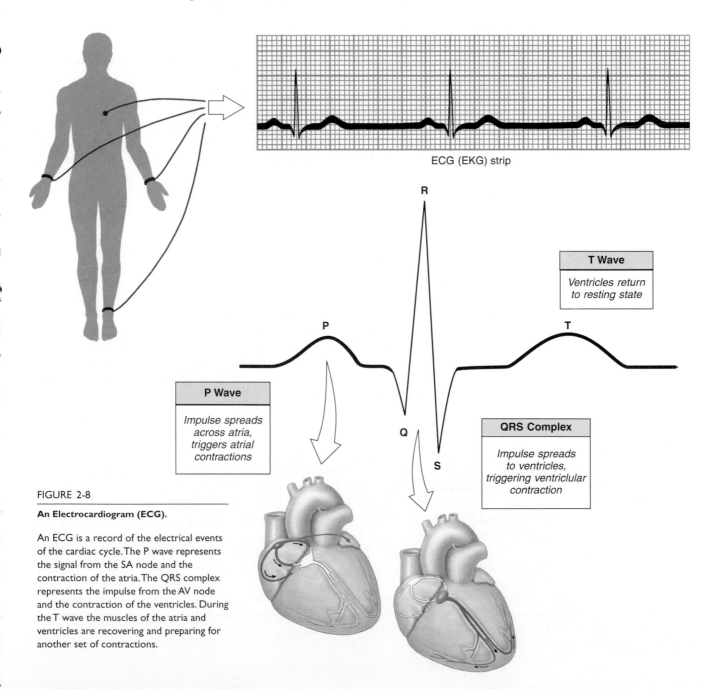

ECG (EKG) strip

R

T Wave

Ventricles return to resting state

P

T

P Wave

Impulse spreads across atria, triggers atrial contractions

Q

S

QRS Complex

Impulse spreads to ventricles, triggering ventriclular contraction

FIGURE 2-8

An Electrocardiogram (ECG).

An ECG is a record of the electrical events of the cardiac cycle. The P wave represents the signal from the SA node and the contraction of the atria. The QRS complex represents the impulse from the AV node and the contraction of the ventricles. During the T wave the muscles of the atria and ventricles are recovering and preparing for another set of contractions.

ECG analysis is especially useful in detecting and diagnosing **cardiac arrhythmias** (a-RITH-mē-as), abnormal patterns of cardiac activity. Momentary arrhythmias are not usually dangerous, and about 5 percent of the normal population experience a few abnormal heartbeats each day. Clinical problems appear when the arrhythmias reduce the pumping efficiency of the heart.

CONTROL OF HEART RATE

The amount of blood ejected by the ventricles (the cardiac output) is precisely regulated so that all the tissues of the body receive an adequate blood supply under a variety of conditions. Although the basic resting heart rate is established by the pacemaker cells of the SA node, this rate can be modified by the autonomic nervous system (ANS). Both the sympathetic and parasympathetic divisions of the ANS have direct connections at the SA and AV nodes and with the myocardium.

Neurotransmitters released by the sympathetic division cause an increase in the heart rate and in the force and degree of cardiac contraction. In contrast, neurotransmitter released by parasympathetic neurons (under control of the vagus nerves) slows the heart rate and decreases the force of cardiac contractions.

Both autonomic divisions are normally active at a steady background level, releasing neurotransmitters both at the nodes and into the myocardium. As a result, cutting the vagus nerves increases the heart rate, and administering drugs that prevent sympathetic stimulation slows the heart rate.

Other factors that can alter the heart rate include ions, hormones, and body temperature. For example, a lower than normal body temperature slows the production of electrical impulses at the SA node, reduces the strength of cardiac contractions, and lowers the heart rate. An elevated body temperature increases the heart rate and strength of cardiac contractions. This is one reason why your heart seems to be racing and pounding when you have a fever.

Concept Questions

✔ Why is it important for the electrical impulses from the atria to be delayed at the AV node before passing into the ventricles?

✔ How does bradycardia differ from a normal heart rate?

▶ BLOOD VESSELS

Propelled by the heart, bood flows to and from the lungs and other body organs through tube-like arteries and veins. The large-diameter **arteries** that carry blood away from the heart branch repeatedly and gradually decrease in size until they become **arterioles** (ar-TĒ-rē-ōlz), the smallest vessels of the arterial system. From the arterioles blood enters the capillary networks that serve local tissues.

Barely larger in diameter than a single red blood cell, capillaries are the smallest blood vessels. It is at the capillaries that the vital functions of the cardiovascular system take place. All the exchanges of chemicals and gases between the blood and interstitial fluid take place across capillary walls.

Blood flowing out of the capillaries first enters the **venules** (VEN-ūlz), the smallest vessels of the venous system. These slender vessels subsequently merge with their neighbors to form small **veins**. Blood then passes through medium-sized and large veins before reaching the heart.

VESSEL STRUCTURE

The walls of arteries and veins contain three distinct layers, or *tunics*. The innermost layer of a blood vessel is made up of a squamous epithelium called an *endothelium*. The middle layer contains smooth muscle tissue in a framework of collagen and elastic fibers. When these smooth muscles contract, the vessel decreases in diameter (an action known as *vasoconstriction*), and when they relax, the diameter increases (an action termed *vasodilation*). The outer layer consists of a stabilizing sheath of connective tissue.

The multiple layers in their vessel walls give arteries and veins considerable strength, and the muscular and elastic components permit controlled alterations in diameter as blood pressure or blood volume changes.

Figure 2-9 shows the differences in structure of an artery, capillary, and vein. Arteries have the thickest walls and contain more smooth muscle and elastic fibers than veins. Note that the walls of capillaries are only one cell thick.

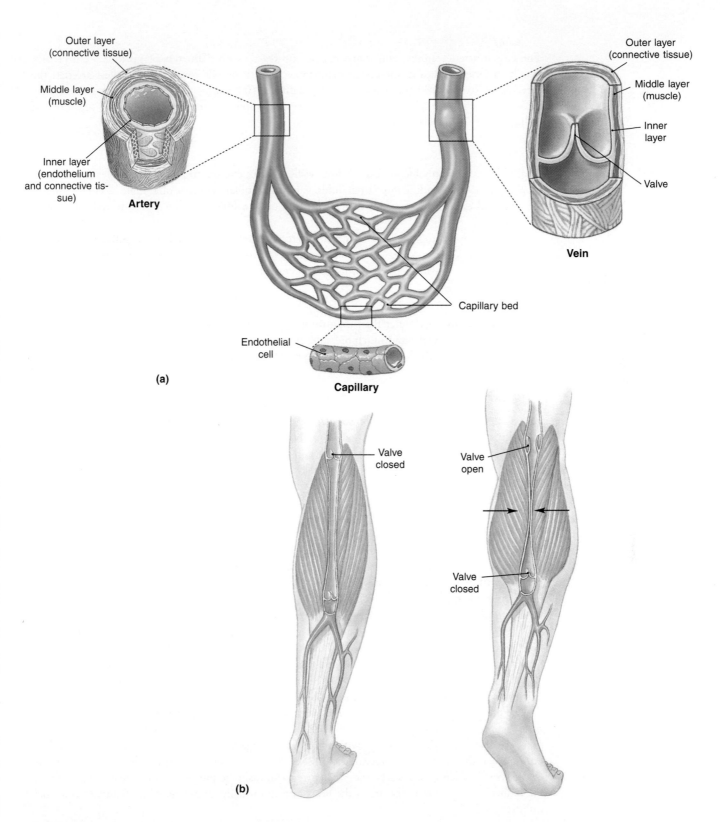

Outer layer
(connective tissue)

Middle layer
(muscle)

Inner layer
(endothelium
and connective tis-
sue)

Artery

Outer layer
(connective tissue)

Middle layer
(muscle)

Inner
layer

Valve

Vein

Capillary bed

Endothelial
cell

(a)

Capillary

Valve
closed

Valve
open

Valve
closed

(b)

FIGURE 2-9

Structure of Blood Vessels.

(a) A comparison of a typical artery, capillary, and vein. Note that the walls of arteries and veins are made up of three layers of tissue, but a capillary wall is only one cell thick. **(b)** Valves in the walls of medium-sized veins prevent the backflow of blood. Squeezing of the veins by the contraction of adjacent skeletal muscles helps maintain venous blood flow.

Arteries

The largest arteries are extremely resilient, elastic vessels with diameters of up to 2.5 cm (1 in.). Smaller arteries are less elastic and contain more smooth muscle tissue. The smallest arteries, the **arterioles**, have an average diameter of about 30 μm (0.03 mm). The smooth muscle cells help these vessels change their diameter. Such changes are important in altering the blood pressure and changing the rate of flow through body tissues.

Capillaries

Capillaries are the only blood vessels whose walls are thin enough to permit exchanges between the blood and the surrounding interstitial fluids. A typical capillary consists of a single layer of endothelial cells and an average diameter that is a mere 8 μm (0. 008 mm), very close to that of a single red blood cell.

Capillaries work together as part of an interconnected network called a **capillary bed**. Upon reaching its target area, a single arteriole usually gives rise to a capillary bed made up of dozens of capillaries that, in turn, merge to form several **venules**, the smallest vessels of the venous system.

Veins

The walls of veins are thinner than than those of arteries. Veins have relatively thin walls because they do not have to withstand much pressure. In the limbs, medium-sized veins contain **valves** that act like the valves in the heart, preventing the backflow of blood (see Figure 2-9b).

BLOOD PRESSURE

The tissues and organs of the cardiovascular system (blood, heart, and blood vessels) work together to maintain an adequate flow of blood to the body's tissues. Adequate blood flow requires enough pressure to push the blood through smaller and smaller arteries, along the capillaries, and back to the heart through the venous system. Generally, blood flow is equal to cardiac output. The higher the cardiac output, the higher the blood flow and pressure, and the lower the cardiac output, the lower the blood flow and pressure.

Two factors affect blood flow: *pressure* and *resistance*. **Blood pressure** is the pressure, or force, that blood exerts against the walls of the blood vessels. Resistance to blood flow primarily results from the length and diameter of blood vessels and the viscosity, or "thickness," of blood. Blood pressure is highest in the larger arteries because they are closest to the heart. Resistance, however, is greatest within the smallest diameter vessels (arterioles and capillaries) because of the friction of blood rubbing against their walls. Because blood is some five times "thicker" than water, it is also harder to push through the blood vessels.

Blood pressure rises and falls in the larger arteries in response to the pumping activities of the heart. Blood pressure is measured in units of millimeters of mercury (mm Hg), a standardized unit of pressure. Blood pressure in the systemic circulation reaches a maximum "normal" level of 120 mm Hg in the largest arteries during ventricular systole. During ventricular diastole, blood pressure falls to about 80 mm Hg. Figure 2-10 shows the basic steps involved in measuring blood pressure.

The difference between the systolic and diastolic pressures is the **pulse pressure.** The pulse pressure becomes smaller as the distance from the heart increases. The usual procedure for feeling the pulse involves squeezing an artery with the fingertips against a relatively solid mass, preferably a bone. When the vessel is compressed, the pulse is felt as a pressure against the fingertips. The inside of the wrist is often used because the *radial artery* can easily be pressed against the distal portion of the radius. The pulse is a measure of the heart rate and usually ranges between 70 and 75 beats per minute at rest.

Capillaries and Fluid Movement

As blood passes through the capillaries, blood pressure drops even further, and the blood flow slows down. Unlike other blood vessels, however, capillaries are permeable to water, ions, and other small solutes (dissolved materials). Diffusion, blood pressure, and osmosis are the primary important

✚ Clinical Note

How Is Blood Pressure Measured?

Blood pressure is determined with a *sphygmomanometer* (sfig-mō-ma-NOM-e-ter). Derived from *sphygmos*, meaning "pulse," and *manometer*, "a device for measuring pressure," this instrument is used to measure *arterial pressure* (the blood pressure in arteries). As shown in Figure 2-10, an inflatable cuff is placed around the arm in such a position that its inflation squeezes the brachial artery. A stethoscope is placed over the artery below the cuff, and the cuff is then inflated. A tube connects the cuff to a glass chamber containing liquid mercury, and as the pressure in the cuff rises, it pushes the mercury up into a vertical column. A scale along the column permits one to determine the cuff pressure in millimeters of mercury. Inflation continues until cuff pressure is roughly 30 mm Hg above the pressure sufficient to completely collapse the brachial artery, stop the flow of blood, and eliminate the sound of the pulse.

The investigator then slowly lets the air out of the cuff with the releasing valve. When the pressure in the cuff falls below systolic pressure, blood can again enter the artery. At first, blood enters only at peak systolic pressures, and the stethoscope picks up the sound of blood pulsing through the artery. As the pressure falls further, the sound changes because the vessel is remaining open for longer and longer periods. When the cuff pressure falls below diastolic pressure, blood flow becomes continuous and the sound of the pulse becomes muffled or disappears completely. Thus the pressure at which the pulse appears corresponds to the peak systolic pressure; when the pulse fades the pressure has reached diastolic levels.

When the blood pressure is recorded, systolic and diastolic pressures are usually separated by a slash mark, as in "120/80" ("one-twenty over eighty") or "110/75." These values are considered normal for young adults. High blood pressure, or *hypertension*, occurs when the systolic pressure is over 140, and the diastolic pressure is over 95 (140/95).

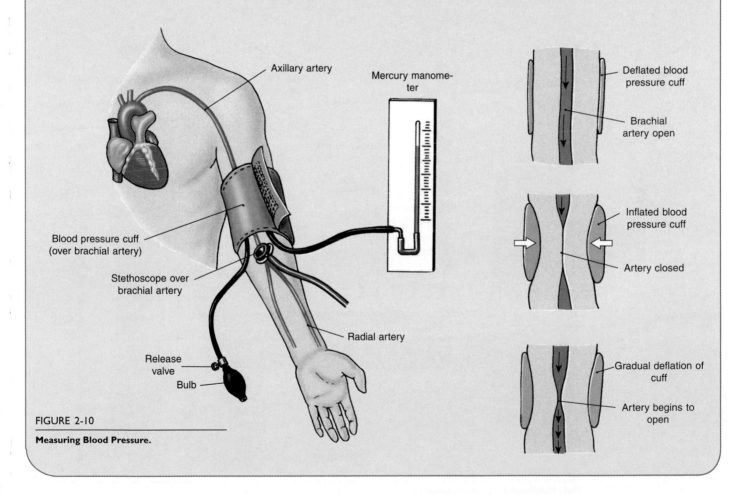

FIGURE 2-10

Measuring Blood Pressure.

forces that cause exchange across the walls of capillaries. Diffusion is the passive movement of dissolved materials from an area of relatively high concentration to an area of relatively low concentration. Diffusion across capillary walls tends to move oxygen and nutrients into the surrounding tissues, whereas carbon dioxide and waste products tend to diffuse from the tissues into the bloodstream.

Blood pressure tends to push water and dissolved substances out of the bloodstream and into the tissues. Osmosis refers to the movement of water between two solutions separated by a selectively permeable membrane, which in this case is the capillary wall. Osmosis always involves water movement into the solution that contains a higher concentration of solutes. As we noted earlier in the chapter, plasma proteins are the primary contributors to the osmotic concentration of the blood. The balance between blood pressure and osmosis tends to shift along a capillary from its start at an arteriole to its end at a venule (Figure 2-11).

At the start of a capillary, blood pressure is relatively high. This tends to force water and other small dissolved materials out of the bloodstream and into the surrounding tissue fluid. When this movement occurs, it increases the solute concentration in the blood, because plasma proteins cannot cross the capillary walls. At first, osmosis cannot eliminate this concentration gradient, because the blood pressure is too high—it is pushing water out of the bloodstream faster than osmosis can pull it back in. However, as blood flows along the capillary, the blood pressure gradually decreases. As the blood nears the end of the capillary, osmosis draws much of the released water and solutes back into the bloodstream. By the time the blood enters the venule, all but about one sixth of the

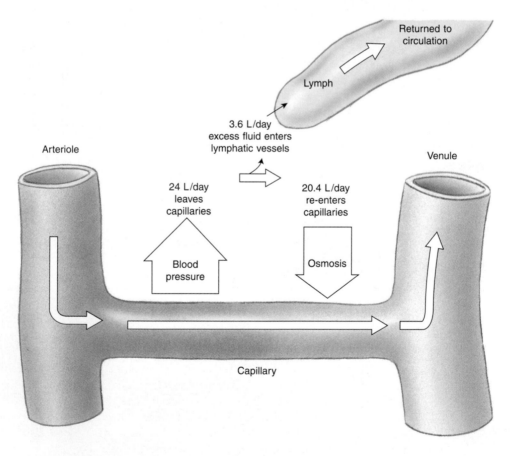

FIGURE 2-11

Fluid Movement Across the Capillaries.

Fluid passes through capillary walls because of differences in osmosis and blood pressure along the length of the capillary. Most of the outflow of fluid from the capillaries is reabsorbed by osmosis. The fluid not immediately reabsorbed into the capillaries flows into lymphatic vessels, which then return it to the venous circulation.

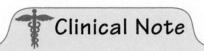

Clinical Note

What Do Red Lips, Dark Circles Under the Eyes, and Blushing Have in Common?

Blood vessels! All these different features are due to blood vessels that lie near the surface of the skin.

For example, lips are reddish in color because of the color of their underlying capillaries. The color is visible through this part of the skin because the lips are covered only by a thin, almost transparent layer of epidermis.

Dark circles under the eyes are due to tiny blood vessels located in those areas. These vessels normally collect blood from the head. When an individual is ill or tired, these vessels become wider, or dilated, and hold larger amounts of blood than normal. As with the lips, the skin in this region is also thin, and so the blood-filled vessels are more easily seen.

Blushing is a brief and sudden reddening of the face and sometimes the neck. It occurs when blood vessels close to the surface of the skin dilate, or widen, in an involuntary response to embarrassment. Blushing also occurs in some women during menopause in response to changes in the levels of sex hormones.

total volume of fluid pushed into the tissues along the capillary has been reabsorbed. In the course of a typical day, 24 L of fluid are forced out of the capillaries into the interstitial fluids, and roughly 21.4 L are reabsorbed. The rest, 3.6 L, mixes with the interstitial fluid, flows through the tissues, and then enters the *lymphatic vessels*. These vessels, part of the lymphatic system, return 3.6 L of fluid, now called *lymph*, to the venous system each day.

▶ REGULATION OF BLOOD FLOW

Body tissues require a constant blood flow to meet their demands for oxygen and nutrients. To meet these needs, homeostatic adjustments may occur in any of the three main variables that affect tissue blood flow: cardiac output, vessel resistance, and blood pressure.

Generally, short-term responses adjust cardiac output and blood vessel resistance to stabilize blood pressure and tissue blood flow. Long-term adjustments mainly involve changes in blood volume.

SHORT-TERM RESPONSES

Tissues can indirectly regulate their own blood flow through capillary networks. The smooth muscles of the arterioles that open into such networks contract and relax in response to varying levels of oxygen and carbon dioxide. When oxygen is abundant in a tissue, the smooth muscles contract and reduce blood flow. In contrast, when carbon dioxide concentration is high, the smooth muscles relax and increase blood flow. Such regulation by local factors provides a rapid response to immediate tissue needs.

The nervous system also provides a rapid response to maintain adequate blood flow. It does this through adjustments of cardiac output and blood vessel resistance. Changes in blood pressure and the levels of blood gases at specific sensory receptors stimulate these responses of the nervous system.

The medulla oblongata of the brain stem contains two important cardiovascular centers: the *cardiac* and *vasomotor centers*. The cardiac centers control cardiac output, and the vasomotor centers control blood vessel resistance. The cardiac centers include a *cardioacceleratory center* and a *cardioinhibitory center*. Sympathetic stimulation of the heart by the cardioacceleratory center increases cardiac output, and parasympathetic stimulation of the heart by the cardioinhibitory center decreases cardiac output.

The vasomotor center primarily controls the diameters of the arterioles. Inhibition of the vasomotor center leads to **vasodilation**, a dilation (widening) of arterioles that reduces vessel resistance. Stimulation of the vasomotor center causes **vasoconstriction**, a narrowing of the arterioles, which increases vessel resistance.

LONG-TERM RESPONSES

Hormones from the endocrine system are associated with both short-term and long-term responses. Epinephrine (E) and norepinephrine (NE) from the adrenal medullae act within seconds of their release to stimulate cardiac output and trigger the vasoconstriction of blood vessels.

Four other hormones—antidiuretic hormone (ADH), angiotensin II, erythropoietin (EPO), and atrial natriuretic peptide (ANP)—are concerned primarily with the long-term regulation of blood volume and blood pressure. All but ANP are stimulated by decreased blood pressure.

Angiotensin II appears in the blood following the release of renin by specialized kidney cells. Angiotensin II causes an extremely powerful vasoconstriction that elevates blood pressure almost at once. It also stimulates the secretion of ADH by the pituitary, and aldosterone by the adrenal cortex. These two hormones help increase blood pressure by increasing the volume of blood. ADH stimulates water conservation at the kidneys, and promotes thirst. Aldosterone stimulates the reabsorption of sodium ions and water at the kidneys, reducing their loss in the urine.

EPO is released at the kidneys in response to low blood pressure or low oxygen content of the blood. This hormone stimulates red blood cell production. Having more red blood cells increases the blood volume and improves the oxygen-carrying capacity of the blood.

ANP is produced by specialized cardiac muscle cells in the atrial walls when they are stretched by excessive amounts of venous blood. Unlike the three previous hormones, ANP reduces blood volume and blood pressure. It acts by increasing water losses at the kidneys, reducing thirst, and stimulating vasodilation. As blood volume and blood pressure decline, the stress on the atrial walls is removed, and ANP production decreases.

► BLOOD VESSELS OF THE BODY

The circulatory system is divided into the pulmonary and systemic circulations. The pulmonary circulation, which transports blood between the heart and the lungs, begins at the right ventricle and ends at the left atrium. From the left ventricle, the arteries of the systemic circulation transport oxygenated blood to all the organs and tissues of the body except the lungs, ultimately returning deoxygenated blood to the right atrium. Figure 2-12 summarizes the primary circulatory routes within the pulmonary and systemic circulations.

PULMONARY CIRCULATION

Blood entering the right atrium is returning from a trip through capillary networks where oxygen was released and carbon dioxide absorbed. After passing through the right atrium and ventricle, blood enters the **pulmonary trunk**, the start of the pulmonary circulation. Along the pulmonary circulation a fresh supply of oxygen enters the blood, carbon dioxide is excreted, and the oxygenated blood is returned to the heart for distribution in the systemic circulation.

Figure 2-13 shows the structure of the pulmonary circulation. The arteries of the pulmonary circulation differ from those of the systemic circulation in that they carry deoxygenated blood. (For this reason, color-coded diagrams usually show the pulmonary arteries in blue, the same color as systemic veins.) The pulmonary trunk gives rise to the **left** and **right pulmonary arteries**. These large arteries enter the lungs before branching repeatedly, giving rise to smaller and smaller arteries. The smallest arterioles provide blood to capillary networks that surround small air pockets or sacs, called *alveoli* (al-VĒ-ol-i). The walls of alveoli are thin enough for gas exchange to occur between the capillary blood and air. As it leaves the alveolar capillaries, oxygenated blood enters venules that in turn unite to form larger vessels carrying blood to the **pulmonary veins**. These four veins, two from each lung, empty into the left atrium.

SYSTEMIC CIRCULATION: ARTERIES

The systemic circulation supplies the capillary beds in all other parts of the body. It begins at the left ventricle and ends at the right atrium. Figure 2-14 indicates the names and relative locations of the major arteries of the body.

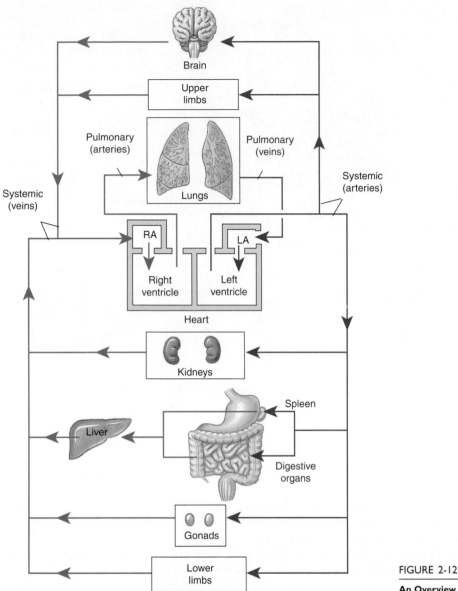

FIGURE 2-12

An Overview of the Pattern of Circulation.

The **ascending aorta** begins at the aortic semilunar valve of the left ventricle. The *left* and *right coronary arteries* originate near its base. The **aortic arch** curves over the top of the heart, connecting the ascending aorta with the **descending aorta**.

Arteries of the Aortic Arch

The three arteries that originate along the aortic arch are the **brachiocephalic** (brā-kē-ō-se-FAL-ik; *brachium,* arm + *cephalon,* head), the **left common carotid**, and the **left subclavian** (sub-KLĀ-vē-an; *sub,* below + *clavis,* a key). They deliver blood to the head, neck, shoulders, and upper limbs. The brachiocephalic artery branches to form the **right common carotid artery** and the **right subclavian artery**.

The Subclavian Arteries

The subclavian arteries supply blood to the upper limbs, chest wall, shoulders, back, and central nervous system. Before a subclavian artery leaves the thoracic cavity it gives rise to an artery that

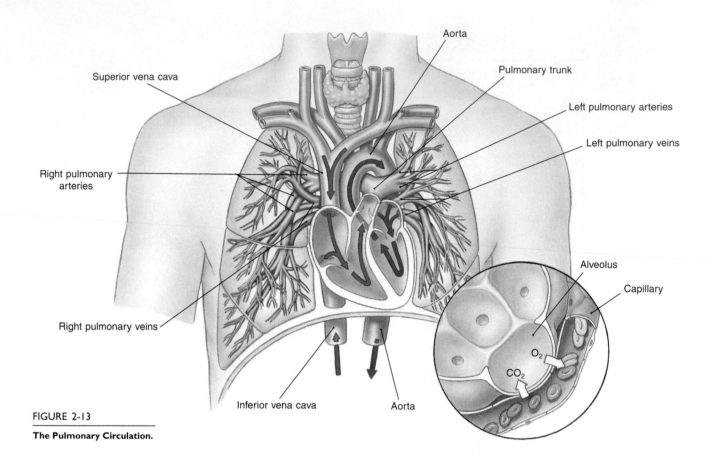

FIGURE 2-13

The Pulmonary Circulation.

supplies the pericardium and anterior wall of the chest, and a **vertebral artery** that supplies blood to the brain and spinal cord.

After passing the first rib, the subclavian gets a new name, the **axillary artery**. The axillary artery crosses the axilla (armpit) to enter the arm, where its name changes again, becoming the **brachial artery**. The brachial artery provides blood to the arm before branching to create the **radial artery** and **ulnar artery** of the forearm. These arteries are interconnected by anastomoses at the palm, from which arteries to the fingers arise. In this way, blood can reach the fingers by various routes.

Arteries Supplying the Brain

The common carotid arteries ascend deep in the tissues of the neck. A carotid artery can usually be located by pressing gently along either side of the trachea until a strong pulse is felt. Each common carotid artery divides into an **external carotid** and an **internal carotid** artery at an expanded chamber, the *carotid sinus*. The external carotids supply blood to the pharynx, larynx, and face. The internal carotids enter the skull to deliver blood to the brain.

The brain is extremely sensitive to changes in its circulatory supply. An interruption of circulation for several seconds will produce unconsciousness, and after 4 minutes there may be some permanent brain damage. Such circulatory problems are rare because blood reaches the brain through the vertebral arteries as well as by way of the internal carotids. Inside the cranium, the vertebral arteries fuse to form a large **basilar artery** that continues along the lower surface of the brain. This gives rise to the vessels indicated in Figure 2-15.

Normally, the internal carotids supply the arteries of the front half of the cerebrum, and the rest of the brain receives blood from the vertebral arteries. But this circulatory pattern can easily change because the internal carotids and the basilar artery are interconnected in a ring-shaped anastomosis, the **cerebral arterial circle**, or *circle of Willis*, that encircles the stalk (infundibulum) of the pituitary gland. With this arrangement, the brain can receive blood from either the carotids or the vertebrals, and the chances for a serious interruption of circulation are reduced.

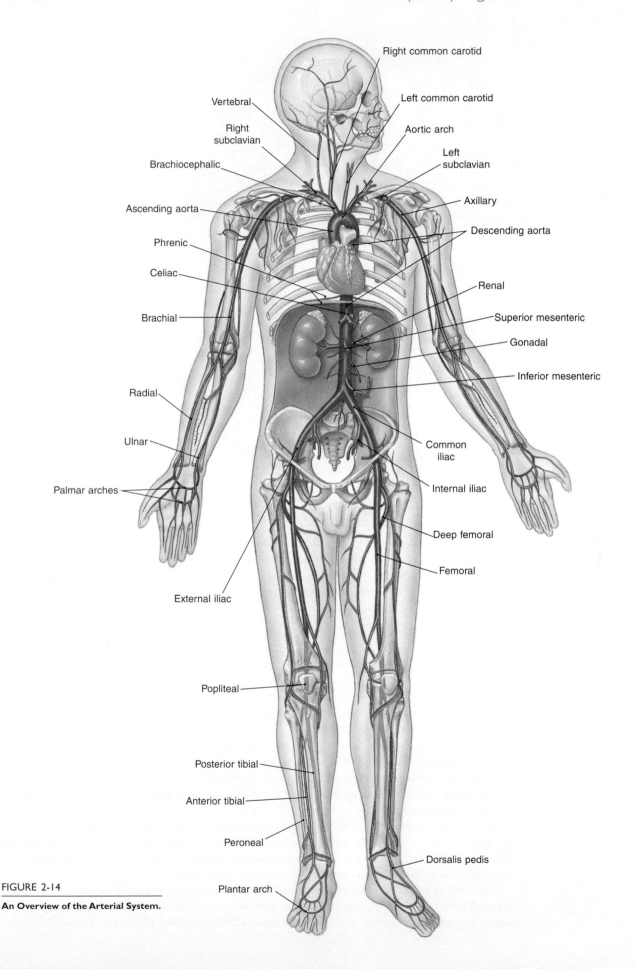

Right common carotid
Left common carotid
Vertebral
Aortic arch
Right subclavian
Left subclavian
Brachiocephalic
Axillary
Ascending aorta
Descending aorta
Phrenic
Renal
Celiac
Superior mesenteric
Brachial
Gonadal
Inferior mesenteric
Radial
Common iliac
Ulnar
Internal iliac
Palmar arches
Deep femoral
Femoral
External iliac
Popliteal
Posterior tibial
Anterior tibial
Peroneal
Dorsalis pedis
Plantar arch

FIGURE 2-14

An Overview of the Arterial System.

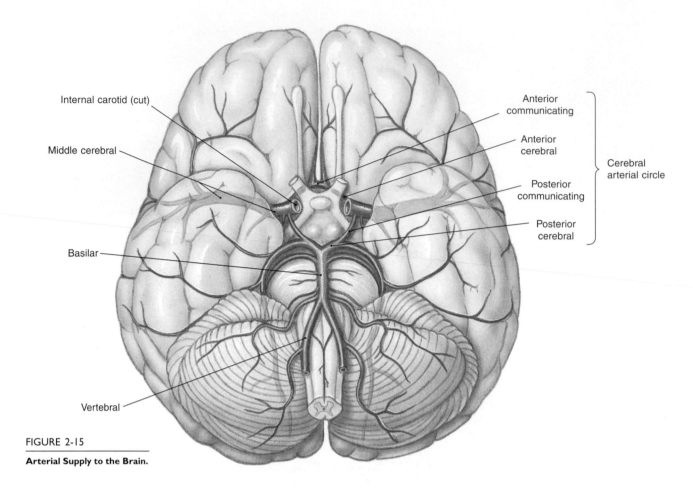

FIGURE 2-15

Arterial Supply to the Brain.

Branches of the Thoracic Aorta

The portion of the descending aorta within the chest is called the *thoracic aorta*. It provides blood to the **intercostal** (*inter*, between + *costa*, rib) **arteries**, which carry blood to the spinal cord and the body wall. Other branches of this artery provide blood to the esophagus and pericardium. The **phrenic** (FREN-ik) **arteries** deliver blood to the muscular diaphragm that separates the thoracic and abdominopelvic cavities.

Branches of the Abdominal Aorta

The portion of the descending aorta inferior to the diaphragm is called the *abdominal aorta*. The abdominal aorta delivers blood to arteries that distribute blood to organs of the digestive system, and to the kidneys and adrenal glands. The **celiac** (SĒ-lē-ak), **superior mesenteric** (mez-en-TER-ik), and **inferior mesenteric arteries** provide blood to all the digestive organs in the abdominopelvic cavity. The celiac divides into three branches that deliver blood to the liver, spleen, and stomach. The superior mesenteric artery supplies the pancreas, small intestine, and most of the large intestine. The inferior mesenteric delivers blood to the last portion of the large intestine and the rectum.

Paired **gonadal** (gō-NAD-al) **arteries** originate between the superior and inferior mesenteric arteries; in males they are called *testicular arteries*; in females, *ovarian arteries*.

The **renal arteries** arise along the sides of the abdominal aorta and provide blood to the adrenal glands and kidneys.

Within the lumbar region, the abdominal aorta divides to form the **common iliac** (IL-ē-ak) **arteries** that carry blood to the pelvis and lower limbs. As it travels along the inner surface of the ilium, each common iliac divides to form an **internal iliac artery** that supplies smaller arteries of the pelvis and an **external iliac artery** that enters the lower limb.

Once in the thigh, the external iliac artery branches, forming the **femoral artery** and the **deep femoral artery**. When it reaches the leg, the femoral artery becomes the **popliteal artery**, which almost immediately branches to form the **anterior tibial**, **posterior tibial**, and **peroneal** arteries.

These arteries are connected by two anastomoses, one on the top of the foot (the *dorsalis pedis*) and one on the bottom (the *plantar arch*).

SYSTEMIC CIRCULATION: VEINS

Figure 2-16 shows the major veins of the body. Arteries and veins supplying and draining the same organs and structures often run side by side, and in many cases they have comparable names. For example, the axillary arteries run alongside the axillary veins. In addition, arteries and veins often travel in the company of nerves that have the same names and innervate the same structures.

One significant exception to this pairing of arteries and veins occurs with the distribution of major veins in the neck and limbs. Arteries in these areas are not found at the body surface; instead, they are deep beneath the skin, protected by bones and surrounding soft tissues. In contrast, there are usually two sets of veins, one superficial and the other deep. The superficial veins are so close to the surface that they can be seen quite easily. This makes them easy targets for obtaining blood samples, and most blood tests are performed on venous blood collected from the superficial veins of the upper limb, usually a *median cubital vein* where it crosses the elbow.

This dual venous drainage helps control body temperature. When body temperature becomes abnormally low, the arterial blood supply to the skin is reduced and the superficial veins are bypassed. Blood entering the limbs then returns to the trunk in the deep veins. When overheating occurs, the blood supply to the skin increases and the superficial veins dilate. This is one reason why superficial veins in the limbs become so visible during periods of heavy exercise, or when sitting in a sauna, hot tub, or steam bath.

Superior Vena Cava

The **superior vena cava** (**SVC**) receives blood from the head and neck and the chest, shoulders, and upper limbs.

Head and neck. Small veins in the nervous tissue of the brain empty into a network of thin-walled channels, the **dural sinuses**. A sinus is a chamber or hollow in a tissue. Most of the blood leaving the brain passes through one of the dural sinuses and enters one of the **internal jugular veins** that descend in the deep tissues of the neck. The more superficial **external jugular veins** collect blood from the overlying structures of the head and neck. **Vertebral veins** drain the cervical spinal cord and the posterior surface of the skull.

Limbs and chest. A network of veins in the palms collects blood from each finger. These vessels drain into the **cephalic vein** and the **basilic vein**. The deeper veins of the forearm are the **radial** and **ulnar veins**. After crossing the elbow, these veins join to form the **brachial vein**. As the brachial vein continues toward the trunk it receives blood from the cephalic and basilic veins before entering the **axillary vein**.

The axillary vein then continues into the trunk, and at the level of the first rib it becomes the **subclavian vein**. After traveling a short distance inside the thoracic cavity, the subclavian meets and merges with the external and internal jugular veins of that side. This merger creates the large **brachiocephalic vein**. Near the heart, the two brachiocephalic veins (one from each side of the body) combine to create the superior vena cava. The superior vena cava receives blood from the thoracic body wall in the **azygos** (AZ-i-gos; unpaired) **vein** before arriving at the right atrium.

Inferior Vena Cava

The **inferior vena cava** (**IVC**) collects most of the venous blood from organs below the diaphragm.

Blood leaving the capillaries in the sole of each foot is collected by the *plantar venous arch,* which provides blood to the **anterior tibial vein**, the **posterior tibial vein**, and the **peroneal vein**, the deep veins of the leg. A *dorsal venous arch* drains blood from capillaries on the superior surface of the foot. This arch is drained by two superficial veins, the **great saphenous vein** (sa-FĒ-nus) and the **small saphenous vein**. The term *saphenous* means "prominent." (Surgeons use segments of the great saphenous vein, the largest superficial vein, as bypass vessels during coronary bypass surgery.) There are extensive interconnections between the plantar arch and the dorsal arch, and the path of blood flow can easily shift from superficial to deep veins.

At the knee, the small saphenous, tibial, and peroneal veins unite to form the **popliteal vein**, which, when it reaches the femur, becomes the **femoral vein**. Immediately before penetrating the

FIGURE 2-16

An Overview of the Venous System.

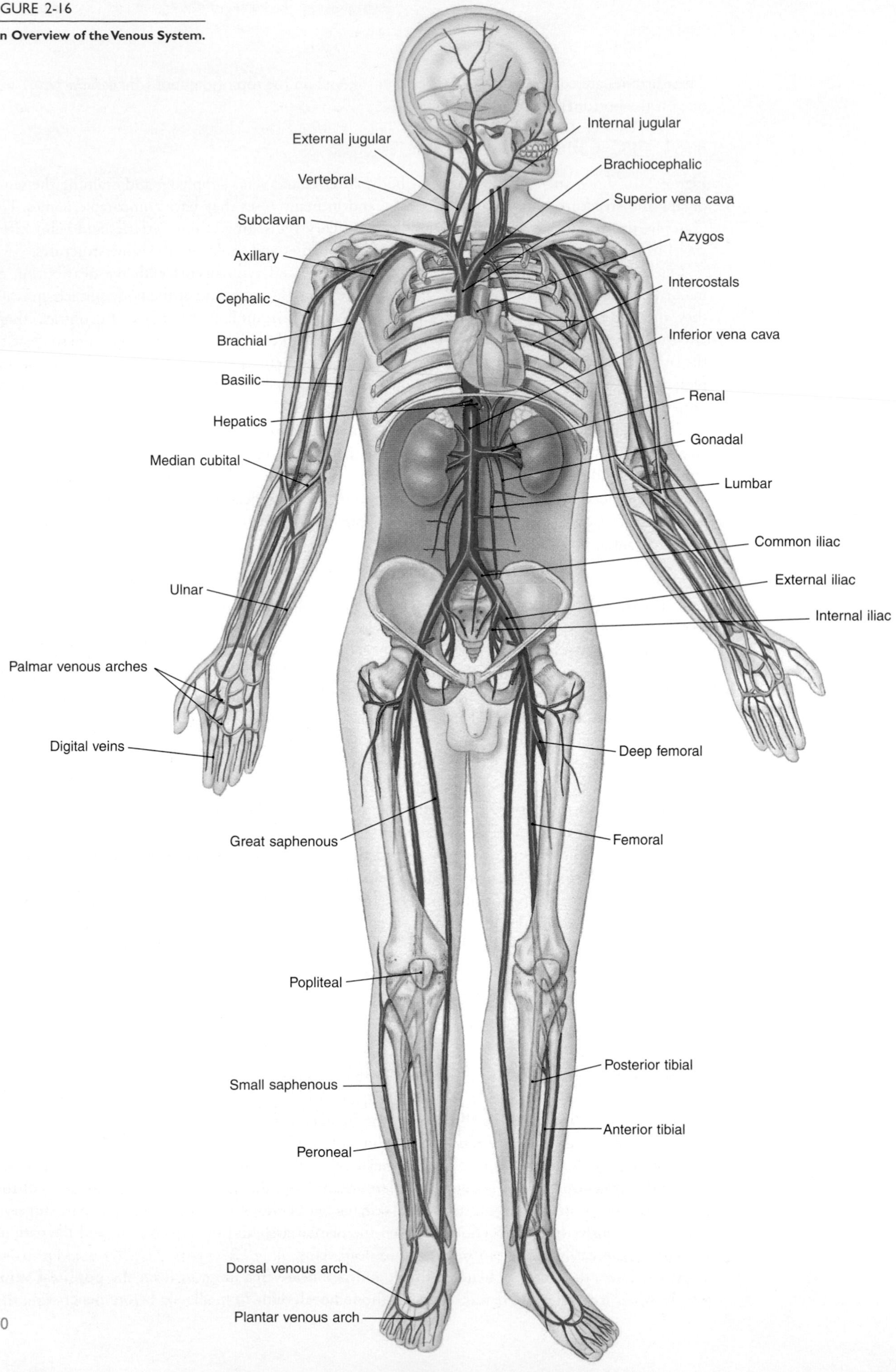

External jugular

Vertebral

Subclavian

Axillary

Cephalic

Brachial

Basilic

Hepatics

Median cubital

Ulnar

Palmar venous arches

Digital veins

Great saphenous

Popliteal

Small saphenous

Peroneal

Dorsal venous arch

Plantar venous arch

Internal jugular

Brachiocephalic

Superior vena cava

Azygos

Intercostals

Inferior vena cava

Renal

Gonadal

Lumbar

Common iliac

External iliac

Internal iliac

Deep femoral

Femoral

Posterior tibial

Anterior tibial

abdominal wall, the femoral, great saphenous, and **deep femoral veins** unite. The large vein that results penetrates the body wall as the **external iliac vein**. The external iliac fuses with the **internal iliac vein**, which drains the pelvic organs. The resulting **common iliac vein** then meets its counterpart from the opposite side to form the inferior vena cava.

Like the aorta, the inferior vena cava lies posterior to the abdominopelvic cavity. As it ascends to the heart it collects blood from several **lumbar veins**, which may also empty into the common iliac vein. In addition, the IVC receives blood from the **gonadal**, **renal**, **suprarenal**, **phrenic**, and **hepatic veins** before reaching the right atrium.

Hepatic Portal System

You may have noticed that the veins just discussed did not include any veins from the digestive organs other than the liver. That is because blood from the capillaries serving the digestive organs does not enter veins that connect with the inferior vena cava. Instead, blood leaving the capillaries supplied by the celiac, superior, and inferior mesenteric arteries flows to the liver through the **hepatic portal system.** (A portal is a gate.) Blood in this system is quite different from that in other veins, because the hepatic portal vessels contain substances absorbed from the digestive tract. For example, levels of blood glucose, amino acids, fatty acids, and vitamins in the hepatic portal vein often exceed those found anywhere else in the cardiovascular system.

A portal system carries blood from one capillary bed to another and, in the process, prevents its contents from dilution by the entire bloodstream. The hepatic portal system begins at capillaries of the digestive tract and ends at capillaries in the liver. The liver regulates the concentrations of nutrients, such as glucose or amino acids, in the arriving blood before it continues into the inferior vena cava. When digestion is under way, the digestive tract absorbs high concentrations of nutrients, along with various wastes and an occasional toxin. The hepatic portal system delivers these compounds directly to the liver, where liver cells absorb them for storage, process them for immediate use, or excrete them. After passing through the liver capillaries, blood collects in the hepatic veins that empty into the inferior vena cava. The liver, then, is in an ideal position to regulate and maintain the composition of the blood in a relatively stable condition.

Figure 2-17 shows the vessels of the hepatic portal system. It begins in the capillaries of the digestive organs. Blood from capillaries along the lower portion of the large intestine enters the **inferior mesenteric vein**. As it nears the liver, veins from the spleen, the stomach, and the pancreas fuse with the inferior mesenteric, forming the **splenic vein**. The **superior mesenteric vein** collects blood from the entire small intestine, two thirds of the large intestine, and a portion of the stomach. The **hepatic portal vein**, which empties into the liver capillaries, forms through the fusion of the superior mesenteric and splenic veins.

FETAL CIRCULATION

There are significant differences in our cardiovascular systems before and after birth. The differences reflect differing sources of respiratory and nutritional support. For example, the lungs of the developing fetus are collapsed and nonfunctional, and the digestive tract has nothing to digest. Before birth, these needs are provided by the placenta.

Placental Blood Supply

Fetal circulation is shown in Figure 2-18a. Blood flow to the placenta is provided by a pair of **umbilical arteries** that arise from the internal iliac arteries and enter the umbilical cord. Blood returns from the placenta in the **umbilical vein**, bringing oxygen and nutrients to the developing fetus. The umbilical vein delivers blood to capillaries within the developing liver and to the inferior vena cava by the **ductus venosus**. At birth, blood flow ceases along the umbilical vessels, and they soon degenerate.

Circulatory Changes at Birth

One of the most interesting aspects of circulatory development occurs at birth. Throughout embryonic and fetal life, the lungs are collapsed; yet following delivery, the newborn infant must be able to extract oxygen from inspired air rather than across the placenta.

Although the septa between the chambers of the heart develop early in fetal life, the interatrial septum contains an opening up to the time of birth. This opening, called the **foramen ovale**, is covered by a flap that acts as a valve. Blood can flow freely from the right atrium to the left atrium,

Concept Questions

✔ Blockage of which branch of the aortic arch would interfere with the blood flow to the left arm?

✔ Why would compression of the common carotid artery cause a person to lose consciousness?

✔ Grace is in an automobile accident and ruptures her celiac artery. What organs would be affected most directly by this injury?

FIGURE 2-17

The Hepatic Portal System.

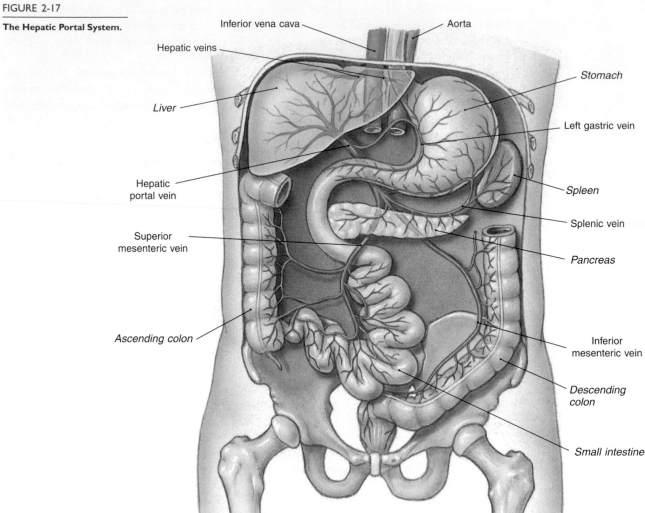

but any backflow will close the valve and isolate the two chambers. This allows blood to enter the heart at the right atrium and bypass the lungs. A second short-circuit exists between the pulmonary and aortic trunks. This connection, the **ductus arteriosus**, consists of a short, muscular vessel.

At birth dramatic changes occur in circulatory patterns (Figure 2-18b). When an infant takes its first breath, the lungs expand, and so do the pulmonary vessels. Within a few seconds, the smooth muscles in the ductus arteriosus contract, isolating the pulmonary and aortic trunks, and blood begins flowing into and out of the lungs. As pressures rise in the left atrium, the valvular flap closes the foramen ovale and completes the circulatory remodeling.

► AGING AND THE CARDIOVASCULAR SYSTEM

The capabilities of the cardiovascular system gradually decline with age. Age-related changes occur in the blood, heart, and blood vessels.

- **Blood.** Age-related changes in the blood may include (1) decreased hematocrit, (2) constriction or blockage of peripheral veins by formation of a thrombus (stationary blood clot), and (3) pooling of blood in the veins of the legs because the valves in these veins are no longer working effectively.

- **Heart.** Major age-related changes in the heart include (1) a reduction in the maximum cardiac output, (2) changes in the activities of the nodal and conducting cells, (3) replacement of damaged cardiac muscle cells by scar tissue, and (4) progressive blood vessel changes that restrict coronary circulation.

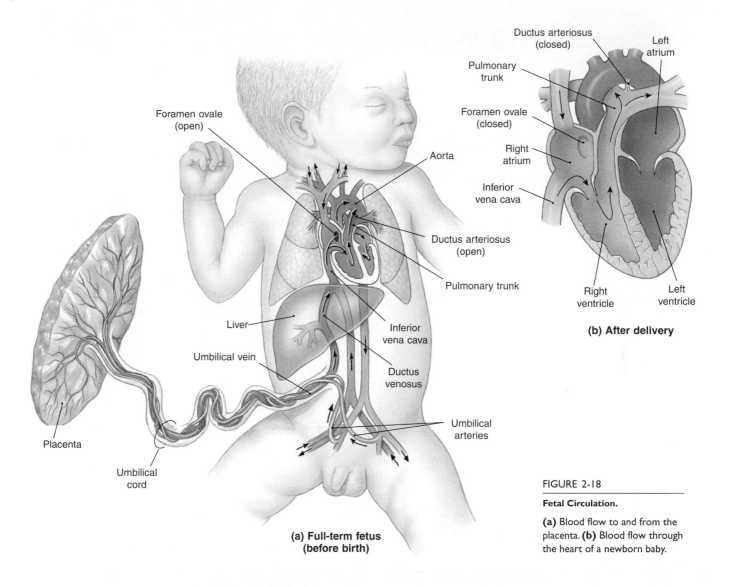

FIGURE 2-18

Fetal Circulation.

(a) Blood flow to and from the placenta. (b) Blood flow through the heart of a newborn baby.

- **The Blood Vessels.** Age-related changes in blood vessels are often related to **arteriosclerosis** (ar-tē-rē-ō-skle-RŌ-sis), a thickening and toughening of arterial walls. **Atherosclerosis** (ath-er-ō-skle-RŌ-sis) is a type of arteriosclerosis characterized by changes in the endothelial lining of blood vessels. Atherosclerosis in coronary vessels restricts circulation through the myocardium and produces symptoms of *coronary artery disease.*

▶ INTEGRATION OF BODY SYSTEMS

The following is an explanation of how the circulatory system is integrated with the other systems in the body:

Circulatory System

The heart is the organ that makes up the circulatory system. The circulatory system also contains the blood, blood vessels, and also the formation that make up the lymphatic system. The responsibility of the heart is to also move blood through the vascular and the arterial system to the body completely, which in turn will provide oxygenation and also remove the necessary waste for the body completely. While this is occurring, the immune/lymphatic system, a subsystem of the circulatory system, will regulate the body's transportation system. The immune/lymphatic system also takes the responsibility for the defense against disease-causing components named pathogens. Also involved are the nervous and muscular system, which control the contractions of the heart.

CHAPTER REVIEW SECTION

KEY WORDS

anastomosis:	The joining of two tubes, usually referring to a connection between two blood vessels without an intervening capillary bed.
arteriole:	A small arterial branch that delivers blood to a capillary network.
atria:	Thin-walled chambers of the heart that receive venous blood from the pulmonary or systemic circulation.
atrioventricular valve:	One of the valves that prevent backflow into the atria during contraction of the ventricles (ventricular systole).
blood pressure:	A force exerted against the vessel walls by the blood, as the result of the push exerted by cardiac contraction and the elasticity of the vessel walls.
capillary:	Small blood vessel between arterioles and venules, whose thin wall permits the diffusion of gases, nutrients, and wastes between the blood plasma and interstitial fluids.
cardiac cycle:	One complete heartbeat, including atrial and ventricular systole and diastole.
cardiac output:	The amount of blood ejected by a ventricle each minute; normally about 5 L.
diastole:	A period of relaxation within the cardiac cycle.
electrocardiogram (ECG, EKG):	Graphic record of the electrical activities of the heart, as monitored at specific locations on the body surface.
endocardium:	The simple squamous epithelium that lines the heart.
epicardium:	Serous membrane covering the outer surface of the heart.
myocardium:	The cardiac muscle tissue of the heart.
pericardium:	The fibrous sac that surrounds the heart.
pulmonary circulation:	Blood vessels between the pulmonary semilunar valve of the right ventricle and the entrance to the left atrium; the circulatory pathway between the heart and the lungs.
systemic circulation:	Vessels between the aortic semilunar valve and the entrance to the right atrium; the blood vessels other than those of the pulmonary circulation.
systole:	A period of contraction within the cardiac cycle.
vasoconstriction:	A reduction in the diameter of arterioles due to the contraction of smooth muscles in the vessel wall.

vasodilation:	An increase in the diameter of arterioles due to the relaxation of smooth muscles in the vessel wall.
venae cavae:	The major veins delivering systemic blood to the right atrium.
venule:	Small, thin-walled vein that receives blood from capillaries.
ventricle:	One of the large, muscular pumping chambers of the heart that discharges blood into the pulmonary or systemic circulations.

STUDY OUTLINE

INTRODUCTION

1. Contractions of the heart power the movement of blood through blood vessels to all parts of the body.

THE HEART AND THE CIRCULATORY SYSTEM

1. The circulatory system can be subdivided into the **pulmonary circulation** (which carries blood to and from the lungs) and the **systemic circulation** (which transports blood to and from the rest of the body). **Arteries** carry blood away from the heart; **veins** return blood to the heart. **Capillaries** are tiny vessels that connect the smallest arteries and the smallest veins. *(Figure 2-1)*
2. The heart has four chambers: the **right atrium** and **right ventricle**, and the **left atrium** and **left ventricle**.

STRUCTURE OF THE HEART

1. The heart is surrounded by the **pericardial cavity** (lined by the **pericardium**); the **visceral pericardium (epicardium)** covers the heart's outer surface, and the **parietal pericardium** lines the inner surface of the pericardial cavity.
2. The widest veins and arteries of the circulatory system are connected to the **base** of the heart; the pointed tip of the heart is the **apex**. *(Figure 2-2)*

INTERNAL ANATOMY OF THE HEART

3. The right atria and ventricle are separated from the left atria and left ventricle by *septa*. The right atrium receives blood from the systemic circuit through two large veins, the **superior vena cava** and **inferior vena cava**. *(Figure 2-3)*
4. Blood flows from the right atrium into the right ventricle via the **right atrioventricular (AV) valve (tricuspid valve)**.
5. Blood leaving the right ventricle enters the **pulmonary trunk** after passing through the **pulmonary semilunar valve**. The pulmonary trunk divides to form the **left** and **right pulmonary arteries**, which go to the lungs. The left and right pulmonary veins return blood from the lungs to the left atrium. Blood leaving the left atrium flows into the left ventricle via the **left atrioventricular (AV) valve (bicuspid valve** or **mitral valve)**. Blood leaving the left ventricle passes through the **aortic semilunar valve** and into the systemic circulation via the *ascending aorta*. *(Figures 2-3, 2-4)*
6. Valves normally permit blood flow in only one direction. *(Figure 2-4)*

THE HEART WALL

7. The bulk of the heart consists of the muscular **myocardium**. The **endocardium** lines the inner surfaces of the heart. *(Figure 2-5)*
8. Cardiac muscle cells are interconnected by **intercalated discs** that convey the force of contraction from cell to cell and conduct action potentials. *(Figure 2-5)*

BLOOD SUPPLY TO THE HEART

9. The **coronary circulation** meets the high oxygen and nutrient demands of cardiac muscle cells. The **coronary arteries** originate at the base of the ascending aorta. Interconnections between arteries called **anastomoses** ensure a constant blood supply. Two **cardiac veins** carry blood from the coronary capillaries to the **coronary sinus**.

THE HEARTBEAT

1. The average heart beats about 100,000 times per day, or about 70 to 80 beats per minute.

CARDIAC CYCLE

2. The **cardiac cycle** consists of **systole** (contraction), followed by **diastole** (relaxation). Both sides of the heart contract at the same time, and they eject equal volumes of blood. *(Figure 2-6)*
3. The amount of blood ejected by a ventricle during a single beat is the **stroke volume**; the amount of blood pumped each minute is the **cardiac output**.

CONDUCTING SYSTEM OF THE HEART

4. The conducting system, composed of **nodal cells** and **conducting cells**, initiates and distributes electrical impulses within the heart. Nodal cells establish the rate of cardiac contraction, and conducting cells distribute the contractile stimulus to the general myocardium.
5. Unlike skeletal muscle, cardiac muscle contracts without neural or hormonal stimulation. **Pacemaker cells** found in the **cardiac pacemaker** (**sinoatrial**, or **SA**, **node**) normally establish the rate of contraction. From the SA node the stimulus travels to the **atrioventricular (AV) node**, then to the **AV bundle**, which divides into **bundle branches**. From here **Purkinje cells** convey the impulses to the ventricular myocardium. *(Figure 2-7)*

THE ELECTROCARDIOGRAM

6. A recording of electrical activities in the heart is an **electrocardiogram** (**ECG** or **EKG**). Important landmarks of an ECG include the **P wave** (atrial impulse and contraction), **QRS complex** (ventricular impulse and contraction), and **T wave** (ventricles recover). *(Figure 2-8)*

CONTROL OF HEART RATE

7. Although the basic heart rate is established by the pacemaker cells of the SA node, it can be modified by the autonomic nervous system (ANS).

BLOOD VESSELS

1. Arteries, veins, and capillaries form a closed system of tubes that carry blood to all the cells of the body. **Arteries** branch repeatedly, decreasing in size until they become **arterioles**; from the arterioles blood enters the capillary networks. Blood flowing from the capillaries enters small **venules** before entering larger veins.

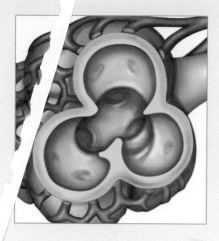

MEDICAL TERMINOLOGY OF THE RESPIRATORY SYSTEM

OBJECTIVES

On completion of this chapter, you should be able to:

- Describe the organs of the respiratory system.

- State the functions of the organs of the respiratory system.

- Define terms that are used by physiologists and respiratory specialists to describe the volume of air exchanged in breathing.

- State the vital function of respiration.

- Provide the respiratory rates for some different age groups.

- Analyze, build, spell, and pronounce medical words that relate to surgical procedures and pathology.

- Identify and give the meaning of selected vocabulary words.

- Identify and define selected abbreviations.

- Review Drug Highlights presented in this chapter.

- Provide the description of diagnostic and laboratory tests related to the respiratory system.

- Successfully complete the study and review section.

▶ ANATOMY AND PHYSIOLOGY OVERVIEW

The respiratory system consists of the *nose, pharynx, larynx, trachea, bronchi,* and *lungs.* The primary function of the respiratory system is to furnish oxygen for use by individual tissue cells and to take away their gaseous waste product, carbon dioxide. See Figure 3–1. This process is accomplished through the act of *respiration.* Respiration consists of external and internal processes. *External respiration* is the process whereby the lungs are ventilated and oxygen and carbon dioxide are exchanged between the air in the lungs and the blood within capillaries of the alveoli. *Internal respiration* is the process whereby oxygen and carbon dioxide are exchanged between the blood in tissue capillaries and the cells of the body.

▶ THE NOSE

The *nose* is the projection in the center of the face and consists of an external and internal portion. The *external portion* is a triangle of cartilage and bone that is covered with skin and lined with mucous membrane. The external entrance of the nose is known as the *nostrils* or *anterior nares.* The *internal portion* of the nose is divided into two chambers by a partition, the *septum,* separating it into a right and a left cavity. These cavities are divided into three air passages: the *superior, middle,* and *inferior conchae.* These passages lead to the pharynx and are connected by openings with the paranasal sinuses, with the ears by the eustachian tube, and with the region of the eyes by the nasolacrimal ducts.

The *palatine bones* separate the nasal cavities from the mouth cavity. When the palatine bones fail to unite during fetal development, a congenital defect known as *cleft palate* occurs. This defect may be corrected by surgery. The nose, as well as the rest of the respiratory system, is lined with mucous membrane, which is covered with *cilia.* The nasal mucosa produces about 946 mL or 1 qt of mucus per day. Four pairs of paranasal sinuses drain into the nose. These are the *frontal, maxillary, ethmoidal,* and *sphenoidal* sinuses (Fig. 3–2).

FUNCTIONS OF THE NOSE

Five functions have been attributed to the nose. These functions are:

1. It serves as an air passageway.
2. It warms and moistens inhaled air.

THE RESPIRATORY SYSTEM

ORGAN/STRUCTURE	PRIMARY FUNCTIONS
The Nose	Serves as an air passageway; warms and moistens inhaled air; its cilia and mucous membrane trap dust, pollen, bacteria, and other foreign matter; contains olfactory receptors, which sort out odors; aids in phonation and the quality of voice
The Pharynx	Serves as a passageway for air and for food; aids in phonation by changing its shape
The Larynx	Production of vocal sounds
The Trachea	Provides an open passageway for air to the lungs
The Bronchi	Provide a passageway for air to and from the lungs
The Lungs	Bring air into intimate contact with blood so that oxygen and carbon dioxide can be exchanged in the alveoli

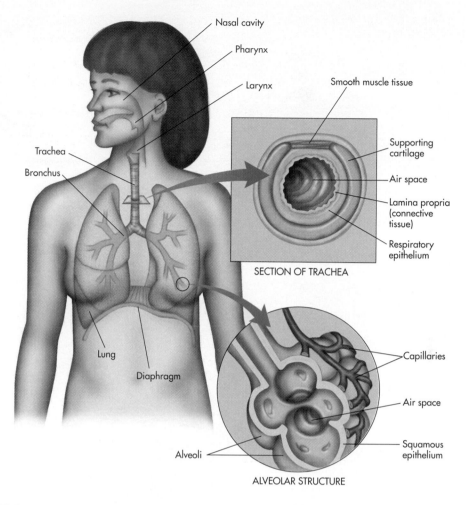

FIGURE 3–1

The respiratory system: nasal cavity, pharynx, larynx, trachea, bronchus, and lung with expanded views of the trachea and alveolar structure.

3. Its cilia and mucous membrane trap dust, pollen, bacteria, and other foreign matter.
4. It contains olfactory receptors, which sort out odors.
5. It aids in phonation and the quality of voice.

▶ THE PHARYNX

The *pharynx* or throat is a musculomembranous tube about 5 inches long that extends from the base of the skull, lies anterior to the cervical vertebrae, and becomes continuous with the esophagus. It is divided into three portions: the *nasopharynx* located behind the nose, the *oropharynx* located behind the mouth, and the *laryngopharynx* located behind the larynx. Seven openings are found in the pharynx: two openings from the eustachian tubes, two openings from the posterior nares into the nasopharynx, the fauces or opening from the mouth into the oropharynx, and the openings from the larynx and the esophagus into the laryngopharynx (Fig. 3–2). Associated with the pharynx are three pairs of lymphoid tissues, which are the *tonsils*. The nasopharynx contains the *adenoids* or *pharyngeal* tonsils. The oropharynx contains the *faucial* or *palatine* tonsils and the *lingual* tonsils. The tonsils are accessory organs of the lymphatic system and aid in filtering bacteria and other foreign substances from the circulating lymph.

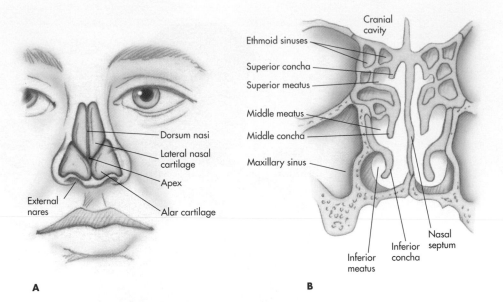

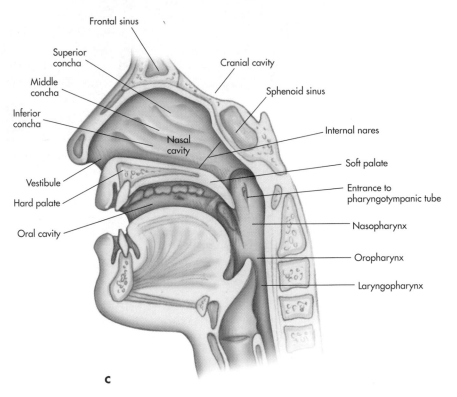

FIGURE 3–2

The nose, nasal cavity, and pharynx: **(A)** nasal cartilages and external structure, **(B)** meatuses and positions of the entrance to the ethmoid and maxillary sinuses, **(C)** sagittal section of the nasal cavity and pharynx.

FUNCTIONS OF THE PHARYNX

The following three functions are associated with the pharynx:

1. It serves as a passageway for air.
2. It serves as a passageway for food.
3. It aids in phonation by changing its shape.

► THE LARYNX

The *larynx* or voicebox is a muscular, cartilaginous structure lined with mucous membrane. It is the enlarged upper end of the trachea below the root of the tongue and hyoid bone (Fig. 3–1).

CARTILAGE OF THE LARYNX

The larynx is composed of nine cartilages bound together by muscles and ligaments. The three unpaired cartilages, each of which is described below, are the *thyroid, cricoid,* and *epiglottic,* and the three paired cartilages are the *arytenoid, cuneiform,* and *corniculate.*

The Thyroid Cartilage

The *thyroid cartilage* is the largest cartilage in the larynx and forms the structure commonly called the *"Adam's apple."* This structure is usually larger and more prominent in men than in women and contributes to the deeper male voice.

The Epiglottic Cartilage

The *epiglottic cartilage* is a small cartilage attached to the superior border of the thyroid cartilage. Known as the *epiglottis,* it covers the entrance of the larynx, and during swallowing, it acts as a lid to prevent aspiration of food into the trachea. When the epiglottis fails to cover the entrance to the larynx, food or liquid intended for the esophagus may enter, causing irritation, coughing, or in extreme cases, choking.

The Cricoid Cartilage

The *cricoid cartilage* is the lowermost cartilage of the larynx. It is shaped like a signet ring with the broad portion being posterior and the anterior portion forming the arch and resembling the ring's band.

   The cavity of the larynx contains a pair of *ventricular folds* (false vocal cords) and a pair of vocal folds or true vocal cords. The cavity is divided into three regions: the vestibule, the ventricle, and the entrance to the glottis. The *glottis* is a narrow slit at the opening between the true vocal folds.

FUNCTION OF THE LARYNX

The function of the larynx is the production of vocal sounds. High notes are formed by short, tense vocal cords. Low notes are produced by long, relaxed vocal cords. The nose, mouth, pharynx, and bony sinuses aid in phonation.

► THE TRACHEA

The *trachea* or windpipe is a cylindrical cartilaginous tube that is the air passageway extending from the pharynx and larynx to the main bronchi. It is about 1 inch wide and 4½ inches (11.3 cm) long. It is composed of smooth muscle that is reinforced at the front and sides by C-shaped rings of cartilage. Mucous membrane lining the trachea contains *cilia,* which sweep foreign matter out of the passageway. The function of the trachea is to provide an open passageway for air to the lungs (see Fig. 3–1).

▶ THE BRONCHI

The *bronchi* are the two main branches of the trachea, which provide the passageway for air to the lungs. The trachea divides into the *right bronchus* and the *left bronchus.* The right bronchus is larger and extends down in a more vertical direction than the left bronchus. When a foreign body is inhaled or aspirated, it frequently lodges in the right bronchus or enters the right lung. Each bronchus enters the lung at a depression, the *hilum.* They then subdivide into the bronchial tree composed of smaller bronchi, bronchioles, and alveolar ducts. The bronchial tree terminates in the *alveoli,* which are tiny air sacs supporting a network of capillaries from pulmonary blood vessels. The function of the bronchi is to provide a passageway for air to and from the lungs (see Fig. 3–1).

▶ THE LUNGS

The *lungs* are cone-shaped, spongy organs of respiration lying on either side of the heart within the pleural cavity of the thorax. They occupy a large portion of the thoracic cavity and are enclosed in the *pleura,* a serous membrane composed of several layers. The six layers of the pleura are the *costal, parietal, pericardiac, phrenic, pulmonalis,* and *visceral. The parietal pleura* extends from the roots of the lungs and lines the walls of the thorax and the superior surface of the diaphragm. The *visceral pleura* covers the surface of the lungs and enters into and lines the interlobar fissures. The pleural cavity is a space between the parietal and visceral pleura and contains a serous fluid that lubricates and prevents friction caused by the rubbing together of the two layers. The thoracic cavity is separated from the abdominal cavity by a musculomembranous wall, the *diaphragm.* The central portion of the thoracic cavity, between the lungs, is a space called the *mediastinum,* containing the heart and other structures.

The lungs consist of elastic tissue filled with interlacing networks of tubes and sacs that carry air and with blood vessels carrying blood. The broad inferior surface of the lung is the *base,* which rests on the diaphragm, while the *apex,* or pointed upper margin, rises from 2.5 to 5 cm above the sternal end of the first rib. The lungs are divided into *lobes* with the right lung having three lobes and the left lung having only two lobes. The left lung has an indentation, the *cardiac depression,* for the normal placement of the heart. In an average adult male, the right lung weighs approximately 625 g and the left about 570 g. In an average adult male, the total lung capacity is 3.6 to 9.4 L, whereas in an average adult female it is 2.5 to 6.9 L. The lungs contain around 300 million *alveoli,* which are the air cells where the exchange of oxygen and carbon dioxide takes place. The main function of the lungs is to bring air into intimate contact with blood so that oxygen and carbon dioxide can be exchanged in the alveoli (see Fig. 3–3).

▶ RESPIRATION

VOLUME

The following terms are used by physiologists and respiratory specialists to describe the volume of air exchanged in breathing:

Tidal Volume. The amount of air in a single inspiration or expiration. In the average adult male, about 500 cc of air enters the respiratory tract during normal quiet breathing.

Supplemental Air. The amount of air that may be forcibly expired after a normal quiet respiration. This is also the expiratory reserve volume and measures approximately 1600 cc.

Complemental Air. The amount of air that may be forcibly inspired over and above a normal inspiration. This is known as the inspiratory reserve volume.

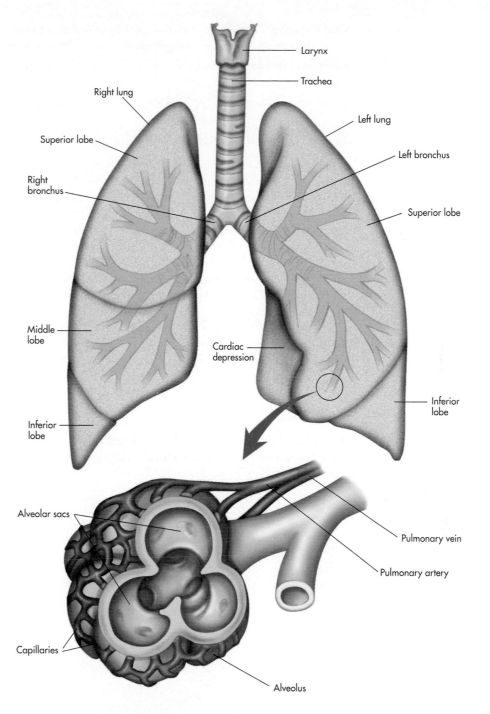

Larynx

Trachea

Right lung

Left lung

Superior lobe

Left bronchus

Right bronchus

Superior lobe

Middle lobe

Cardiac depression

Inferior lobe

Inferior lobe

Alveolar sacs

Pulmonary vein

Pulmonary artery

Capillaries

Alveolus

FIGURE 3–3

The larynx, trachea, bronchi, and lungs with an expanded view showing the structures of an alveolus and the pulmonary blood vessels.

Residual Volume. The amount of air remaining in the lungs after maximal expiration—about 1500 cc.

Minimal Air. The small amount of air that remains in the alveoli. After death, if the thorax is opened and the lungs collapse, the minimal air pressure will allow the lungs to float.

Vital Capacity. The volume of air that can be exhaled after a maximal inspiration. This amount equals the sum of the tidal air, complemental air, and the supplemental air.

Functional Residual Capacity. The volume of air that remains in the lungs at the end of a normal expiration.

Total Lung Capacity. The maximal volume of air in the lungs after a maximal inspiration.

THE VITAL FUNCTION OF RESPIRATION

Temperature, pulse, respiration, and *blood pressure* are the vital signs that are essential elements for determining an individual's state of health. A deviation from normal of one or all of the vital signs denotes a state of illness. Evaluation of an individual's response to changes occurring within the body can be measured by taking his or her vital signs. Through careful analysis of these changes in the vital signs, a physician may determine a diagnosis, a prognosis, and a plan of treatment for the patient. The variations of certain vital signs signify a typical disease process and its stages of development. For example, in a patient who has pneumonia the temperature is elevated from 101° to 106°F, and pulse and respiration increase to almost twice their normal rates. When the patient's temperature falls, he or she will perspire profusely and his or her pulse and respiration will begin to return to normal rates.

The process of *respiration* is interrelated with other systems of the body. The *medulla oblongata* and the *pons* of the central nervous system regulate and control respiration. The rate, rhythm, and depth of respiration are controlled by nerve impulses from the medulla oblongata and the pons via the spinal cord and nerves to the muscles of the diaphragm, abdomen, and rib cage.

RESPIRATORY RATES

Individuals of different ages breathe at different respiratory rates. *Respiratory rate* is regulated by the respiratory center located in the medulla oblongata. The following are respiratory rates for some different age groups:

Newborn	30 to 80 per minute
1st year	20 to 40 per minute
5th year	20 to 25 per minute
15th year	15 to 20 per minute
Adult	15 to 20 per minute

LIFE SPAN CONSIDERATIONS

▶ THE CHILD

At 12 weeks' gestation the lungs of the fetus have a definite shape. At 20 weeks the fetus is able to suck its thumb and swallow amniotic fluid. The cellular structure of the **alveoli** of the lungs are complete. At 24 weeks the nostrils open, respiratory movements occur, and alveoli begin the production of **surfactant.** Surfactant is a substance in the lung that regulates the amount of surface tension of the fluid lining the alveoli. In preterm infants the lack of surfactant contributes to respiratory distress syndrome.

During fetal life gaseous exchange occurs at the placental interface. The lungs do not function until birth. The respiratory rate of the newborn is 30 to 80 per minute. During the first year it is 20 to 40 per minute and at age 5 it is 20 to 25 per minute. Around the 15th year the respiratory rate is 15 to 20, the same as the average, healthy adult rate. Diaphragmatic abdominal breathing is common in infants. Accessory muscles of respiration are not as strong in infants as in older children and adults.

Oxygen consumption and metabolic rate are higher in children than in adults. Airway diameter is smaller in children, thereby increasing the potential for airway obstruction. The mucous membranes of children are vascular and susceptible to trauma, edema, and spasm.

▶ THE OLDER ADULT

With advancing age, the respiratory system is vulnerable to injuries caused by infections, environmental pollutants, and allergic reactions. Age-related changes include a decline in the protection normally provided by intact mucous barrier, a decrease in the effectiveness of the bronchial cilia, and changes in the composition of the connective tissues of the lungs and chest. Older adults rely more on the **diaphragm** for inspiration, and when lying down, breathing requires more effort. **Vital capacity** declines with age; there is a decline in the elastic recoil of the lungs and an increase in the stiffness of the chest wall. This makes it more difficult for the older adult to inspire or expire air.

In the pharynx and larynx muscle atrophy can occur, with slackening of the vocal cords and loss of elasticity of the laryngeal muscles and cartilages. These changes may cause a gravelly, softer voice with a rise in pitch, making communication more difficult, especially if there is impaired hearing.

TERMINOLOGY

WITH SURGICAL PROCEDURES & PATHOLOGY

TERM	WORD PARTS			DEFINITION
aerophore (air′ ō-for)	aero phore	CF S	air bearing	An apparatus for inflating the lungs of stillborn infants
aeropleura (air′ ō-ploo″ rǎ)	aero pleura	CF R	air pleura	Air in the pleural cavity
alveolus (ăl-vē′ ō-lǔs)	alveol us	R S	small, hollow air sac pertaining to	Pertaining to a small air sac in the lungs
anosmia (ăn-ŏz′ mǐ-ă)	an osm ia	P R S	lack of smell condition	A condition in which there is a lack of the sense of smell
anoxia (ăn-ŏks′ ǐ-ă)	an ox ia	P R S	lack of oxygen condition	A condition in which there is a lack of oxygen
anthracosis (ăn″ thrǎ-kō′ sǐs)	anthrac osis	R S	coal condition of	Black lung; a lung condition caused by inhalation of coal dust and silica
aphonia (ǎ-fō′ nǐ-ă)	a phon ia	P R S	lack of voice condition	A condition of inability to produce vocal sounds
aphrasia (ǎ-frā-′ zǐ-ă)	a phras ia	P R S	lack of speech condition	A condition of inability to speak
apnea (ăp′ -nē ă)	a pnea	P S	lack of breathing	Temporary cessation of breathing

TERMINOLOGY SPOTLIGHT

Apnea is defined as a temporary cessation of breathing. **Sleep apnea** is cessation of breathing during sleep. The disruption of sleep patterns due to an obstruction of airways affects about 10 million Americans. To be so classified, the apnea must last for at least 10 seconds and occurs 30 or more times during a 7-hour period of sleep. This definition may not apply to older adults in whom periods of sleep apnea are increased. Sleep apnea is classified according to the mechanism involved.

Terminology - continued

TERM	WORD PARTS		DEFINITION

- Obstructive apnea is caused by obstruction to the upper airway. This condition generally occurs in middle-aged men who are obese and have a history of excessive daytime sleepiness. It is associated with loud snorting, snoring, and gasping sounds.
- Central apnea is marked by absence of respiratory muscle activity. A person with this type of apnea may exhibit excessive daytime sleepiness, but the snorting and gasping sounds during sleep are absent.
- Mixed apnea begins with absence of respiratory effort followed by upper airway obstruction.

Sleep deprivation can make a person tired, sluggish, irritable, prone to accidents, and less productive. Although the amount of sleep needed is different for every person, adults need at least 7 hours of sleep in a 24-hour time period, children under the age of 10 need 11 to 13 hours of sleep, and teenagers need 10 to 12 hours of sleep.

TERM	WORD PARTS			DEFINITION
atelectasis (ăt″ ĕ-lĕk′ tă-sĭs)	atel ectasis	R S	imperfect dilation, expansion	A condition of imperfect dilation of the lungs; the collapse of an alveolus, a lobule, or a larger lung unit
bronchiectasis (brŏng″ kĭ-ĕk′ tă-sĭs)	bronchi ectasis	CF S	bronchi dilation, expansion	Dilation of the bronchi
bronchiolitis (brŏng″ kĭ-ō-lī′ tĭs)	bronchiol itis	R S	bronchiole inflammation	Inflammation of the bronchioles
bronchitis (brŏng-kī′ tĭs)	bronch itis	R S	bronchi inflammation	Inflammation of the bronchi
bronchomycosis (brŏng″ kō-mī-kō′ sĭs)	broncho myc osis	CF R S	bronchi fungus condition of	A fungus condition of the bronchi
bronchoplasty (brŏng′ kō-plăs″ tē)	broncho plasty	CF S	bronchi surgical repair	Surgical repair of the bronchi
bronchoscope (brŏng′ kō-skōp)	broncho scope	CF S	bronchi instrument	An instrument used to examine the bronchi
cyanosis (sī″ăn-ō′ -sĭs)	cyan osis	R S	dark blue condition of	A dark blue condition of the skin and mucous membrane caused by oxygen deficiency
diaphragmalgia (dī″ ă-frăg-măl′ jĭ-ă)	dia phragm algia	P R S	through partition pain	Pain in the diaphragm

continued

Terminology - continued

TERM	WORD PARTS			DEFINITION
diaphragmatocele (dī″ă-frăg-măt′ ō-sēl)	dia phragmato cele	P CF S	through partition hernia	A hernia of the diaphragm
dysphonia (dĭs-fō′ nĭ-ă)	dys phon ia	P R S	difficult voice condition	A condition of difficulty in speaking
dyspnea (dĭsp-nē′ ă)	dys pnea	P S	difficult breathing	Difficulty in breathing
endotracheal (ĕn″ dō-trā′ kē-ăl)	endo trache al	P CF S	within trachea pertaining to	Pertaining to within the trachea
eupnea (ūp-nē′ ă)	eu pnea	P S	good, normal breathing	Good or normal breathing
exhalation (ĕks″ hə-lā′ shən)	ex halat ion	P R S	out breathe process	The process of breathing out
expectoration (ĕk-spĕk″ tə′ rā′ shən	ex pectorat ion	P R S	out breast process	The process by which saliva, mucus, or phlegm is expelled from the air passages
hemoptysis (hē-mŏp′ tĭ-sĭs)	hemo ptysis	CF S	blood to spit	The spitting up of blood
hemothorax (hē″ mō-thō-răks)	hemo thorax	CF R	blood chest	Blood in the chest cavity
hyperpnea (hī″ pĕrp-nē′ ă)	hyper pnea	P S	excessive breathing	Excessive or rapid breathing
hypoxia (hī-pŏks′ ĭ-ă)	hyp ox ia	P R S	below, deficient oxygen condition	A condition of deficient amounts of oxygen in the inspired air
inhalation (ĭn″ hă-lă′ shŭn)	in halat ion	P R S	in breathe process	The process of breathing in
laryngeal (lăr-ĭn′ jĭ-ăl)	larynge al	CF S	larynx pertaining to	Pertaining to the larynx
laryngectomy (lăr″ ĭn-jĕk′ tō-mē)	laryng ectomy	R S	larynx excision	Surgical excision of the larynx

Terminology - continued

TERM	WORD PARTS			DEFINITION
laryngitis (lăr″ ĭn-jī′ tĭs)	laryng itis	R S	larynx inflammation	Inflammation of the larynx
laryngoplasty (lăr-ĭn′ gō-plăs″ tē)	laryngo plasty	CF S	larynx surgical repair	Surgical repair of the larynx
laryngoscope (lăr-ĭn′ gō-skōp)	laryngo scope	CF S	larynx instrument	An instrument used to examine the larynx
laryngostenosis (lăr-ĭng″ gō-stĕ- nō′sĭs)	laryngo sten osis	CF R S	larynx narrowing condition of	A condition of narrowing of the larynx
laryngostomy (lăr″ ĭn-gŏs′ tō-mē)	laryngo stomy	CF S	larynx new opening	Establishing a new opening in the larynx
lobectomy (lō-bĕk′ tō-mē)	lob ectomy	R S	lobe excision	Surgical excision of a lobe of any organ or gland, such as the lung
nasomental (nā″ zō-mĕn′ tăl)	naso ment al	CF R S	nose chin pertaining to	Pertaining to the nose and chin
nasopharyngitis (nā″ zō-făr′ ĭn-jī′ tĭs)	naso pharyng itis	CF R S	nose pharynx inflammation	Inflammation of the nose and pharynx
orthopnea (or″ thŏp-nē′ ă)	ortho pnea	CF S	straight breathing	Inability to breathe unless in an upright or straight position
palatoplegia (păl″ă-tō-plē′ jĭ-ā)	palato plegia	CF S	palate stroke, paralysis	Paralysis of the muscles of the soft palate
pharyngalgia (făr″ ĭn-găl′ jĭ-ă)	pharyng algia	R S	pharynx pain	Pain in the pharynx
pharyngitis (făr″ ĭn-jī′ tĭs)	pharyng itis	R S	pharynx inflammation	Inflammation of the pharynx
pleuritis (ploo-rī′ tĭs)	pleur itis	R S	pleura inflammation	Inflammation of the pleura
pleurodynia (ploo″ rō-dĭn′ ĭ-ă)	pleuro dynia	CF S	pleura pain	Pain in the pleura

continued

Terminology - continued

TERM	WORD PARTS			DEFINITION
pneumoconiosis (nū″ mō-kō″ nĭ-ō′ sĭs)	pneumo coni osis	CF R S	lung dust condition of	A condition of the lung caused by the inhalation of dust
pneumonitis (nū″ mō-nī′ tĭs)	pneumon itis	R S	lung inflammation	Inflammation of the lung
pneumothorax (nū″ mō-thō′ răks)	pneumo thorax	CF R	air chest	A collection of air in the chest cavity
pulmometer (pŭl-mŏm′ ĕ-tĕr)	pulmo meter	CF S	lung instrument to measure	An instrument used to measure lung capacity
pulmonectomy (pŭl″ mō-nĕk′ tō-mē)	pulmon ectomy	R S	lung excision	Surgical excision of the lung or a part of a lung
pyothorax (pī″ ō-thō′ răks)	pyo thorax	CF R	pus chest	Pus in the chest cavity
rhinoplasty (rī′ nō-plăs″ tē)	rhino plasty	CF S	nose surgical repair	Surgical repair of the nose
rhinorrhagia (rī″ nō-ră′ jĭ-ă)	rhino rrhagia	CF S	nose bursting forth	The bursting forth of blood from the nose
rhinorrhea (rī″ nō-rē′ ă)	rhino rrhea	CF S	nose flow, discharge	Discharge from the nose
rhinostenosis (rī″ nō-stĕn-ō′ sĭs)	rhino sten osis	CF R S	nose narrowing condition of	A condition of narrowing of the nasal passages
rhinotomy (rī-nŏt′ ō-mē)	rhino tomy	CF S	nose incision	Incision of the nose
sinusitis (sī″ nūs-ī′ tĭs)	sinus itis	R S	a curve, hollow inflammation	Inflammation of a sinus
spirogram (spī′ rō-grăm)	spiro gram	CF S	breath a mark, record	A record made by a spirograph showing respiratory movements
spirometer (spī-rŏm′ ĕt-ĕr)	spiro meter	CF S	breath instrument to measure	An instrument used to measure the volume of respired air

Terminology - continued

TERM	WORD PARTS			DEFINITION
tachypnea (tăk″ ĭp-nē′ ă)	tachy pnea	P S	fast breathing	Fast breathing
thoracocentesis (thō″ răk-ō-sĕn-tē′ sĭs)	thoraco centesis	CF S	chest surgical puncture	Surgical puncture of the chest for removal of fluid
thoracopathy (thō″ răk-ŏp′ ă-thē)	thoraco pathy	CF S	chest disease	Any disease of the chest
thoracoplasty (thō′ ră-kō-plăs″ tē)	thoraco plasty	CF S	chest surgical repair	Surgical repair of the chest
thoracotomy (thō″ răk-ŏt′ ō-mē)	thoraco tomy	CF S	chest incision	Incision of the chest
tonsillectomy (tŏn″ sĭl-ĕk′ tō-mē)	tonsill ectomy	R S	almond, tonsil excision	Surgical excision of the tonsils
tonsillitis (tŏn″ sĭl-ī′ tĭs)	tonsill itis	R S	almond, tonsil inflammation	Inflammation of the tonsils
tracheal (trā′ kē-ăl)	trache al	R S	trachea pertaining to	Pertaining to the trachea
trachealgia (trā″ kē-ăl′ jĭ-ă)	trache algia	R S	trachea pain	Pain in the trachea
tracheitis (trā″ kē-ī′ tĭs)	trache itis	R S	trachea inflammation	Inflammation of the trachea
tracheolaryngo-tomy (trā″ kē-ō-lăr″ ĭn-gŏt′ ō-mē)	tracheo laryngo tomy	CF CF S	trachea larynx incision	Incision into the larynx and trachea
tracheostomy (trā″ kē-ŏs′ tō-mē)	tracheo stomy	CF S	trachea new opening	New opening into the trachea

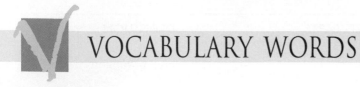

VOCABULARY WORDS

Vocabulary words are terms that have not been divided into component parts. They are common words or specialized terms associated with the subject of this chapter. These words are provided to enhance your medical vocabulary.

WORD	DEFINITION
artificial respiration (ăr″ tĭ-fĭsh′ ăl rĕs″ pĭr-ā′ shŭn)	The process of using artificial means to cause air to flow into and out of an individual's lungs when breathing is inadequate or ceases
asphyxia (ăs-fĭk′ sĭ-ă)	A condition in which there is a depletion of oxygen in the blood with an increase of carbon dioxide in the blood and tissues. First-aid treatment is by artificial respiration.
aspiration (ăs″ pĭ-rā′ shŭn)	The process of taking substances in or out by means of suction
asthma (ăz′ mă)	A disease of the bronchi characterized by wheezing, dyspnea, and a feeling of constriction in the chest
carbon dioxide (kăr bən dī-ŏk′ sīd)	A colorless, odorless gas used with oxygen to stimulate respiration
Cheyne-Stokes respiration (chān′ stōks′ rĕs″ pĭr-ā′ shŭn)	A rhythmic cycle of breathing with a gradual increase in respiration followed by apnea (which may last from 10 to 60 sec), then a repeat of the same cycle
coryza (kŏr-rī′ ză)	The common cold characterized by sneezing, nasal discharge, coughing, and malaise
cough (kawf)	Sudden, forceful expulsion of air from the lungs. It is an essential protective response that clears irritants, secretions, or foreign objects from the trachea, bronchi, and/or lungs.
croup (croop)	A respiratory disease characterized by a "barking" cough, dyspnea, hoarseness, and laryngeal spasm
cystic fibrosis (sĭs′ tĭk fī-brō′ sĭs)	An inherited disease that affects the pancreas, respiratory system, and sweat glands. The etiology is unknown, and the prognosis is generally poor.
emphysema (ĕm″ fĭ-sē′ mă)	A chronic pulmonary disease in which the bronchioles become obstructed with mucus

Vocabulary - continued

WORD	DEFINITION
empyema (ĕm″ pī-ē′ mă)	Pus in a body cavity, especially the pleural cavity
epistaxis (ĕp″ ĭ-stăk′ sĭs)	Nosebleed
Heimlich maneuver (hīm′ lĭk)	A technique for removing a foreign body (usually a bolus of food) that is blocking the trachea
hyperbaric oxygenation (hī″ pĕr-băr′ ĭk ŏk″ sĭ-jĕn-ā′ shŭn)	The process of administering oxygen in a closed chamber at a pressure greater than one and one-half to three times absolute atmospheric pressure
hyperventilation (hī″ pĕr-vĕn″ tĭ-lā′ shŭn)	The process of excessive ventilating, thereby increasing the air in the lungs beyond the normal limit
influenza (ĭn″ flū-ĕn′ ză)	An acute, contagious respiratory infection caused by a virus. Onset is usually sudden, and symptoms are fever, chills, headache, myalgia, cough, and sore throat.
Kussmaul's breathing (koos′ mowiz brēth′ ĭng)	A distressing, deep gasping type of breathing associated with metabolic acidosis and coma; also called air hunger
legionnaire's disease (lē jə naerz′ dĭ-zēz′)	A severe pulmonary pneumonia caused by *Legionella pneumophilia*
mesothelioma (mĕs″ ō-thē″ lĭ-ō′ mă)	A malignant tumor of mesothelium (serous membrane of the pleura) caused by the inhalation of asbestos
nares (nā′ rĕs)	The nostrils
olfaction (ŏl-făk′ shŭn)	The process of smelling
oropharynx (or″ ō-făr′ ĭnks)	The central portion of the throat that lies between the soft palate and upper portion of the epiglottis
palatopharyn-goplasty (păl″ ăt-ō-făr″ ĭn′ gō-plăs″ tē)	A type of surgery that cures snoring and sleep apnea by removing the uvula and the tonsils and reshaping the lining at the back of the throat to enlarge the air passageway

continued

Vocabulary - continued

WORD	DEFINITION
pertussis (pĕr-tŭs′ ĭs)	An acute, infectious disease characterized by coryza, an explosive paroxysmal cough ending in a "crowing" or "whooping" sound; *also called whooping cough*
pleurisy (ploo′ rĭsē)	Inflammation of the pleura caused by injury, infection, or a tumor
pneumonia (nū-mō′ nĭ-ă)	Inflammation of the lung caused by bacteria, viruses, or chemical irritants
pollinosis (pŏl-ĭn-ō′ sĭs)	Hay fever; nasal congestion of mucous membranes caused by an allergic reaction to a pollen or pollens
polyp (pŏl′ ĭp)	A tumor with a stem; may occur where there are mucous membranes, such as the nose, ears, mouth, uterus, and intestines
rale (rahl)	An abnormal sound heard on auscultation of the chest; a crackling, rattling, or bubbling sound
respirator (rĕs′ pĭ-rā″ tor)	A type of machine used for prolonged artificial respiration
respiratory distress syndrome (hyaline membrane disease) (rĕs′ pĭ-ră-tō″ rē dĭs-trĕs′ sĭn′ drōm)	A condition that may occur in a premature infant in which the lungs are not matured to the point of manufacturing lecithin, a pulmonary surfactant. This results in collapse of the alveoli, which leads to cyanosis and hypoxia.
rhinovirus (rī″ nō-vī′ rŭs)	One of a subgroup of viruses that causes the common cold in humans
rhonchus (rŏng′ kŭs)	A rale or rattling sound in the throat or bronchial tubes caused by a partial obstruction
sarcoidosis (sar″ koyd-ō′ sĭs)	A chronic granulomatous condition that may involve almost any organ system of the body. The lungs are usually involved and this causes dyspnea on exertion. With multisystem involvement the patient may experience fatigue, fever, anorexia, weight loss, joint pain, and skin changes, including erythemanodosum, plaques, maculopapular eruptions, and subcutaneous nodules. See Figures 3–4 and 3–5.
sputum (spū′ tŭm)	Substance coughed up from the lungs; may be watery, thick, purulent, clear, or bloody and may contain microorganisms
stridor (strī′ dōr)	A high-pitched sound caused by obstruction of the air passageway

Vocabulary - continued

WORD	DEFINITION
tuberculosis (tū-běr″ kū-lō′ sĭs)	An infectious disease caused by the tubercle bacillus, *Mycobacterium tuberculosis*
wheeze (hwēz)	A whistling sound caused by obstruction of the air passageway

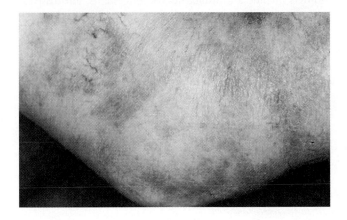

FIGURE 3–4

Sarcoidosis. *(Courtesy of Jason L. Smith, MD.)*

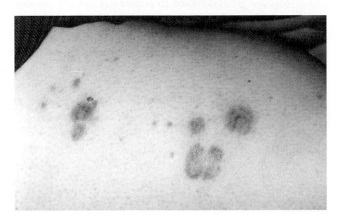

FIGURE 3–5

Sarcoidosis. *(Courtesy of Jason L. Smith, MD.)*

ABBREVIATIONS

ABGs	arterial blood gases	**IPPB**	intermittent positive-pressure breathing
AFB	acid-fast bacilli	**IRDS**	infant respiratory distress syndrome
ARD	acute respiratory disease	**IRV**	inspiratory reserve volume
ARDS	adult respiratory distress syndrome	**MBC**	maximal breathing capacity
CF	cystic fibrosis	**MV**	minute volume
CO$_2$	carbon dioxide	**MVV**	maximal voluntary ventilation
COLD	chronic obstructive lung disease	**O$_2$**	oxygen
COPD	chronic obstructive pulmonary disease	**PEEP**	positive end-expiratory pressure
CXR	chest x-ray	**PND**	postnasal drip
ENT	ear, nose, and throat	**PPD**	purified protein derivative
ERV	expiratory reserve volume	**R**	respiration
ET	endotracheal	**RD**	respiratory disease
FEF	forced expiratory flow	**RDS**	respiratory distress syndrome
FEV	forced expiratory volume	**SIDS**	sudden infant death syndrome
HBOT	hyperbaric oxygen therapy	**SOB**	shortness of breath
HMD	hyaline membrane disease	**T & A**	tonsillectomy and adenoidectomy

TB	tuberculosis	**URI**	upper respiratory infection
TLC	total lung capacity	**VC**	vital capacity
TV	tidal volume		

DRUG HIGHLIGHTS

Drugs that are generally used in respiratory system diseases and disorders include antihistamines, decongestants, antitussives, expectorants, mucolytics, bronchodilators, inhalational corticosteroids, and antituberculosis agents.

Antihistamines
Act to counter the effects of histamine by blocking histamine 1 (H_1) receptors. They are used in the treatment of allergy symptoms, for preventing or controlling motion sickness, and in combination with cold remedies to decrease mucus secretion and produce bedtime sedation.
Examples: Benadryl (diphenhydramine HCl), Hismanal (astemizole), and Dimetane (brompheniramine maleate).

Decongestants
Act to constrict dilated arterioles in the nasal mucosa. These agents are used for the temporary relief of nasal congestion associated with the common cold, hay fever, other upper respiratory allergies, and sinusitis.
Examples: Sudafed (pseudoephedrine HCl), Coricidin (phenylephrine HCl), Sinutab Long-Lasting Sinus Spray (xylometazoline HCl), and Afrin (oxymetazoline HCl).

Antitussives
May be classified as non-narcotic and narcotic.

Non-narcotic agents
Anesthetize the stretch receptors located in the respiratory passages, lungs, and pleura by dampening their activity and thereby reducing the cough reflex at its source.
Examples: Tessalon (benzonatate), Benylin (diphenhydramine HCl), and dextromethorphan hydrobromide.

Narcotic agents
Depress the cough center that is located in the medulla, thereby raising its threshold for incoming cough impulse.
Examples: codeine and Codimal (hydrocodone bitartrate).

Expectorants
Promote and facilitate the removal of mucus from the lower respiratory tract.
Examples: Robitussin (guaifenesin) and terpin hydrate.

Mucolytics
Break chemical bonds in mucus, thereby lowering its thickness.
Example: Mucomyst (acetylcysteine).

Bronchodilators
Are used to improve pulmonary airflow.
Examples: Adrenalin (epinephrine), Proventil (albuterol), ephedrine sulfate, aminophylline, and Tedral SA (theophylline).

Inhalational Corticosteroids
Used in the treatment of bronchial asthma, and in seasonal or perennial allergic conditions when other forms of treatment are not effective.
Examples: Decadron (dexamethasone phosphate), Beclovent (beclomethasone dipropionate), and Azmacort (triamcinolone acetonide).

Antituberculosis Agents
Used in the long-term treatment of tuberculosis (9 months to 1 year). They are often used in *combination of two or more drugs and the primary drug regimen for active tuberculosis combines the drugs Myambutol (ethambutol HCl); INH, Nydrazid (isoniazid); and Rifadin, Rimactane (rifampin).*

DIAGNOSTIC AND LABORATORY TESTS

Test	Description
acid-fast bacilli (AFB) (ăs ĭd-făst″ bă-sĭl′ ī)	A test performed on sputum to detect the presence of *Mycobacterium tuberculosis,* an acid-fast bacilli. Positive results indicate tuberculosis.
antistreptolysin O (ASO) (ăn″ tĭ-strĕp-tŏl′ ī-sĭn)	A test performed on blood serum to detect the presence of streptolysin enzyme O, which is secreted by beta-hemolytic streptococcus. Positive results indicate streptococcal infection.
arterial blood gases (ABGs) (ăr-tē′ rē-ăl blod găs′ ĕs)	A series of tests performed on arterial blood to establish acid–base balance. Important in determining respiratory acidosis and/or alkalosis, metabolic acidosis and/or alkalosis.
bronchoscopy (brŏng-kŏs′ kō-pē)	Visual examination of the larynx, trachea, and bronchi via a flexible bronchoscope. With the use of biopsy forceps, tissues and secretions can be removed for further analysis.
culture, sputum (kŭl′ tūr, spū′ tŭm)	Examination of the sputum to determine the presence of microorganisms. Abnormal results may indicate tuberculosis, bronchitis, pneumonia, bronchiectasis, and other infectious respiratory diseases.
culture, throat (kŭl′ tūr, thrōt)	A test done to identify the presence of microorganisms in the throat, especially beta-hemolytic streptococci.
laryngoscopy (lăr″ ĭn-gŏs′ kō-pē)	Visual examination of the larynx via a laryngoscope.
nasopharyngography (nā″ zō-făr-ĭn-ŏg′ ră-fē)	X-ray examination of the nasopharynx.
pulmonary function test (pŭl′ mō-nĕ-rē fŭng′ shŭn test)	A series of tests performed to determine the diffusion of oxygen and carbon dioxide across the cell membrane in the lungs. Tests included are: tidal volume (TV), vital capacity (VC), expiratory reserve volume (ERV), inspiratory capacity (IC), residual volume (RV), forced inspiratory volume (FIV), functional residual capacity (FRC), maximal voluntary ventilation (MVV), total lung capacity (TLC), and flow volume loop (F-V loop). Abnormal results may indicate various respiratory diseases and conditions.
rhinoscopy (rī-nŏs′ kō-pē)	Visual examination of the nasal passages.

COMMUNICATION ENRICHMENT

This segment is provided for those who wish to enhance their ability to communicate in either English or Spanish.

▶ Related Terms

English	Spanish	English	Spanish
asthma	asma (*ăs*-mă)	nosebleed	hemorragia nasal (ĕ-mōr-*nă*-hĭ-ă *nă*-săl)
breath	aliento; respiro (ă-lĭ-*ĕn*-tō; rĕs-pĭ-rō)	phlegm	flema (flĕ-*mă*)
bronchitis	bronquitis (brōn-*kĭ*-tĭs)	pneumonia	neumonía; pulmonía (nĕ-ū-*mō*-nĭ-ă; pūl-*mō*-nĭ-ă)
chest	pecho (*pĕ*-chō)	pollen	polen (pō-*lĕn*)
cough	tos (tōs)	throat	garganta (găr-*găn*-tă)
deep breath	rispire profundo (rĕs-*pĭ*-rĕ *prō*-fūn-dō)	sore throat	dolor de garganta (*dō*-lōr dĕ găr-*găn*-tă)
diaphragm	diafragma (dĭ-*ă*-frăg-mă)	tuberculosis	tuberculosis (tŭ-*bĕr*-kū-lōs-ĭs)
difficulty in breathing	dificultad en respirar (dĭ-*fĭ*-cŭl-tăd ĕn rĕs-pĭ-răr)	voice	voz (vōz)
dust	polvo (*pōl*-vō)	whooping cough	tosferina (tōs-*fĕ*-rĭ-nă)
hoarseness	ronquedad; ronquera (rōn-*kĕ*-dăd; rōn-*kay*-ră)	respiration	respiración (rĕs-pĭ-*nă*-sĭ-ōn)
lungs	pulmónes (pŭl-*mō*-nĕs)	thorax	tórax (*tō*-răx)
nose	nariz (*nă*-riz)	hoarse	ronco (*rōn*-kō)
		snore	ronquido (rōn-*kĭ*-dō)
		influenza	gripe (*grĭ*-pĕ)

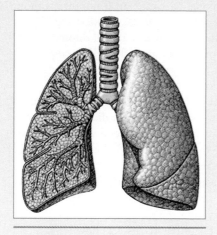

4

ANATOMY AND PHYSIOLOGY OF THE RESPIRATORY SYSTEM

OBJECTIVES

On completion of this chapter, you should be able to:

- Describe the primary functions of the respiratory system.

- Explain how the delicate respiratory exchange surfaces are protected from pathogens, debris, and other hazards.

- Relate respiratory functions to the structural specializations of the tissues and organs in the system.

- Describe the process of breathing.

- Describe the actions of respiratory muscles on respiratory movements.

- Describe how oxygen and carbon dioxide are transported in the blood.

- Describe the major factors that influence the rate of respiration.

- Describe the changes that occur in the respiratory system with aging.

Breathing is more essential to our lives than eating or drinking. In fact, 5 to 6 minutes without breathing will likely prove fatal. This is because the cells of our body must keep generating ATP to support their maintenance, growth, and replication. This cellular energy is obtained through chemical reactions that require oxygen, and we get that oxygen from the air around us. The same chemical reactions that consume oxygen generate carbon dioxide as a waste product. A constant supply of oxygen and a reliable method for removing the carbon dioxide are thus vital to our cells.

Every time we inhale we bring additional oxygen into our lungs, where it can be absorbed by the blood and distributed to our cells. Every time we exhale we eliminate carbon dioxide. The lungs provide the huge surface area needed for the exchange of gases between our blood and the external atmosphere. How huge is huge? In order to meet our oxygen demand, the total exchange surface of the lungs is at least 35 times larger than the total surface area of the body.

The *respiratory system* includes the lungs, the air-filled passageways leading to the lungs, and the skeletal muscles that move air into and out of the lungs. The following discussion of the organs of the respiratory system will follow the flow of air as it travels from the exterior toward the delicate exchange surfaces of the lungs. We will then consider how breathing occurs and how oxygen and carbon dioxide are transported and exchanged between the air and the blood, and between the blood and other body tissues.

▶ SYSTEM BRIEF

Respiration is the exchange of gases between living cells and the environment. Respiration involves three different steps or activities:

1. **Pulmonary ventilation**: breathing, or the movement of air into and out of the lungs.
2. **Gas exchange**: the diffusion of oxygen and carbon dioxide between the lungs and blood (*external respiration*), and the diffusion of oxygen and carbon dioxide between blood and cells in the body tissues (*internal respiration*).
3. **Gas pickup and transport**: the transport of oxygen and carbon dioxide within the blood.

The eventual use of oxygen within cells for the production of energy is called *cellular respiration*.

The major function of the respiratory system is to move air to and from the lungs, where diffusion can occur between air and circulating blood. Additional functions include providing a defense against pathogenic invasion, producing sounds for speaking, assisting in the regulation of blood volume and pressure, and assisting in the control of body fluid pH.

▶ STRUCTURE OF THE RESPIRATORY SYSTEM

The **respiratory system** includes the nose, nasal cavity, and sinuses; the pharynx (throat); the larynx (voice box); the trachea (windpipe); the bronchi and bronchioles (conducting passageways); and the lungs (Figure 4-1). The bronchioles end at air sacs within the lungs called *alveoli* (al-VE-o-li); singular: *alveolus*. The walls of the alveoli are the gas-exchange surfaces of the lungs.

THE NOSE

Air normally enters the respiratory system through the paired **nostrils**, which open into the **nasal cavity**. Coarse hairs within the nostrils guard the nasal cavity from large airborne particles such as sand, dust, and insects.

The nasal cavity is divided into left and right compartments by the *nasal septum*. The bony nasal septum and the walls of the nasal cavity are formed by bones of the cranium and face. The *superior, middle*, and *inferior nasal conchae* project toward the nasal septum from the sides of the nasal cavity. The nasal conchae cause the incoming air to swirl, much like water flows turbulently over rapids. Because this movement slows down the passage of air, there is additional time for it to be

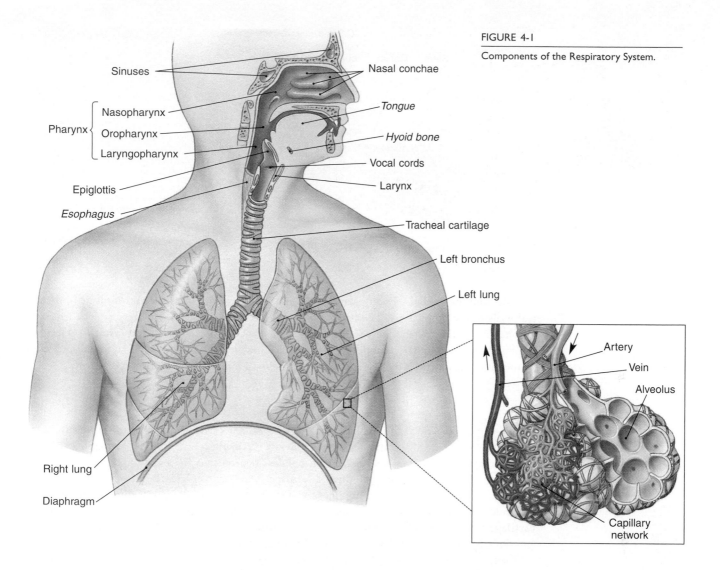

FIGURE 4-1

Components of the Respiratory System.

warmed and humidified. In addition, the air is cleaned of small airborne particles as they come in contact with the mucus that coats the lining of the nasal cavity.

A bony **hard palate** forms the floor of the nasal cavity and separates it from the underlying oral cavity. A fleshy **soft palate** extends behind the hard palate. The area above the soft palate is the **nasopharynx** (nā-zō-FAR-inks), which lies between the nasal cavity and the portion of the pharynx connected to the oral cavity.

The nasal cavity and the lower air- conducting passageways are lined by a mucous membrane made up of a ciliated epithelium that contains many mucus-producing *goblet cells* (Figure 4-2). The cilia sweep mucus and any trapped particles or microorganisms toward the pharynx, where they can be swallowed and exposed to the acids and enzymes of the stomach. The nasal cavity is also flushed by mucus produced in the *paranasal sinuses* (air-filled chambers in the facial bones) and by tears flowing through the *nasolacrimal duct*. Exposure to toxic vapors, large quantities of dust and debris, allergens, or pathogens usually causes a rapid increase in the rate of mucus production, and a "runny nose" develops.

THE PHARYNX

The **pharynx** is a chamber shared by the digestive and respiratory systems. Its three subdivisions are shown in Figure 4-1. The upper portion, the **nasopharynx**, is lined by a ciliated epithelium. This region contains the pharyngeal tonsil and the entrances to the auditory tubes. The **oropharynx**

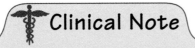

Ciliated columnar epithelial cell

Stem cell

Goblet cell

Mucus layer

Movement of mucus to pharynx

Loose connective tissue

FIGURE 4-2

Ciliated Respiratory Epithelium.

Mucus is transported to the pharynx by ciliated respiratory epithelium within the nasal cavity and the lower air-conducting passageways.

extends from the level of the soft palate to the base of the tongue. The palatine tonsils lie in the lateral walls of the oropharynx. The narrow **laryngopharynx** (la-rin-gō-FAR-inks) extends from the oropharynx to the entrance to the esophagus. Food and liquids entering the digestive tract pass through both the oropharynx and laryngopharynx. These regions are lined by a stratified squamous epithelium that can resist mechanical abrasion, chemical attack, and pathogenic invasion.

THE LARYNX

Incoming air passes through the pharynx and then through a narrow opening, the **glottis** (GLOT-is), which is surrounded and protected by the **larynx** (LAR-inks), or voice box. The larynx contains nine cartilages that are stabilized by ligaments and/or skeletal muscles (Figure 4-3). The two largest cartilages are the epiglottis and the thyroid cartilage. The elastic **epiglottis** (ep-i-GLOT-is) projects above the glottis. During swallowing the epiglottis folds back over the glottis, preventing the entry of liquids or solid food into the larynx and lower air passageways. The shield-shaped **thyroid cartilage** forms much of the anterior and lateral surfaces of the larynx. A prominent ridge on the anterior surface of this cartilage forms the "Adam's apple."

Two pairs of ligaments extend across the larynx, between the thyroid cartilage and other, smaller cartilages. The upper pair, known as the *false vocal cords*, help prevent foreign objects from entering the glottis and protect the more delicate lower folds, which are the true **vocal cords**.

✚ Clinical Note

Lung Cancer

Lung cancer accounts for one-third of all U.S. cancer deaths, making it the primary cause of all U.S. cancer deaths. Although treatment and survival statistics have improved for other cancers, this has not been the case for lung cancer. Even with early detection, the 5-year survival rates are only 30 percent for men and 50 percent for women, and most lung cancer patients die within 1 year of diagnosis. It is well documented that cigarette smoking causes 85 to 90 percent of all lung cancers. Before about 1970, lung cancer affected primarily middle-aged men, but as the number of women smokers has increased, so has the number of women who die from lung cancer.

Smoking changes the quality of the inhaled air, making it drier and contaminating it with several cancer-causing compounds (carcinogens) and fine particles that damage the cells lining the respiratory system. The development of lung cancer appears to be related to the total cumulative exposure to such contaminated air. The more cigarettes smoked, the greater the risk. Fortunately, changes in the respiratory epithelium are usually reversible. If an individual quits smoking before lung cancer develops, the respiratory epithelium gradually repairs itself. As the repair process continues, the risk of developing lung cancer gradually declines to that of nonsmokers.

FIGURE 4-3

Structure of the Larynx and Vocal Cords.

(a) Anterior view of the larynx.
(b) Posterior view of the larynx.
(c) Superior view of the larynx with the glottis open. **(d)** Superior view of the larynx with the glottis closed.

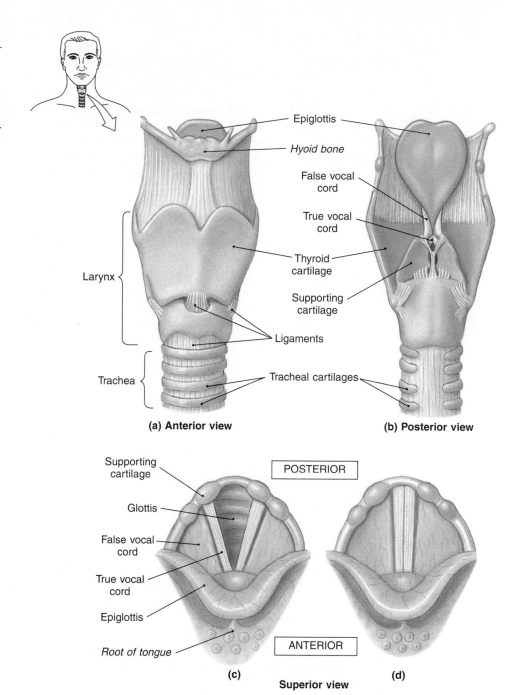

FIGURE 4-3

Structure of the Larynx and Vocal Cords.

(a) Anterior view of the larynx.
(b) Posterior view of the larynx.
(c) Superior view of the larynx with the glottis open. **(d)** Superior view of the larynx with the glottis closed.

(a) Anterior view

(b) Posterior view

(c)   (d)

Superior view

The vocal cords vibrate when air passes through the glottis. These vibrations generate sound waves. As on a guitar or violin, short, thin strings vibrate rapidly, producing a high-pitched sound and large, long strings vibrate more slowly, producing a low-pitched tone. Because children of both sexes have slender, short vocal cords, their voices tend to be high-pitched. At puberty the larynx of a male enlarges more than that of a female. The true vocal cords of an adult male are thicker and longer and they produce lower tones than those of an adult female.

The pitch of the voice is regulated by the amount of tension in the vocal cords. The volume depends on the force of the air movement through the vocal cords. Further amplification and resonance occur within the pharynx, the oral cavity, the nasal cavity, and the paranasal sinuses. The final production of distinct words further depends on voluntary movements of the tongue, lips, and cheeks.

THE TRACHEA

The **trachea** (TRĀ-ke-a), or windpipe, is a tough, flexible tube about 2.5 cm (1 in.) in diameter and 11 cm (4.0 in.) long. The walls of the trachea are supported by about 20 **tracheal cartilages**. These C-shaped structures stiffen the tracheal walls and protect the airway. As you can see in Figure 4-3b, the open portions of the tracheal cartilages face posteriorly, toward the esophagus. As a result, the posterior tracheal wall distorts easily, and this is important when large masses of food pass along the esophagus. The diameter of the trachea is adjusted by the ANS, which controls contractions of smooth muscle in its walls. Stimulation by the sympathetic nervous system increases the diameter of the trachea and makes it easier to move large volumes of air along the respiratory passageways.

THE BRONCHI

The trachea branches to form the **right** and **left primary bronchi** (BRONG-ki). The right primary bronchus is larger and more vertical than the left bronchus. As a result, accidentally inhaled objects, such as pieces of food, most often enter (and get stuck in) the right primary bronchus.

Each primary bronchus enters its lung at a groove or depression called the **hilus**. Pulmonary blood vessels, nerves, and lymphatic vessels also enter the lung at the hilus. Each primary bronchus branches as it enters the lung, giving rise to *secondary bronchi* that enter the lobes of the lung. In each lung, the secondary bronchi divide to form 10 *tertiary bronchi* in each lung, which then branch repeatedly. The primary bronchi and their branches form a network that is called the *respiratory tree*, or *bronchial tree*.

The cartilages surrounding the secondary bronchi are quite massive, but they decrease in size as the branches of the "tree" become smaller and smaller. When the diameter of the passageway has narrowed to around 1 mm, the cartilage rings disappear completely. This narrow passage represents a **bronchiole**.

All portions of the trachea and the various bronchi are lined by the same type of pseudostratified ciliated columnar epithelium found within the nasal cavity and nasopharynx. The beating of the cilia moves mucus and any foreign particles toward the pharynx for elimination by swallowing, coughing, or sneezing.

THE BRONCHIOLES

The walls of bronchioles contain more smooth muscle than the wider air-conducting passageways discussed above. Contraction and relaxation of the smooth muscle of the bronchioles is under autonomic control. Varying the diameter of the bronchioles regulates the amount of resistance to airflow and the distribution of air in the lungs. For example, impulses from the sympathetic nervous system can cause the smooth muscles in the walls of bronchioles to relax, thereby increasing the diameter of the respiratory passageways. This helps prepare us for intense activity by making it easier to move air quickly to and from the lungs. Extreme contraction of these smooth muscles can almost completely close the bronchioles, and this can make breathing difficult or even impossible. Significant reductions in the diameter of bronchioles accompany a severe asthma attack or an acute allergic reaction.

Bronchioles continue to divide until they form the **terminal bronchioles,** the end of the air-conducting portion of the respiratory system (Figure 4-4). The terminal bronchioles branch to form passageways that open into clusters of *alveoli*.

THE ALVEOLI

Each lung contains approximately 150 million alveoli. The total gas-exchange area of all the alveoli in both lungs is about 140 m^2—roughly the size of a tennis court. Gas exchange at an alveolus is highly efficient because of its unusually thin epithelium. Figure 4-4b shows the **alveolar macrophages** (*dust cells*) that patrol this epithelium, engulfing dust or debris that has reached the alveolar surfaces. **Surfactant** (sur-FAK-tant) **cells** produce an oily secretion, or **surfactant**, that

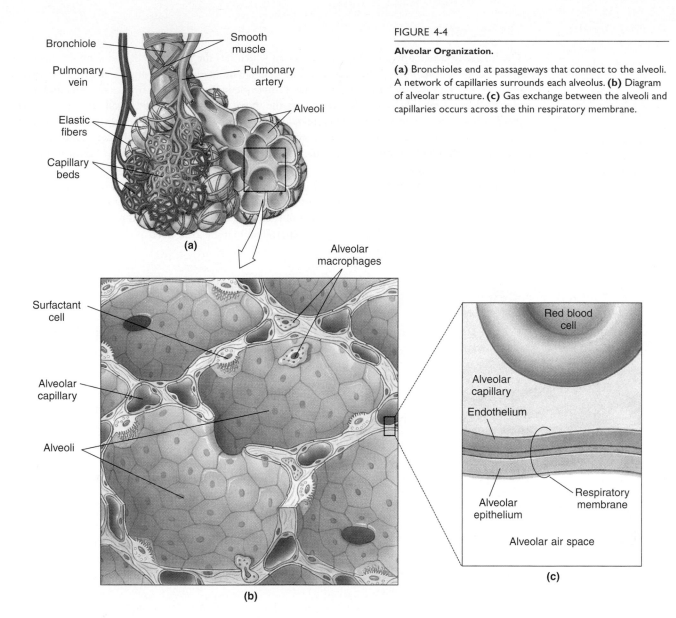

FIGURE 4-4

Alveolar Organization.

(a) Bronchioles end at passageways that connect to the alveoli. A network of capillaries surrounds each alveolus. **(b)** Diagram of alveolar structure. **(c)** Gas exchange between the alveoli and capillaries occurs across the thin respiratory membrane.

forms a thin coating over the alveolar epithelium. Surfactant is important because it reduces surface tension within the alveolus. Surface tension results from the pull or attraction between water molecules at an air–water boundary. The alveolar walls are so delicate that without surfactant, they would collapse like deflating balloons.

The respiratory exchange surfaces receive blood from arteries of the pulmonary circulation. The pulmonary arteries enter the lungs and branch, following the bronchi to the alveoli. Each cluster of alveoli receives an arteriole and a venule, and a network of capillaries surrounds each alveolus (Figure 4-4a). The walls of the alveoli, like the walls of capillaries, are made up of a single layer of epithelium. Together, these two epithelia make up the *respiratory membrane* that separates the alveolar air and the blood (Figure 4-4c). Because it is so thin, as little as one ten-thousandth of a millimeter (0.1 μm), the exchange of respiratory gases by diffusion can occur very rapidly. After passing through the pulmonary venules, venous blood enters the pulmonary veins that deliver it to the left atrium.

Concept Questions

✔ When the tension in the vocal cords increases, what happens to the pitch of the voice?

✔ Why are the cartilages that reinforce the trachea C-shaped instead of complete circles?

✔ What would happen to the alveoli if surfactant were not produced?

THE LUNGS

The lungs are situated within the thoracic cavity, which has the shape of a broad cone. Its walls are the rib cage, and its floor is the muscular diaphragm. The mediastinum divides the thoracic cavity into two pleural cavities. Each lung occupies a single pleural cavity, lined by a serous membrane, or **pleura** (PLOO-ra). The *parietal pleura* covers the inner surface of the body wall and extends over the diaphragm and mediastinum. The *visceral pleura* covers the outer surfaces of the lungs. Because the parietal and visceral layers are in close contact with each other, the pleural cavity is not an open chamber. A thin layer of fluid between these layers lubricates and reduces friction between them as the lungs expand and contract.

The left and right lungs (Figure 4-1) occupy the left and right pleural cavities. Each lung has distinct **lobes** separated by deep grooves, or fissures. The right lung has three lobes and the left lung has two. Because most of the actual volume of each lung consists of air-filled passageways and alveoli, the lung has a light and spongy consistency. The many elastic fibers give the lungs the ability to tolerate large changes in volume.

▶ PHYSIOLOGY OF RESPIRATION

The process of respiration involves exchanges of gases between the air and the lungs, the lungs and the blood, the blood and body tissue fluids and cells, and the transport of gases by the blood. Problems that affect any of these steps will ultimately affect the gas concentrations of the tissue fluids and body cells.

PULMONARY VENTILATION

Pulmonary ventilation, or breathing, is the physical movement of air into and out of the lungs. A single breath, or *respiratory cycle*, consists of an **inhalation**, the movement of air into the lungs, and an **exhalation**, the movement of air out of the lungs. The movement of air into and out of the lungs during each breath is controlled by differences in air pressure between the lungs and the external environment.

Changes in the volume of the lungs are due to changes in the volume of their surrounding pleural cavities. Fluid in the pleural cavities causes the surface of each lung to stick to the inner wall of the chest and the superior surface of the diaphragm, much like the strong bond between the bottom of a wet glass and smooth table. As a result, when the diaphragm and chest wall move, the volume of the lungs changes.

When relaxed, the diaphragm has the shape of a dome and projects upward into the thoracic cavity, compressing the lungs. When the diaphragm contracts, it flattens and increases the volume of the thoracic cavity, expanding the lungs. Figure 4-5a shows how the thoracic cavity enlarges when the diaphragm contracts. Any change in volume has an effect on pressure. If you have ever watched a physician using a syringe, you are already aware of this. When the plunger is drawn back, the volume inside the syringe increases, and this lowers the internal pressure and pulls air or fluid into the syringe. When the plunger is pushed in, the volume inside decreases, and the air or fluid is pushed out of the syringe. The same principle is responsible for moving air in and out of the lungs.

Inhalation

At the start of a breath, pressures inside and outside the lungs are identical and there is no movement of air. When the thoracic cavity enlarges, the pressure inside the lungs drops, and air enters the respiratory passageways (Figure 4-5b). Enlargement of the thoracic cavity involves the contractions of the diaphragm, aided by the external intercostal muscles.

The external intercostals elevate the rib cage. Because of the way the ribs and the vertebrae articulate, this movement increases the volume of the thoracic cavity. During heavy breathing, other muscles, such as the sternocleidomastoid, help the external intercostals elevate the ribs. This increases the amount of air moved into the lungs while reducing the time spent in inhalation.

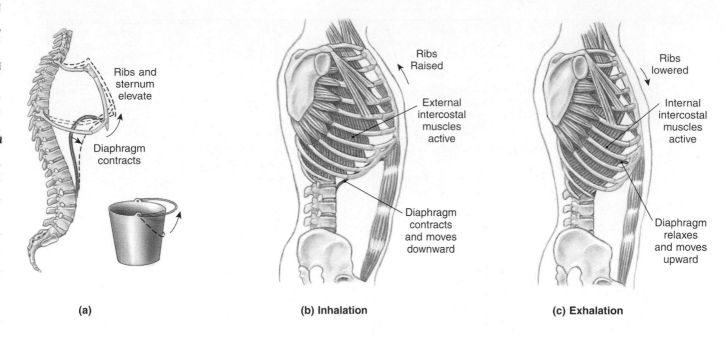

(a)

(b) Inhalation

(c) Exhalation

FIGURE 4-5

Breathing (Pulmonary Ventilation).

(a) Raising the curved bucket handle increases the amount of space between it and the bucket. Similarly, the volume of the thoracic cavity is increased when the diaphragm contracts. **(b)** Inhalation: As the thoracic cavity increases in volume, pressure within the lungs falls and air flows in. **(c)** Exhalation: When the rib cage returns to its resting position, the volume of the thoracic cavity decreases. Pressure rises, and air moves out of the lungs.

Exhalation

Downward movement of the rib cage and upward movement of the relaxed diaphragm reverse the process and reduce the size of the lungs. Pressure inside the lungs now rises, and air moves out of the lungs (Figure 4-5c).

During quiet breathing, as when sitting and reading, exhalation is a passive process. That is, when the respiratory muscles used during inhalation relax, gravity pulls the ribs downward, the stretched elastic fibers of the lungs recoil, and air is forced out of the lungs. When breathing heavily, contractions of the internal intercostal muscles and the abdominal muscles assist gravity in pulling the ribs downward and forcing the diaphragm into the thoracic cavity. These muscles increase the rate of exhalation as well as the amount of air moved out of the lungs.

Movement of Air

An inhalation, or *inspiration*, at rest does not completely fill the lungs with air. In fact, during a quiet respiratory cycle, about 500 ml of air is inhaled and 500 ml is exhaled. This amount of air movement is called the **tidal volume**. Only about two-thirds of the inspired air reaches the alveolar exchange surfaces within the lungs. The rest never gets farther than the conducting passageways, and thus does not participate in gas exchange with the blood. The volume of air in the conducting passages is known as the **dead space** of the lungs.

We can increase the tidal volume by inhaling more vigorously and exhaling more completely. Measurements of such increased volumes of air are used to evaluate how well an individual's respiratory system is functioning. For example, the **inspiratory reserve volume** is the amount of air that can be taken in over and above the resting tidal volume. Because lungs are larger in males, the inspiratory reserve volume averages 3300 ml in males versus 1900 ml in females. On the other hand, a forced exhalation, or *expiration*, at the end of a tidal cycle will push out an additional 1000 ml of air in males (700 ml in females). This is the **expiratory reserve volume**.

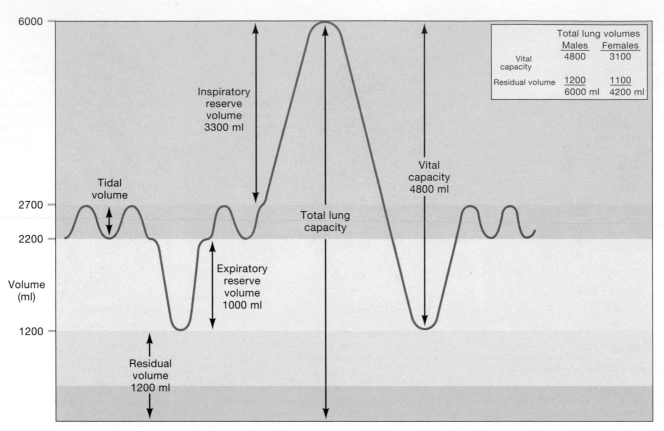

FIGURE 4-6

Respiratory Volumes and Capacities.

The graph diagrams the relationships among the respiratory volumes and capacities of an average male. The table compares the values for males and females.

Concept Questions

✔ How does contraction and relaxation of the diaphragm affect the volume of the thoracic cavity?

✔ What is meant by vital capacity?

The sum of the inspiratory reserve volume, the expiratory reserve volume, and the tidal volume is the **vital capacity**. This is the maximum amount of air that can be moved into and out of the respiratory system in a single respiratory cycle.

Roughly 1100–1200 ml of air remains in the respiratory passageways and alveoli, even after exhausting the expiratory reserve volume. This amount of air, called the **residual volume**, remains because the lungs are held against the thoracic wall, preventing them from contracting further.

The sum of the vital capacity and the residual volume is the **total lung capacity**. The average total lung capacity of males is about 6000 ml, and 4200 ml in females. Figure 4-6 shows the relationships among these different lung volumes and capacities in a male.

GAS EXCHANGE

The exchange of respiratory gases occurs across the membranes of living cells through the process of diffusion. External respiration is the diffusion of gases between the blood and alveolar air across the single cell layers (respiratory membrane) of the alveoli and lung capillaries. Internal respiration is the diffusion of gases between the blood and tissue fluid across the one-cell-thick capillary wall. The directions in which oxygen and carbon dioxide move by diffusion depend on their relative concentrations in air, blood, and tissue fluid.

External Respiration

The air we inhale contains 20.8 percent oxygen and 0.04 percent carbon dioxide, and exhaled air contains about 15 percent oxygen and 3.7 percent carbon dioxide. These differences are due to the

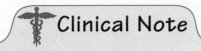

Clinical Note

The Heimlich Maneuver

Choking on food that becomes lodged in the larynx or trachea is a common accident. In most cases, coughing expels the food, the airway clears, and no emergency measures need to be taken. Unfortunately, this is not always the case. In the United States, it is estimated that at least eight such choking events end in death every year.

If a person does get food stuck in the airway and cannot inhale or exhale, a procedure called the **Heimlich** (HĪM-lik) **maneuver**, or abdominal thrust, can save a life. This procedure relies on compressing the chest so forcefully that the remaining air in the lungs will blow the food mass out of the airway. In this procedure, a rescuer compresses the abdomen just beneath the diaphragm with a strong, upward squeeze. Figure 4-7 shows the placement of the rescuer's fist below the ribs and above the navel, and the direction of the upward thrust. Care must be taken to avoid damage to the ribs and underlying organs.

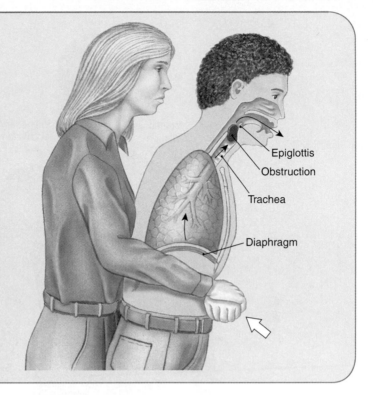

FIGURE 4-7

The Heimlich Maneuver.

uptake of oxygen by the blood and the removal of carbon dioxide from blood in the lung capillaries. The upper portion of Figure 4-8 shows the opposite directions in which oxygen and carbon dioxide diffuse between the alveoli and pulmonary capillaries in the lungs. Each gas diffuses independently from its area of relatively high concentration to its respective area of relatively low concentration.

Internal Respiration

Body cells are constantly using oxygen and generating carbon dioxide. As a result, oxygen concentrations are low within cells and carbon dioxide concentrations are high. The lower portion of Figure 4-8 shows the gas-exchange process during internal respiration; oxygen diffuses out of the capillaries, and carbon dioxide diffuses in until its concentration is the same as in the surrounding tissues.

GAS TRANSPORT

Oxygen and carbon dioxide do not readily dissolve in blood plasma. So how do body cells obtain adequate oxygen and eliminate enough carbon dioxide to survive? The answer lies in their red blood cells. The extra oxygen and carbon dioxide diffuse into the red blood cells, where the gas molecules are either tied up (in the case of oxygen) or used to make other chemical compounds (in the case of carbon dioxide). The important thing about these reactions is that they are completely reversible.

Oxygen Transport

Almost all the oxygen that diffuses into the pulmonary capillaries is bound to hemoglobin (Hb) molecules in red blood cells. The amount of oxygen held onto by hemoglobin depends primarily on the concentration of oxygen in the surrounding tissue. Therefore, the lower the oxygen content of a tissue, the more oxygen will be released by hemoglobin molecules as they circulate through the region.

FIGURE 4-8

External and Internal Respiration.

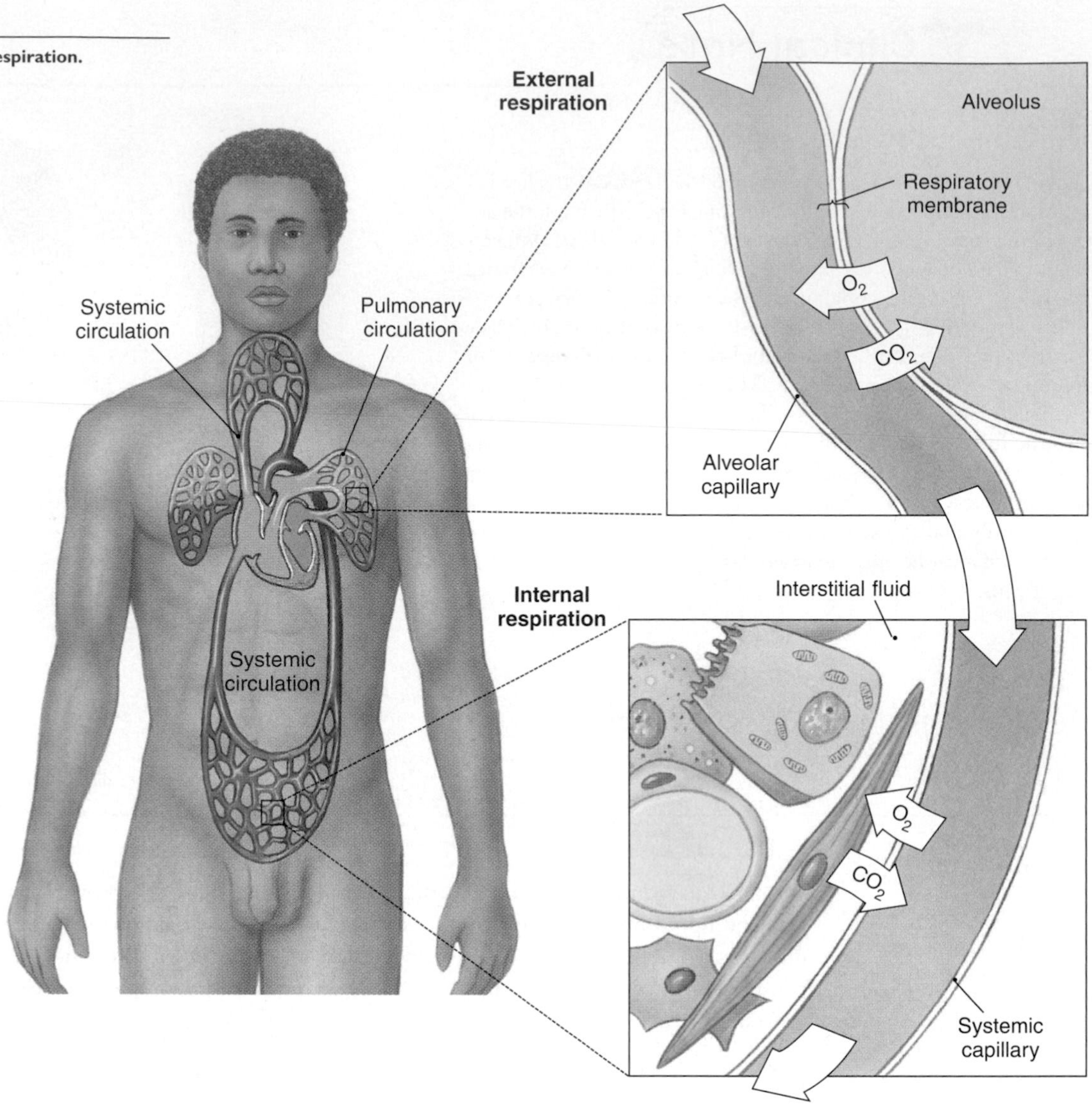

Carbon Dioxide Transport

Carbon dioxide molecules enter the bloodstream and are transported to the lungs three different ways. As Figure 4-9 shows, most of the carbon dioxide enters red blood cells, and only a small amount (7 percent) actually dissolves in the blood plasma. Within the red blood cells, some 23 percent of the carbon dioxide binds directly to hemoglobin, and 70 percent is rapidly converted to *bicarbonate ions* (HCO_3^-).

The bicarbonate ions form in a two-step process. First, the carbon dioxide molecules combine with water to form carbonic acid. Second, the enzyme *carbonic anhydrase* catalyzes the rapid breakdown of carbonic acid molecules into bicarbonate ions and hydrogen ions. The newly formed bicarbonate ions move out of the red blood cells and into the blood plasma. The hydrogen ions produced by this reaction are bound to hemoglobin molecules inside the RBC.

On arrival at the pulmonary capillaries in the lungs, the dissolved carbon dioxide diffuses out of the blood plasma and into the alveoli. As this occurs, the hemoglobin-bound carbon dioxide is released, and bicarbonate and hydrogen ions combine into carbonic acid, which breaks apart into water and carbon dioxide. As this carbon dioxide enters the plasma it diffuses into the alveoli.

The pH of blood is affected by the amount of carbon dioxide that is transported. Some of the CO_2 dissolved in the blood plasma combines with water, forming carbonic acid that releases hydrogen ions and bicarbonate ions. The more CO_2 enters the blood, the more hydrogen ions are released,

Concept Questions

✔ In what form is most of the carbon dioxide transported to the lungs?

✔ In what part of the body does external respiration take place?

FIGURE 4-9

Carbon Dioxide Transport in the Blood.

Most of the carbon dioxide absorbed into the systemic capillaries enters red blood cells. Part of the carbon dioxide binds with hemoglobin, and the rest is converted to bicarbonate ions and released into the plasma. At the alveolar capillaries within the lungs, the carbon dioxide uptake processes are reversed, and carbon dioxide is released.

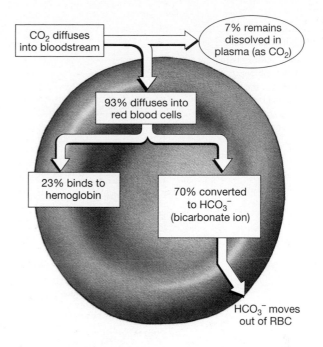

CO_2 diffuses into bloodstream

7% remains dissolved in plasma (as CO_2)

93% diffuses into red blood cells

23% binds to hemoglobin

70% converted to HCO_3^- (bicarbonate ion)

HCO_3^- moves out of RBC

lowering the pH and increasing blood acidity. At the lungs, as CO_2 diffuses from the blood, hydrogen and bicarbonate ions recombine, and blood pH increases. The presence of bicarbonate ions in body fluids is essential for the control of body fluid pH.

► CONTROL OF BREATHING

Under normal conditions the rates of gas exchange between the body cells and tissue capillaries, and between the alveoli and capillaries in the lungs are equal. If these rates become seriously unbalanced, problems soon develop. For example, if body cells are absorbing oxygen faster than it is being absorbed at the alveolar capillaries, tissues will soon become oxygen-starved. To prevent this the activities of the cardiovascular and respiratory systems must be adjusted.

RESPIRATORY CONTROL CENTERS

Normal breathing occurs automatically, without conscious control. Breathing is controlled by the **respiratory centers**, three groups of neurons in the brain stem. Two of these groups are located in the pons, and the other lies in the medulla oblongata. These respiratory centers regulate contraction of the respiratory muscles, control the **respiratory rate** (number of breaths per minute), and adjust the depth of breathing. The normal adult respiratory rate at rest ranges from 12 to 18 breaths per minute. Children breathe more rapidly, at around 18 to 20 breaths per minute.

The respiratory center within the medulla oblongata sets the basic pace for respiration by direct control of the respiratory muscles. The respiratory centers in the pons alter the basic rhythm established by the medulla oblongata. For example, the pons may adjust the respiratory rate and the depth of respiration in response to sensory stimuli, emotional states, or speech patterns. Figure 4-10 summarizes the factors involved in the involuntary control of respiration.

The activities of the respiratory centers can be affected by any factor that affects the metabolism of nervous tissues. For example, elevated body temperatures or central nervous system stimulants, such as amphetamines or even caffeine, increase the respiratory rate. Decreased body temperature or CNS depressants, such as barbiturates or opiates, reduce the respiratory rate.

FIGURE 4-10

The Control of Breathing.

Various types of sensory receptors in the lungs, medulla oblongata, internal carotid arteries, and the ascending aorta can alter the rate and depth of breathing set by control centers in the medulla oblongata.

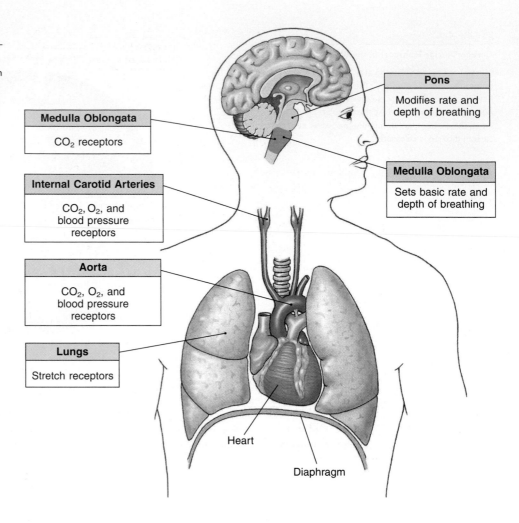

SENSORY RECEPTORS AND RESPIRATION

The respiratory centers constantly receive messages from mechanical (stretching and pressure) and chemical sensory receptors that can alter the rate of respiration.

Stretch Receptors

The *inflation reflex* prevents the lungs from overexpanding as one breathes more deeply during strenuous activity. The receptors involved are stretch receptors that are stimulated when the lungs expand. Sensory fibers leaving these receptors travel within the vagus nerves to reach the respiratory centers in the medulla oblongata.

Pressure Receptors

Blood pressure receptors are located in the walls of the ascending aorta near the heart and at the bases of the internal carotid arteries of the neck. Nerve impulses from these sensory receptors affect the respiratory centers as well as the cardiac and vasomotor centers that control the heart and blood vessels. When blood pressure falls, the respiratory rate increases; when blood pressure rises, the respiratory rate declines. This adjustment results from stimulation or inhibition of the respiratory centers by sensory fibers in the glossopharyngeal (IX) and vagus (X) nerves.

Chemical Receptors

Chemoreceptors respond to chemical changes in the blood and cerebrospinal fluid. Receptors near the carotid arteries (close to the pressure receptors) and the aorta (near the aortic pressure receptors) are sensitive to the concentrations of carbon dioxide and oxygen in arterial blood; receptors in the medulla oblongata respond to the concentration of carbon dioxide in the surrounding cerebrospinal fluid (CSF).

Under normal conditions, carbon dioxide levels have a much more powerful effect on respiratory activity than does oxygen because the oxygen level in the arteries seldom declines enough to activate the oxygen receptors. But when oxygen levels do fall, the two types of receptors cooperate. Carbon dioxide is generated during oxygen consumption, so when oxygen concentrations are falling rapidly, carbon dioxide levels are usually increasing.

Chemoreceptor reflexes are extremely powerful respiratory stimulators, and they cannot be consciously suppressed. For example, you can hold your breath before diving into a swimming pool and thereby prevent the inhalation of water, but you cannot commit suicide by holding your breath "until you turn blue." Once the concentration of carbon dioxide rises to critical levels, you will be forced to take a breath. Inexperienced divers often provide an example of the significance of the carbon dioxide level. In order to hold their breath longer underwater they may take a series of deep, full breaths. This process is called *hyperventiliation*. Although most believe that their increased breath-holding ability is due to "extra oxygen," it is really due to the loss of carbon dioxide. If the carbon dioxide level is reduced low enough, breath-holding ability may increase to the point that the individual becomes unconscious from oxygen starvation in the brain without ever feeling the urge to breathe.

Concept Questions

✔ Where are the automatic control centers for respiration located?

✔ Are the carotid and aortic chem-oreceptors more sensitive to carbon dioxide levels or to oxygen levels?

VOLUNTARY AND INVOLUNTARY INFLUENCES

Higher centers in the brain can influence respiration by affecting the respiratory centers of the pons, and by the direct control of respiratory muscles. For example, the contractions of respiratory muscles can be voluntarily suppressed or exaggerated; this must be done while talking or singing. Respiration can also be affected by activities of the limbic system. For example, activation of centers involved with rage, feeding, or sexual arousal will change the pattern of respiration.

▶ AGING AND THE RESPIRATORY SYSTEM

Many factors interact to reduce the efficiency of the respiratory system in elderly individuals. For example,

1. With increasing age, elastic tissue throughout the body breaks down. This deterioration reduces the resilience of the lungs and lowers the vital capacity.
2. Movements of the chest cage become restricted because of arthritic changes in the rib joints and less flexible rib cartilages.
3. Some degree of *emphysema* is normally found in individuals age 50 to 70. Emphysema is a condition characterized by shortness of breath. It is caused by the destruction of the surfaces of alveoli, which, in turn, reduces the area available for gas exchange in the lungs. However, the degree of emphysema varies widely depending on the lifetime exposure to cigarette smoke and other respiratory irritants. Comparative studies of nonsmokers and those who have smoked for varying lengths of time clearly show the negative effect of smoking on respiratory performance.

Integration of Body Systems

The following is an explanation of how the immune system and respiratory system are integrated with the other systems in the body:

Immune System

The immune system protects the body from all types of bacteria, parasites, and microbes. These pathogens do not enter the body when the immune system is working properly. Every body system is prone to bacteria, parasites, and microbes, therefore the immune system is directly related to all body systems.

Respiratory System

There are many responsibilities that the respiratory system holds, but the primary function is the supply blood with oxygen to that blood can transport it to the entire body. This is done primarily simply by breathing. Whenever humans breathe, we inhale oxygen and then we exhale carbon dioxide. Since blood is transported by oxygen, the circulatory system is directly connected with the respiratory system.

CHAPTER REVIEW SECTION

KEY WORDS

alveolus/alveoli (al-VĒ-o-lī): Air sacs within the lungs; the sites of gas exchange with the blood.

bronchiole: The finest subdivisions of the conducting passageways in the lungs.

diaphragm (DĪ-a-fram): The respiratory muscle that separates the thoracic cavity from the abdominopelvic cavity.

larynx (LAR-inks): A complex cartilaginous structure that surrounds and protects the glottis and vocal cords; the upper margin is bound to the hyoid bone, and the lower margin is bound to the trachea.

lungs: Paired organs of respiration that occupy the left and right pleural cavities.

nasal cavity: A chamber in the skull that extends between the nostrils and the nasopharynx.

paranasal sinuses: Air-filled chambers within bones of the skull; they are lined by a respiratory epithelium and they open into the nasal cavity.

pharynx: The throat; a muscular passageway shared by the digestive and respiratory tracts.

pleural cavities: Subdivisions of the thoracic cavity that contain the lungs.

respiration: Exchange of gases between living cells and the environment.

surfactant (sur-FAK-tant): Lipid secretion that coats alveolar surfaces and prevents their collapse.

trachea (TRĀ-kē-a): The windpipe; an airway extending from the larynx to the primary bronchi.

vital capacity: The maximum amount of air that can be moved in or out of the respiratory system; the sum of the inspiratory reserve, the expiratory reserve, and the tidal volume.

STUDY OUTLINE

INTRODUCTION

1. To continue functioning, body cells must obtain oxygen and eliminate carbon dioxide.

SYSTEM BRIEF

1. The process of **respiration** includes pulmonary ventilation (breathing), gas exchange, and gas transport. *Cellular respiration* refers to the cellular use of the oxygen obtained through respiration.
2. The functions of the respiratory system include providing for the gas exchange between air and circulating blood, defending the respiratory system from pathogens, permitting vocal communication, and aiding in the regulation of blood pressure and body fluid pH.

STRUCTURE OF THE RESPIRATORY SYSTEM

1. The **respiratory system** includes the nose, nasal cavity and sinuses, pharynx, larynx, trachea, and conducting passageways leading to the gas-exchange surfaces of the lungs (*alveoli*). *(Figure 4-1)*

THE NOSE

2. Air normally enters the respiratory system through the **nostrils**, which open into the **nasal cavity**.
3. The **hard palate** separates the oral and nasal cavities. The **soft palate** separates the superior **nasopharynx** from the rest of the pharynx. *(Figure 4-1)*
4. Much of the respiratory epithelium is ciliated and produces mucus that traps incoming particles. *(Figure 4-2)*

THE PHARYNX

5. The **pharynx** is a chamber shared by the digestive and respiratory systems. The nasopharynx contains the pharyngeal tonsil and the entrances to the auditory tubes. The **oropharynx** is continuous with the oral cavity; **laryngopharynx** includes the narrow zone between the oropharynx and the entrance to the esophagus. *(Figure 4-1)*

THE LARYNX

6. Inhaled air passes through the **glottis** on its way to the lungs; the **larynx** surrounds and protects the glottis. The **epiglottis** projects into the pharynx. *(Figure 4-3a,b)*
7. Two pairs of folds span the glottal opening: the relatively inelastic *false vocal cords* and the more delicate true **vocal cords**. Air passing through the glottis causes the true vocal cords to vibrate and produce sound. *(Figure 4-3c,d)*

THE TRACHEA

8. The **trachea** ("windpipe") is a tough, flexible tube. The tracheal wall contains C-shaped **tracheal cartilages** that protect the airway. The posterior tracheal wall can distort to permit passage of large masses of food along the esophagus.

THE BRONCHI

9. The trachea branches to form the **right** and **left primary bronchi**.

THE BRONCHIOLES

10. The primary bronchi and their branches are supported by cartilage rings or plates. The smallest bronchi are connected to smaller passageways called bronchioles. The bronchioles lack cartilage and have relatively larger amounts of smooth muscle than bronchi.
11. Each **terminal bronchiole** delivers air to clusters of alveoli. *(Figure 4-4)*

THE ALVEOLI

12. The alveoli are the respiratory exchange surfaces of the lungs. *(Figure 4-4)*
13. The alveolar lining consists of a simple squamous epithelium; **surfactant cells** scattered in it produce an oily secretion that keep the alveoli from collapsing. **Alveolar macrophages** patrol the epithelium and engulf foreign particles or pathogens. *(Figure 4-4)*
14. Each alveolus is surrounded by a network of capillaries, which make up the respiratory exchange region of the pulmonary circulation. Pulmonary veins collect and deliver the venous blood to the left atrium.

THE LUNGS

15. Each lung occupies a single pleural cavity lined by a **pleura** (a serous membrane).

PHYSIOLOGY OF RESPIRATION

1. Respiratory physiology focuses on three integrated processes: *pulmonary ventilation*, or breathing (movement of air into and out of the lungs); gas exchange between the lungs, circulating blood, and body cells; and gas transport in the blood.

PULMONARY VENTILATION

2. A single breath, or *respiratory cycle*, consists of an **inhalation** (*inspiration*) and an **exhalation** (*expiration*).
3. Contractions of the diaphragm and the *external* and *internal intercostal* muscles of the rib cage alter the volume of the thoracic cavity and lungs. Increased volume lowers the air pressure within the lungs, and air enters the lungs; decreased volume increases air pressure within the lungs, causing air to be exhaled. *(Figure 4-5)*
4. The **vital capacity** is the **tidal volume** plus the **expiratory reserve** and the **inspiratory reserve volumes**. The air left in the lungs at the end of maximum expiration is the **residual volume**. *(Figure 4-6)*

GAS EXCHANGE

5. The directions in which oxygen and carbon dioxide diffuse across cell membranes depend on their concentrations in air, blood, and tissue fluid.
6. Inhaled and exhaled air differ in composition.
7. **External respiration** takes place in the lungs; oxygen diffuses into the blood, and carbon dioxide diffuses into the alveoli. **Internal respiration** takes place at tissue capillary beds; oxygen diffuses into interstitial fluid and body cells, and carbon dioxide diffuses into the blood. *(Figure 4-8)*

GAS TRANSPORT

8. Blood entering systemic capillaries delivers oxygen and absorbs carbon dioxide. The transport of oxygen and carbon dioxide in the blood involves reactions that are completely reversible.
9. Almost all the oxygen is transported attached to hemoglobin molecules within red blood cells.
10. Roughly 7 percent of the CO_2 transported in the blood is dissolved in the plasma, another 23 percent is bound to hemoglobin, and the rest is converted to carbonic acid, which breaks down into hydrogen ions and bicarbonate ions. *(Figure 4-9)*

CONTROL OF BREATHING

1. Large-scale changes in the rates of gas exchange requires homeostatic adjustments by the cardiovascular and respiratory systems.

30. You spend the night at a friend's house during the winter and his hot-air furnace lacks a humidifier. When you wake up in the morning you have a fair amount of nasal congestion and think you may be coming down with a cold. After a steamy shower and some juice at breakfast, the nasal congestion disappears. Explain.

ANSWERS TO CONCEPT CHECK QUESTIONS

(p. 120) **1.** Increased tension in the vocal cords will cause a higher pitch in the voice. **2.** The tracheal cartilages are C-shaped to allow room for expansion of the esophagus when large portions of food or liquid are swallowed. **3.** Without surfactant, surface tension in the thin layer of water that moistens their surfaces would cause the alveoli to collapse.

(p. 122) **1.** During contraction the diaphragm flattens and increases the volume of the thoracic cavity, which expands lung volume. During relaxation the diaphragm projects upward and decreases the volume of thoracic cavity and, in turn, lung volume. **2.** Vital capacity is the maximum amount of air that can be moved into and out of the respiratory system in a single respiratory cycle. It is the sum of the inspiratory reserve volume, the expiratory reserve volume, and the tidal volume.

(p. 124) **1.** Most of the carbon dioxide released by body tissues enters red blood cells, where it is converted into bicarbonate ions that then diffuse into the blood plasma. At the lungs the bicarbonate ions are converted back into carbon dioxide within the red blood cells and released into the alveoli. **2.** External respiration refers to the diffusion of gases between the blood in the lung capillaries and air in the alveoli of the lungs.

(p. 127) **1.** The respiratory control centers are located in the medulla oblongata and the pons. The respiratory center within the medulla oblongata sets the basic pace for respiration by sending involuntary nerve impulses to the respiratory muscles. The respiratory centers in the pons can alter the basic rhythm established by the medulla oblongata. **2.** Carbon dioxide levels have a much more powerful effect on the carotid and aortic chemoreceptors than does oxygen because, under normal conditions, the oxygen level in the arteries does not usually decline enough to activate the oxygen receptors.

Section Two
CLINICAL LABORATORY PROCEDURES

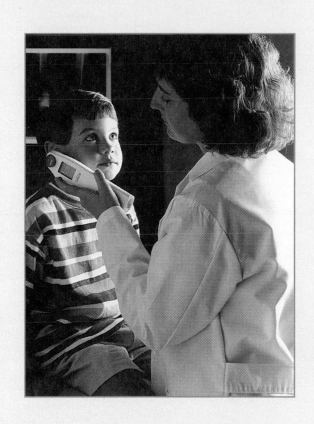

MEDICAL ASSISTANT ROLE DELINEATION CHART

Highlight indicates material covered in this chapter

ADMINISTRATIVE

ADMINISTRATIVE PROCEDURES

- Perform basic clerical functions
- Schedule, coordinate, and monitor appointments
- Schedule inpatient/outpatient admissions and procedures
- Understand and apply third party guidelines
- Obtain reimbursement through accurate claims submission
- Monitor third-party reimbursement
- Perform medical transcription
- Understand and adhere to managed care policies and procedures
- *Negotiate managed care contracts (adv)*

PRACTICE FINANCES

- Perform procedural and diagnostic coding
- Apply bookkeeping principles
- Document and maintain accounting and banking records
- Manage accounts receivable
- Manage accounts payable
- Process payroll
- *Develop and maintain fee schedules (adv)*
- *Manage renewals of business and professional insurance policies (adv)*
- *Manage personal benefits and maintain records (adv)*

CLINICAL

FUNDAMENTAL PRINCIPLES

- Apply principles of aseptic technique and infection control
- Comply with quality assurance practices
- Screen and follow up patient test results

DIAGNOSTIC ORDERS

- Collect and process specimens
- Perform diagnostic tests

PATIENT CARE

- Adhere to established triage procedures
- Obtain patient history and vital signs
- Prepare and maintain examination and treatment areas
- Prepare patient for examinations, procedures, and treatments
- Assist with examinations, procedures, and treatments
- Prepare and administer medications and immunizations
- Maintain medication and immunization records
- Recognize and respond to emergencies
- Coordinate patient care information with other health care providers

GENERAL (TRANSDISCIPLINARY)

PROFESSIONALISM

- Project a professional manner and image
- Adhere to ethical principles
- Demonstrate initiative and responsibility
- Work as a team member
- Manage time efficiently
- Prioritize and perform multiple tasks
- Adapt to change
- Promote the CMA credential
- Enhance skills through continuing education

COMMUNICATION SKILLS

- Treat all patients with compassion and empathy
- Recognize and respect cultural diversity
- Adapt communications to individual's ability to understand
- Use professional telephone technique
- Use effective and correct verbal and written communications
- Recognize and respond to verbal and non-verbal communications
- Use medical terminology appropriately
- Receive, organize, prioritize, and transmit information
- Serve as liaison
  Promote the practice through positive public relations

LEGAL CONCEPTS

- Maintain confidentiality
- Practice within the scope of education, training, and personal capabilities
- Prepare and maintain medical records
- Document accurately
- Use appropriate guidelines when releasing information
- Follow employer's established policies dealing with the health care contract
- Follow federal, state, and local legal guidelines
- Maintain awareness of federal and state health care legislation and regulations
- Maintain and dispose of regulated substances in compliance with government guidelines
- Comply with established risk management and safety procedures
- Recognize professional credentialing criteria
- Participate in the development and maintenance of personnel, policy, and procedure manuals
- *Develop and maintain personnel, policy, and procedure manuals (adv)*

INSTRUCTION

- Instruct individuals according to their needs
- Explain office policies and procedures
- Teach methods of health promotion and disease prevention
- Locate community resources and disseminate information
- *Orient and train personnel (adv)*
- *Develop educational materials (adv)*
- *Conduct continuing education activities (adv)*

OPERATIONAL FUNCTIONS

- Maintain supply inventory
- Evaluate and recommend equipment and supplies
- Apply computer techniques to support office operations
- *Supervise personnel (adv)*
- *Interview and recommend job applicants (adv)*
- *Negotiate leases and prices for equipment and supply contracts (adv)*

SOURCE: Reprinted by permission of the American Association of Medical Assistants from the *AAMA Role Delineation Study: Occupational Analysis of the Medical Assisting Profession.*

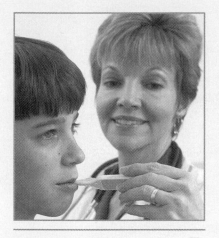

- Temperature
- Pulse
- Respiration
- Blood Pressure (BP)
- Measuring Height and Weight
- Skin-fold Fat Measurement
- Legal and Ethical Issues
- Patient Education

VITAL SIGNS AND MEASUREMENT

OBJECTIVES

After completing this chapter, you should:

1. Define and spell the glossary terms for this chapter.

2. State the normal values of temperature, pulse, respiratory rates, and blood pressure.

3. List 10 conditions which cause the body temperature to increase or decrease.

4. State 3 situations in which measuring an oral, rectal, and axillary temperature should be avoided.

5. List and describe the 7 pulse sites.

6. State 9 factors that can affect the pulse rate.

7. Describe the respiratory rate range for the various age groups.

8. Discuss the 5 phases of the Korotkoff sounds.

9. Explain the 4 physiological factors that affect blood pressure.

10. Discuss the aneroid and mercury sphygmomanometers.

11. Describe the procedure for measuring temperature, pulse, apical-radial pulse, respiration, blood pressure, height, and weight.

12. Explain 10 causes of errors in blood pressure readings.

13. Convert temperature readings from degrees Fahrenheit (F) to degrees Centigrade (C) (and vice versa).

14. Convert weight in pounds to kilograms (and vice versa).

15. Convert height from inches to centimeters (and vice versa).

CLINICAL PERFORMANCE COMPETENCIES

After completing this chapter, you should perform the following tasks:

1. Demonstrate the correct procedures for measuring oral, tympanic, rectal, and axillary temperature using the correct equipment.

2. Correctly determine pulse rate of the adult.

3. Determine pulse rate of infants and children.

4. Identify Korotkoff sounds.

5. Measure height and weight of infants, children, and adults.

6. Demonstrate the correct procedure for measuring a patient's respiration.

7. Demonstrate the correct procedure for measuring respirations noting the rate, rhythm, and depth.

8. Demonstrate the correct procedure for measuring blood pressure of an adult using both mercury and aneroid equipment.

9. Correctly chart all vital signs.

10. Demonstrate the correct procedure for cleaning and disinfecting a glass thermometer.

Glossary

alveoli   Minute air sacs in lungs through which gas exchange takes place between alveolar air and pulmonary capillary blood.

anthropometry   Science of measuring the human body as to size of component parts, height, and weight.

antecubital fossa/space   Area formed at the inside bend of the elbow.

antipyretic   Substance that reduces fever.

arrhythmia   Irregular pulse or heart rate.

asymptomatic   Without having any symptoms; symptom free.

atypical   Unusual; out of the ordinary.

aural   Pertaining to the ear or hearing.

auscultatory gap   Total loss of sound during phase II of the Korotkoff sounds while taking blood pressure. The sound later reoccurs. This is considered abnormal.

axillary   Pertaining to the armpit or area under the arm.

blood stasis   Lack of circulation due to a stoppage of blood flow.

cardiac cycle   Time from the beginning of one beat of the heart to the beginning of the next beat, including the systole (contraction) and diastole (relaxation).

centigrade or Celsius   Scale for measurement of temperature in which 0° C is the freezing point of water and 100° C is the boiling point of water at sea level.

croup   An acute viral infection of the upper and lower respiratory tract in children which may result in difficult, noisy breathing.

cyanosis   Bluish discoloration of the skin and mucous membranes due to oxygen deprivation.

diaphragm   Musculofibrous partition that separates the thoracic and abdominal cavities.

diastole   Period in the cardiac cycle during which the heart is relaxed and the heart cavities are being refilled with blood.

emphysema   Abnormal pulmonary condition with loss of lung elasticity resulting in overinflation of the lungs and difficulty exhaling—"barrel chest."

Fahrenheit   Scale for measurement of temperature in which the boiling point of water is 212° F and the freezing point of water is 32° F at sea level.

frenulum linguae   Longitudinal fold of mucous membrane connecting the floor of the mouth to the underside of the tongue.

heart sounds   Normal noise produced within the heart during the cardiac cycle.

homeostasis   The human body in balance.

hypertension   Elevated blood pressure.

hypotension   Blood pressure which is below normal.

hypothalamus   Portion of brain in the lateral wall of the third ventricle which controls autonomic nervous system functions such as body temperature, sleep, and appetite.

intermittent pulse   Skipping an occasional heart beat.

kilograms   Metric weight.

lumen   Space/cavity within an object or organ.

manometer   Device for taking a measurement (for example, pressure).

medulla oblongata   Most vital part of the brain which contains the respiratory, cardiac, and vasomotor centers of the brain.

pulse deficit   Difference between the rate of the apical pulse and the radial pulse. Normally there is no difference.

palpatory method   To determine by using the sense of touch.

pulse pressure   Difference between systolic and diastolic readings of blood pressure.

pyrexia   Abnormally elevated body temperature; fever.

reading   Interpretation of data.

sublingual(ly)   Under the tongue.

subnormal   Abnormally lowered body temperature.

systole   Period during the cardiac cycle when the atria and ventricles contract and eject the blood out of the heart.

thready   Pulse rate that is barely perceptible.

tympanic membrane   Thin semitransparent membrane separates the outer ear and the middle ear. Also called eardrum.

WARNING!

For all patient contact, adhere to Standard Precautions.
Wear protective equipment as indicated.

A healthy human body regulates itself. Vital signs are indicators of the body's ability to maintain **homeostasis.** Temperature (T), along with pulse (P), respiration (R), and blood pressure (BP) measurements are considered vital signs since they measure some of the body's vital functions and provide necessary information about the patient's physical well being. Vital signs are routinely measured by medical assistants before physical examinations. Care must be taken to be accurate and efficient so the readings or results reflect a true picture of the patient's condition.

Along with the physiology behind body temperature, pulse rate, respirations, blood pressure, and measurement of weight and height, this chapter discusses the normal or average readings for all vital signs at varying ages. Different methods and types of equipment for measuring temperature, pulse rate, respirations, and blood pressure are discussed along with guidelines and ways for choosing the best methods and equipment.

When temperature, pulse, and respirations are measured at the same time it is referred to as TPR. During some office visits only one of the vital signs may be measured, for example blood pressure in a patient with hypertension. Factors influencing readings and procedures with step-by-step instructions for accurately and efficiently measuring vital signs are thoroughly presented.

Note: All health care professionals are required to use Standard Precautions to maintain infection control while measuring vital signs. The details of Standard Precautions will not be repeated for each procedure.

► TEMPERATURE

An understanding of the way the body maintains a balance between the amount of heat produced and the amount of heat lost is important for the medical assistant. Other factors that inform and assist the medical assistant to measure temperature accurately include knowledge of normal readings, factors that influence readings, how to select and use the proper thermometer, and how to clean and care for equipment.

PHYSIOLOGY OF BODY TEMPERATURE

Since body temperature is regulated through balancing the amount of heat produced in the body with the amount of heat lost from the body, there is normally only a 1-2 degree **Fahrenheit** (F) variance throughout the day. The **hypothalamus,** a portion of the brain that controls autonomic nervous system functions, is able to adjust the body temperature as the need for more or less heat production occurs during the day. For example, when a jogger is running on a hot day the body's cooling mechanism reacts to this by creating perspiration which removes some of the excess heat the jogger experiences.

Med Tip: Always be alert for all causes of changes in body temperature. For example, an infant's elevated temperature during an examination may be due to the infant's crying and not due to an illness. Always ask whether the patient has taken aspirin or Tylenol which lower the temperature. Older adults who normally have body temperatures below normal, may be ill even when their temperature is within a normal range for adults.

TEMPERATURE READINGS

The body temperature of a healthy person is 98.6°F or 37°C, and may vary by 1°F (0.6°C) either up or down during the day. While a slight variance in body temperature is not a cause for alarm, it is

Cause	Description
Time of Day	Body temperature is lower in the morning upon wakening when metabolism is still slow. The lowest body temperature is between 2 a.m. and 6 a.m. The highest body temperature usually occurs in the evening between 5 and 8 p.m. Daily variation in oral temperature can range from 97.6° to 99.6°F (36.4° to 37.3°C).
Age	Infants and children normally have a higher body temperature due to immature heat-regulation. Children often spike a fever late in the day. Older adults usually have a lower than normal body temperature.
Gender	Women may experience a slight increase in body temperature at the time of ovulation.
Physical exercise	Body temperature will rise with exercise due to increased muscle contractions causing an increase in metabolism.
Emotions	Emotions, such as crying and anger, can cause an increase in body temperature.
Pregnancy	An increase in metabolism during pregnancy may cause the body temperature to rise.
Environmental changes	Hot weather can cause serious consequences in older adults whose bodies are unable to regulate body temperature due to a decreased metabolism. Exposure to cold may lower the body temperature.
Infection	An elevated temperature, or fever, may be one of the first signs of an infection. A fever is the body's way of fighting or "killing off" infectious organisms.
Drugs	Drugs may increase muscular activity or metabolism which in turn increases temperature. Antipyretic (fever reducing) drugs, such as aspirin, lower the above-normal temperature.
Food	The process of eating may also raise the body temperature. Fasting decreases metabolism which will cause a lowering of body temperature.

TABLE 5-1

Variations in Body Temperature

important to remember that greater body temperature variations from normal are often the first sign of illness or disease. Table 5-1 describes causes of variations in body temperature.

Fever

Fever, or **pyrexia,** is a body temperature above 100.4°F (38°C). At this point it can be stated that the body is producing greater heat than it is losing and is febrile. When the body temperature exceeds 105.8°F (41°C), a serious condition known as hyperpyrexia develops. A body temperature above 109.4°F (43°C) is usually fatal. It can be a result of hyperthermia. Temperatures at this level may result in seizures in infants and small children. See Table 5-2 for a classification of fevers.

Hypothermia

The reverse of a fever is a **subnormal** temperature or hypothermia. This occurs when the temperature falls below 97°F (36°C). At this point, the body is losing more heat than it is producing. This occurs in cases of exposure and near-drowning in cold water. In general a temperature below 93.2°F (34°C) is fatal.

Fever Level	Fahrenheit (F)	Celsius/Centigrade (C)
Slight	99.6°–100.9°	37.6°–38.3°
Moderate	101.0°–101.9°	38.3°–38.8°
Severe	102.0°–104.0°	38.9°–40.0°
Dangerous	104.1°–105.8°	40.1°–41.0°
Fatal	106.0°–109.4° +	41.1°–43.0° +

TABLE 5-2

Classification of Fevers (oral reading)

TEMPERATURE TAKING SITES

Body temperature can be taken in a variety of ways including oral (mouth), aural (ear), axillary (under the arm), and rectal (rectum). The normal temperature—based on statistical averages—for each of these sites is:

- Oral   98.6°F (37°C)
- Rectal   99.6°F (37.6°C)
- Axillary   97.6°F (36.4°C)
- Ear (aural)   98.6°F (37°C)

As the above figures indicate, the temperature obtained through the rectal method registers 1°F (or 0.6°C) higher than the oral temperature. Axillary temperatures register 1°F (0.6°C) lower than oral temperatures. The medical assistant must document if the temperature was taken rectally by the symbol "R" or axillary by the symbol "AX."

Oral

The oral method of temperature measurement is the most commonly used. There is a potential for error with this method since the patient may not form a tight closure over the thermometer. This allows air to enter the mouth and give a false temperature reading. In recording this measurement, no designation needs to be used to indicate it was taken by the oral route. The thermometer is inserted under the tongue on either side of the **frenulum linguae.** This is the longitudinal fold of mucous membrane. For an accurate measurement, the patient must be advised not to talk during the procedure.

Aural (eardrum)

One of the newest technologies for accurate temperature measurement involves the **aural** site. This method uses the area at the end of the external auditory canal for an instantaneous temperature measurement. The tympanic thermometer provides a closed cavity within the easily accessible ear. The aural method is now considered to be the most accurate means of temperature measurement due to the eardrum's proximity to a blood supply and to the hypothalamus. This method also poses the least problems with Standard Precautions.

Axillary (under the arm)

The **axillary** method has proven to be the least accurate of the four temperature measurement sites. It is the recommended site for small children unable to understand how to hold an oral thermometer, if a tympanic membrane thermometer is not available. The axillary site is recommended for patients who have had oral surgery, any situation in which the patient may bite the oral thermometer, and mouth-breathing patients. The axillary temperature reading is affected by perspiration. The underarm area should be dry for an accurate reading.

Rectal

The rectal route is considered more reliable than the oral method. The mucous membrane lining of the rectum does not come into contact with air, which could interfere with accuracy, as do the oral and axillary routes. The rectal route is advised for unconscious patients, infants, small children, and mouth-breathing patients. The rectal method is avoided whenever possible due to possible perforation of the rectal wall.

Use the guidelines that follow to determine which method to use when measuring a patient's body temperature.

FAHRENHEIT/CELSIUS CONVERSIONS

The Fahrenheit (F) scale of temperature measurement is widely used throughout the United States. However, some physicians wish to use the **Centigrade** (C) or **celsius** (C) scale. Figure 5-1 shows examples of Fahrenheit and Celsius in non-mecury thermometers. To convert Fahrenheit (F) to Celsius (C), subtract 32, then multiply by 5/9. To convert degrees Celsius (C) to Fahrenheit (F), multiply by 9/5, and then add 32. See Figure 5-2 for a Fahrenheit/centigrade conversion chart and Table 5-3 for temperature scale conversion formulas and examples.

Scale	Conversion Formula	Example
Centigrade	$(°F - 32)\ 5/9 = °C$	$101°F - 32 = 69 \times 5/9 = 38.3°C$
Fahrenheit	$(°C \times 9/5) + 32 = °F$	$38.3°C \times 9/5 = 69 + 32 = 101°F$

TABLE 5-3

Temperature Scale Conversion Formulas

Guidelines: Selecting a Method for Measuring Body Temperature		
Method	**Advisable**	**Inadvisable**
Oral	Most adults and children who are able to follow instructions	Patients who have had oral surgery, mouth sores, dyspnea
		Uncooperative patients
		Patients receiving oxygen
		Infants and small children
		Patients with facial paralysis
		Patients with nasal obstruction
Rectal	Infants, small children	Active children
	Patients who have had oral surgery	Fragile newborns
	Mouth-breathing patients	
	Unconscious patients	
Axillary	Small children	Patients who cannot form an airtight seal around thermometer
Tympanic (aural)	Infants, children, adults	Patient with in-the-ear-canal hearing aids

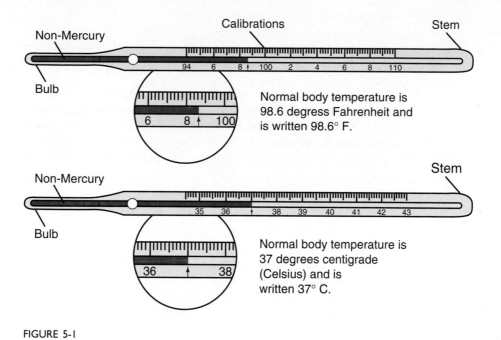

FIGURE 5-1

Fahrenheit and centigrade thermometers.

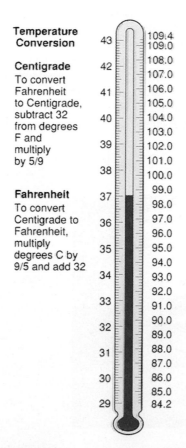

FIGURE 5-2

Fahrenheit/Centigrade conversion chart.

TYPES OF THERMOMETERS

Four types of thermometers are available for measuring body temperature: non mercury glass thermometers, electronic thermometers, tympanic membrane thermometers, and chemical thermometers (Figure 5-3).

Note: Mercury thermometers are no longer widely used in the health care environment due to the potential danger of mercury and the frequency of breakage. Mercury is toxic and can be harmful to humans and animals. Several cities have banned the sale of mercury thermometers and some areas have thermometer exchange programs. An individual brings in a mercury thermometer and is given a non mercury one in exchange. This publication will use non mercury thermometers which may be glass or plastic in its discussion of assessing body temperatures.

Non Mercury Glass Thermometers

Non Mercury glass thermometers are available in two shapes to measure temperature using the oral, rectal, and axillary methods. Mercury has been replaced by safer chemicals and glass has been replaced by plastic in many cases. The oral thermometer has a long, slender tip which fits easily under the tongue. A thermometer with a stubby or pear shaped tip is available which can be used for oral, axillary, and rectal temperature taking. On some thermometers there may be a blue dot indicating the thermometer is for oral use or a red dot indicating rectal use.

The shaft or stem of the thermometer is calibrated in tenths (0.2, 0.4, 0.6, and so on) of degrees each short line represents 0.2 of a degree. A whole degree is marked with a long line. The even-numbered degrees are printed on the thermometer. The average normal body temperature (98.6°F) is pointed out with an arrow on the thermometer.

When reading the thermometer, it should be held between the thumb and index finger, at eye level, by the stem end (Figure 5-4). While looking at the edge of the thermometer, keep the lines at the top of the edge and the numbers at the bottom. The stem is then gently rotated until the silver column can be seen in the middle of the lines and numbers. The point where the silver line stops is read for the body temperature at each two-tenths of a degree. When the silver line appears between two markings it is read at the next higher two-tenths of a degree.

The temperature reading is then recorded. The temperature must be carefully charted with absolute accuracy. Each short line of the thermometer is read as two-tenths of a degree. Always record tenths of degrees of temperature in even numbers when using a non mercury glass thermometer.

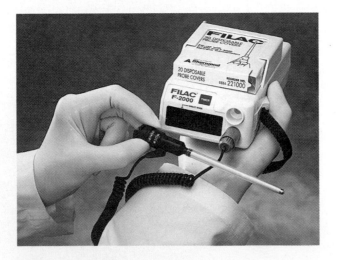

FIGURE 5-3

Digital electronic thermometer.

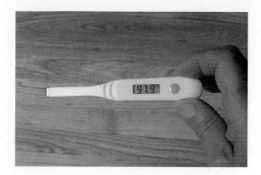

FIGURE 5-4

Example of a digital oral thermometer. (*Source:*
Courtesy of Tom Pantages)

Med Tip: Note the difference between a temperature of 100.4 and 104.0. These two temperatures are read as "one hundred and four-tenths" and "one hundred and four point *0.*" Careful attention is needed when recording temperature to avoid a serious mistake.

Thermometer Sheaths Plastic disposable slip-on sheaths are available to use with both the oral and rectal glass thermometers (Figure 5-5). The sheath comes in a small paper envelope and slips over the tip of the thermometer. The sheath provides a sanitary protective covering and is discarded after use. When using a rectal thermometer, a lubricant is always used over the sheath for ease of insertion into the rectum.

The sheath is removed from the thermometer by pulling on the tear tab which inverts the plastic thus protecting the medical assistant's hands from coming into contact with contamination. Remove and properly dispose of sheath in a hazardous waste container. After the temperature is read, clean and disinfect the thermometer since mucous membranes may still come into contact with the thermometer.

Figure 5-6 illustrates the steps followed in taking an oral temperature. Also see the Procedure for instructions on measuring an oral temperature using a non mercury thermometer. Figure 5-7 provides an example of how to chart temperature readings.

A rectal thermometer has a small, round bulb that inserts gently into the rectum. This thermometer may be marked "for rectal use" on its stem and have a red dot indicating the rectal route should be used. It is not safe to use an oral thermometer to take a rectal temperature since the long slender tip may injure tender rectal mucous membranes or can break off in the rectum. Also see the Procedure: Measuring Rectal Temperature with a Using a Rectal Non Mercury Glass Thermometer.

Cleaning and Storing Glass Thermometers

The non mercury glass thermometer must be cleaned and soaked in a disinfectant after each use. The thermometer is then stored in a proper container. See the following procedure for cleaning and storing glass thermometers.

Electronic Thermometers

The electronic thermometer is becoming very popular. It is considered accurate, easy to read, sanitary, fast, and requires no cleaning or disinfection. These electronic thermometers are battery-

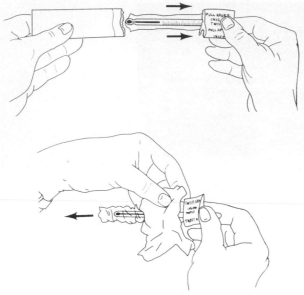

FIGURE 5-5

Using a thermometer sheath.

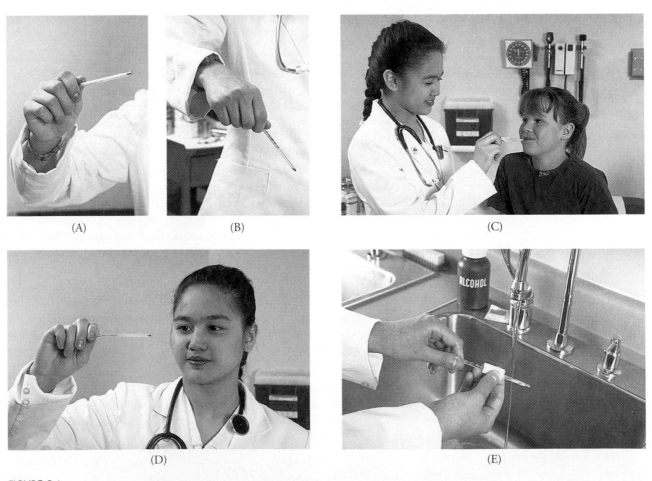

(A)   (B)   (C)

(D)   (E)

FIGURE 5-6

(A) Taking an oral temperature. (B) Shake down the thermometer. (C) Place the thermometer under the tongue. (D) Medical assistant reads the thermometer. (E) Thermometer is washed with soap and water.

PROCEDURE: Oral Temperature Using a Glass/Non Mercury Thermometer

**Terminal Performance
Competency:** Student must be able to accurately perform all steps of procedure and provide a temperature reading within 0.2° of the instructor's reading, unless otherwise instructed.

Equipment and Supplies

Oral glass non mercury thermometer

Disposable plastic thermometer sheath

Watch with second hand

Biohazardous waste container

Patient's record

Paper and pen/pencil

Procedural Steps

1. Wash hands.

2. Apply gloves.

3. Identify patient *Note:* To avoid error call patient by name and check against the name on the patient's record.

4. Ask if patient has recently taken a hot or cold drink or smoked within last 30 minutes. *Rationale:* Hot and cold liquids will affect temperature in the mouth. Wait 10 minutes before taking oral temperature.

5. Take thermometer out of container. Do not touch bulb end with fingers. If thermometer is stored in a disinfectant then rinse thoroughly under cool water.

6. Inspect thermometer for any chipped areas or other defects. Discard if damaged.

7. Read the thermometer. If it is not at 95°F, then shake down to that point by firmly holding the end of the glass shaft between the thumb and index finger. Firmly snap the wrist to shake.

8. Place plastic sheath on thermometer. Make sure that sheath is tightly in place on thermometer.

9. Place bulb end of thermometer encased in plastic sheath **sublingually** (under the tongue) in patient's mouth. *Rationale:* The space on either side of the frenulum linguae is in close proximity to numerous small blood vessels which will provide an accurate indication of body temperature.

10. Ask the patient to close his or her mouth over the thermometer and hold it in place without biting down. It helps to tell the patient to suck the thermometer rather than to clamp it between their teeth.

11. Leave the thermometer in place for at least 3 minutes. *Rationale:* It takes at least 3 minutes for an accurate oral reading to take place. The medical assistant can use this time to take the pulse and respiratory rate.

12. Remove and read the thermometer. If thermometer reads less than 97°F, shake down the thermometer and reinsert for an additional few minutes.

13. Reread the thermometer and write the reading on a piece of paper.

14. Holding tightly by the stem end of the glass shaft pull the plastic sheath off thermometer and discard sheath in biohazardous waste container. *Rationale:* The plastic sheath has come into contact with the patient's mucous membranes.

15. Follow the procedure for temporary storage of soiled thermometers.

16. Remove gloves and place in biohazard waste container.

17. Wash hands.

18. Record temperature in patient's record.

19. Follow procedure for cleaning and disinfecting soiled thermometers.

Charting Example

10/23/XX 4:00 p.m. 99°F M. King, CMA (AAMA)

operated with digital windows for easy viewing and reading (Figure 5-8). They can accurately register body temperature within a few seconds.

The electronic thermometer consists of a metal probe which is color-coded: blue for oral and red for rectal. The probe is attached to the battery unit by a flexible cording. A non-flexible plastic dispos-

PROCEDURE: Measuring a Rectal Temperature Using a Rectal Non Mercury Glass Thermemoter

Terminal Performance

Competency: Student must be able to accurately perform all steps of procedure and provide a temperature reading within 0.2° of the instructor's reading, unless otherwise instructed.

Equipment and Supplies

Rectal non mercury glass thermometer

Disposable thermometer sheath

Disposable gloves

Patient's record

Paper and pen/pencil

Tissue

Watch with second hand

Water soluble lubricant

Biohazardous waste container

Procedural Steps

1. Wash hands.

2. Apply gloves.

3. Identify patient. *Note:* To avoid error call the patient by name and check against the name on the patient's record.

4. Explain procedure. If patient is a child, explain the procedure to both parent and child.

5. Place small amount of lubricant on a tissue. *Rationale:* Tissue will serve to keep work area clean and also as a temporary receptacle for prepared thermometer.

6. Remove rectal thermometer from container by holding stem end only.

7. Inspect thermometer for any cracks or defects. Discard if damaged.

8. Read the thermometer. If it is not at 95°F, then shake down to that point by firmly holding the end of the glass shaft between the thumb and index finger. Firmly snap the wrist to shake down.

9. Place plastic sheath on thermometer, making sure that it is tightly in place.

10. Apply lubricant to thermometer by rolling bulb end in lubricant on tissue. Leave thermometer on the tissue. *Rationale:*

Lubricant allows the thermometer to be inserted easily with reduced chance for injury to mucous membranes. Tissue provides a clean surface for temporary storage of prepared thermometer.

Adult Patient:

a. Instruct patient to remove appropriate clothing so that rectal area can be accessed. Provide privacy for patient.

b. Assist patient onto examining table and cover with sheet/drape. *Rationale:* Protect patient's modesty.

c. Instruct patient to lie on left side with top leg bent (Sims position).

d. With one hand raise the upper buttock to expose the anus or anal opening. If unable to see the anal opening, ask the patient to bear down slightly. This will expose the opening.

e. With other hand, gently insert lubricated thermometer 1 1/2 inches into anal canal. Do not force the thermometer into the anal canal. Rotating the thermometer may make insertion easier.

Infant and Child:

a. Ask the parent to prepare the child by removing diaper or underwear.

b. Place the child in a secure position. Place an infant on his or her back. With one hand firmly grasp the ankles and lift them up. This will expose the infant's anus. An older child is more easily controlled when placed on his or her stomach. The parent may assist in holding the child securely. An infant—lying on his or her stomach with legs hanging down—can be placed across the parent's lap.

c. Gently insert the bulb end of a well-lubricated rectal thermometer one inch into the anal canal.

(Continued on next page)

PROCEDURE: Measuring a Rectal Temperature *(Continued)*

11. Hold the thermometer in place for 5 minutes.
12. Withdraw thermometer.
13. Dispose of the plastic sheath in biohazardous waste container.
14. Read thermometer.
15. Reread thermometer and write the reading on a piece of paper.
16. Place thermometer back on tissue or in a temporary storage container. Never place soiled thermometer on unprotected surface.
17. Wipe anus from front to back removing any excess lubricant.
18. Ask parent to re-diaper and dress infant or child.

19. Assist an adult patient from the examination table. Instruct the patient to dress and assist the patient if necessary.
20. Follow the procedure for temporary storage of soiled thermometers.
21. Remove gloves and place in biohazardous waste container.
22. Wash hands
23. Record temperature in patient's record using (R) to indicate a rectal reading.
24. Follow procedure for cleaning and disinfecting soiled thermometers.

Charting Example

2/14/XX   4:00 p.m.   Temp. 99.6°R

M. King, CMA (AAMA)

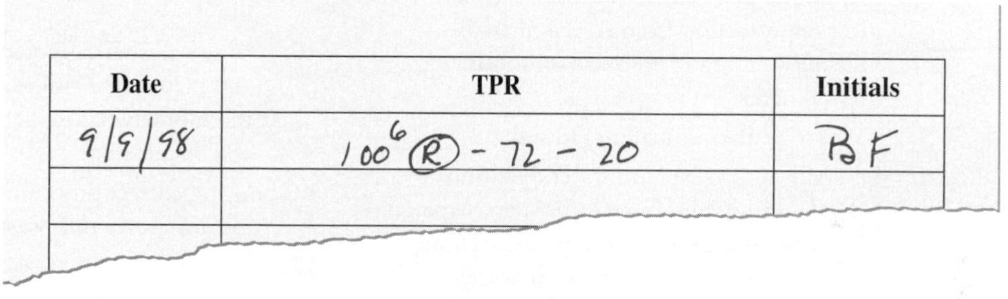

Date	TPR	Initials
9/9/98	100⁶ℝ - 72 - 20	BF

FIGURE 5-7

Charting temperature.

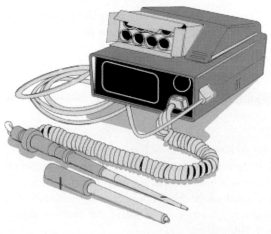

FIGURE 5-8

Battery-operated electronic thermometers have large digital windows making it easy to read.

PROCEDURE: Cleaning and Storing Non Mercury Glass Thermometers

Terminal Performance Competency: Student must correctly clean, inspect, disinfect and store non mercury glass thermometers with 100% accuracy, observing aseptic and safety precautions as prescribed by Standard Precautions.

Equipment and Supplies

70% isopropyl alcohol or other disinfectant for thermometer use

Container with soiled thermometer(s)

Cotton Balls

Soap

Utility or disposable gloves

Water

Biohazardous waste container

Procedural Steps

1. Wash hands.
2. Apply gloves according to office policy. ***Rationale:*** universal precautions are used to provide protection from contaminated mucous membrane products on soiled thermometer.
3. Take soiled thermometer(s) to sink.
4. Liberally apply soap and water to cotton balls. Holding thermometer by stem, wipe from stem end to bulb by applying friction and rotating the glass stem. ***Rationale:*** Friction will assist in dislodging contamination from calibrated markings.
5. Discard cotton balls into container.
6. Hold stem of thermometer while rinsing under cool running water.
7. Inspect thermometer for cleanliness. Note condition of thermometer and discard if damaged. If soil remains, repeat steps 4 through 6.
8. Holding the stem tightly between thumb and index finger shake down to at least 95.0°F by a quick snapping motion of the wrist. ***Rationale:*** Wet thermometer may slip out of hand while shaking down. Thermometer needs to be prepared for next use
9. Place thermometer in a container filled with disinfectant. ***Rationale:*** Thermometer must be completely covered with disinfectant and allowed to remain in solution for at least 20 minutes to be considered disinfected. *Note:* Disinfection in liquid cannot take place without thorough soap and water cleaning first.
10. When all thermometers have been cleaned and placed in disinfectant, then clean soiled thermometer container using soap, water, and disinfectant.
11. Using correct procedure, remove and discard gloves into waste container.
12. Wash hands.
13. Set timer for 20 minutes. ***Rationale:*** Timer should not be touched until hands have been washed to avoid contamination of timer.
14. After 20 minutes has elapsed, wash hands, rinse thermometers under cool water, and place in sterile storage container.

able cover fits over the probe to provide each patient with a sanitary thermometer (Figure 5-9). This plastic covered probe is inserted under the patient's tongue or rectally like a mercury thermometer.

The medical assistant will hold the thermometer in place since the reading is performed quickly. The unit will emit a signal when the temperature has registered. The plastic probe shield is then popped into a biohazardous waste container and the probe is replaced into the battery-powered storage unit (Figure 5-10).

The electronic thermometer can be used for oral, rectal, and axillary body temperature readings. The blue oral probe is generally used for taking oral and axillary temperatures. Rectal temperatures, taken using the red probe, require lubrication onto the tip of the probe. The rectal probe is inserted

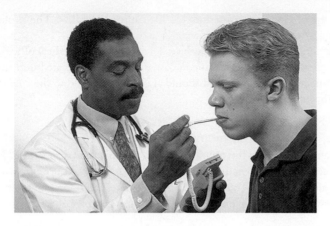

FIGURE 5-9

The disposable cover, also referred to as a sheath, provides sanitary benefits for the patient.

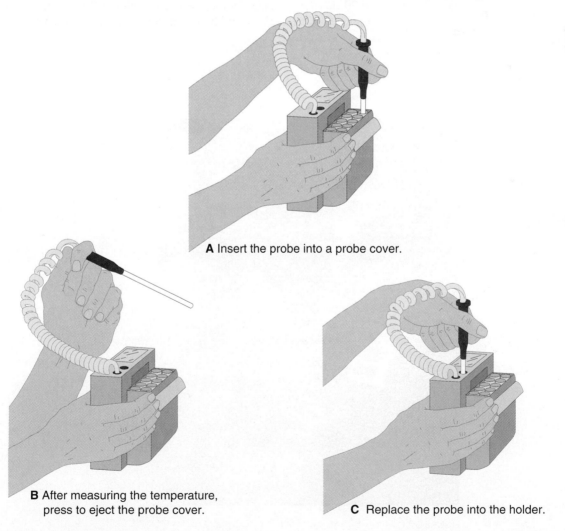

A Insert the probe into a probe cover.

B After measuring the temperature, press to eject the probe cover.

C Replace the probe into the holder.

FIGURE 5-10

Using the electronic thermometer.

1/2 inch into the adult rectum and 1/4 inch into the child's. The probe may have to be angled slightly to ensure contact with the rectal mucosa.

These units are time-saving but expensive. They are used in medical offices, hospitals, and clinics but rarely by patients in their homes due to cost. The battery-operated unit must be readjusted at intervals to maintain accuracy. The unit should always be returned to the charging stand after each use to maintain the battery.

Tympanic Membrane Thermometers

The tympanic membrane thermometer is used for an aural temperature. The **tympanic membrane** or aural thermometer is so named because it is able to detect heat waves within the ear canal and near the tympanic membrane. The thermometer calculates the body temperature from the energy generated by these heat waves. Figures 5-11 and 5-12 are examples of tympanic membrane thermometers.

▶ PULSE

Pulse rate is a measurement of the number of times the heart beats in a minute (BPM). Normally the heart beats around 70 times per minute. An increase in circulation will result in a faster heart beat and, thus, a faster pulse rate. A rate above 100 BPM is tachycardia; a rate below 60 BPM is referred to as bradycardia.

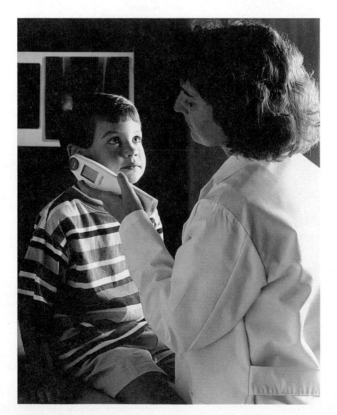

FIGURE 5-11

Tympanic membrane thermometers are particularly helpful when measuring the temperature of a child.

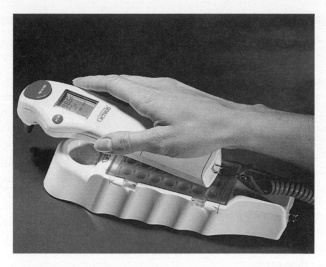

FIGURE 5-12

Filac tympanic thermometer.

The pulse rate is influenced by several factors including exercise, age, gender, size, physical conditions, disease states, medications and feelings such as depression, fear, anxiety, and anger. See Table 5-4 for a description of factors influencing pulse rate and Table 5-5 for a list of average pulse rates for different age groups.

PROCEDURE: Using an Aural (Tympanic Membrane) Thermometer

Terminal Performance Competency: Student must accurately perform all steps of the procedure and provide a temperature reading with 100% accuracy.

Equipment and Supplies
Tympanic membrane thermometer
Disposable protective probe cover
Paper and pen/pencil
Patient record
Biohazardous waste container

Procedural Steps
1. Wash hands.
2. Identify patient. *Note:* To avoid error call patient by name and check against the name on the patient's record.
3. Explain procedure to patient.
4. Remove thermometer from its base. The display will read "ready."
5. Attach disposable probe cover to the ear

piece. ***Rationale:*** The probe cover will assist in keeping probe contamination-free.

6. With one hand gently pull upward on the patient's outer ear if an adult or pull downward if an infant or child. ***Rationale:*** This pulling mechanism will straighten the ear canal for ease of insertion.

7. Gently insert the plastic-covered tip of the probe into ear canal. ***Rationale:*** The ear canal opening is then sealed so that air will not enter and affect the temperature reading.

(Continued on next page)

PROCEDURE: Using an Aural (Tympanic Membrane) Thermometer *(Continued)*

8. Press scan button which activates the thermometer. ***Rationale:*** An infrared beam is activated which measures the heat waves in one to two seconds.

9. Observe the temperature reading in the display window.

10. Gently withdraw the thermometer.

11. Eject the used probe cover into a biohazardous waste container by pressing the eject button. ***Rationale:*** The medical assistant's hands should not come in contact with the contaminated probe cover.

12. Record temperature using the designation (T) indicating a tympanic temperature. *Note:* Tympanic thermometers can be set to correlate with either an oral or rectal reading. Generally, the oral mode in which 98.6°F is considered normal is used.

13. Return tympanic thermometer to its base.

Charting Example

10/23/XX	4:00 p.m.	Temp. 99.2°F
		M. King, CMA (AAMA)

PROCEDURE: Measuring Axillary Temperature

Terminal Performance

Competency: Student must be able to accurately perform all steps of procedure and provide a temperature reading within 0.2° of the instructor's reading, unless otherwise instructed.

Equipment and Supplies

Oral mercury glass thermometer

Paper and pen/pencil

Patient's record

Tissue

Watch with second hand

Biohazardous waste container

Procedural Steps

1. Wash hands.

2. Identify patient. *Note:* To avoid error call patient by name and check against the name on the patient's record.

3. Explain procedure. If patient is a child then explain procedure to both parent and child.

4. Take thermometer out of container. Do not touch bulb end with fingers. If thermometer is stored in a disinfectant then rinse thoroughly under cool water.

5. Inspect thermometer for any chipped areas or other defects. Discard if damaged.

6. Read the thermometer. If it is not at 95°F, then shake down to that point by firmly holding the end of the glass shaft between the thumb and index finger. Firmly snap the wrist to shake down the mercury within the thermometer.

7. Ask patient to expose axilla. If patient is an infant or child, ask parent to take child's arm out of clothing to expose axilla.

8. Using tissue pat axilla dry of perspiration. ***Rationale:*** Perspiration will interfere with thermometer coming into tight contact with skin.

9. Place bulb end of thermometer into the axillary space. Make sure the bulb comes into contact with patient's skin. ***Rationale:*** Temperature cannot register unless patient's skin touches thermometer.

10. Ask patient to remain still and hold the arm tightly next to the body while the temperature registers. Caution patient not to apply so much pressure that the thermometer breaks.

PROCEDURE: Measuring Axillary Temperature *(Continued)*

11. Leave thermometer in place for 8-10 minutes. Children need to be carefully monitored during this time. Do not leave any patient unattended.

12. Medical assistant can take pulse and respirations while patient is holding thermometer under axilla.

13. Remove thermometer after ten minutes have elapsed and wipe dry with tissue. *Note:* If thermometer reads less than 96°F, shake down the mercury and reinsert for an additional few minutes.

14. Read thermometer.

15. Reread thermometer and write the reading on a piece of paper.

16. Follow the procedure for temporary storage of soiled thermometers.

17. Wash hands.

18. Record temperature in patient's record.

19. Follow procedure for cleaning and disinfecting soiled thermometers.

Charting Example

2/14/XX   4:00 p.m.   Temp. 97.0° AX
                                        M. King, CMA (AAMA)

Factor	Effect on Pulse Rate
Exercise	Activity increases body's requirements. Rate may increase 20-30 beats per minute.
Age	As age increases, pulse rate decreases. Infants and children have a faster pulse rate than adults.
Gender	Female pulse rate is around 10 BPM higher than a male of the same age.
Size	Pulse rate is proportionate to the size of the body. Heat loss is greater in a small body resulting in the heart pumping faster to compensate. Larger males will have slower pulse rates than smaller males.
Physical condition	Athletes and people in good physical condition have lower pulse rate. Lower rate is due to more efficient circulatory system. Pulse rate of 60 or below can be normal for athletes. During sleep and rest the pulse rate may drop to 50–60 BPM.
Disease conditions	Increased pulse rate in thyroid disease, fever, and shock due to increased metabolism.
Medications	Many medications can either raise or lower the pulse rate. Medications such as digoxin are given to regulate the heart beat. Caffeine and nicotine can increase the heart rate in certain people.
Depression	May lower the pulse rate.
Fear, anxiety, anger	May raise the pulse rate.

TABLE 5-4

Factors Influencing Pulse Rate

Age	Pulse Rate
Less than 1 year	120–160
2–6 years	80–120
6–10 years	80–100
11–16 years	70–90
Adult	60–80
Older adult	50–65

TABLE 5-5

Average Pulse Rates by Age

CHARACTERISTICS OF PULSE

Three characteristics need to be noted and recorded when observing pulse rate: volume, rhythm and condition of arterial wall.

1. *Volume* is the force or strength of the pulse. This is noted as full, strong, normal, bounding, weak, feeble, or **thready** (barely perceptible). Volume is influenced by the forcefulness of the heart beat, the condition of the arterial walls, and dehydration. A variance in intensity of the pulse may indicate heart disease.
2. *Rhythm* refers to the regularity, or equal spacing of all the beats, of the pulse. Normally, the intervals between each heart beat are the same duration. It is not considered abnormal if the heart occasionally skips a beat. This is referred to as **intermittent pulse.** Exercise or drinking a caffeine rich beverage may cause this to occur. An **arrhythmia** is a pulse lacking in regularity. When this occurs on a consistent basis it may indicate heart disease and should be brought to the attention of the physician.
3. The *condition of the arterial wall* should be felt as elastic and soft. A pulse taken in a blood vessel that feels hard and rope-like is considered abnormal and may indicate heart disease such as arteriosclerosis.

PULSE SITES

There are several areas in the body in which the pulse can be easily measured since the artery is located close to the surface of the skin. These pulse sites are: radial, brachial, carotid, temporal, femoral, popliteal, and dorsalis pedis (Figure 5-13). Table 5-6 describes the 7 common pulse sites.

Figure 5-14 shows a medical assistant measuring a patient's radial pulse as described in the procedure measuring radial pulse rate.

APICAL HEART RATE

The apical heart rate is the heart rate counted at the apex of the heart. It can only be heard with a stethoscope placed over the apex. This is considered to be a very accurate heart rate. The apical rate is taken in infants and young children. The physician may also request an apical rate taken when a patient is on heart medications.

An apical-radial pulse rate may be taken to determine if there is a difference between the pulse rate taken at the two sites. An apical-radial pulse must be taken for a full minute. The difference between the two readings is called the **pulse deficit.** The procedure for taking an apical-radial pulse follows. This measurement requires two people: one to take the radial pulse and one to take the apical pulse. When only one person is doing the procedure, the apical pulse is taken first and then the radial pulse rate.

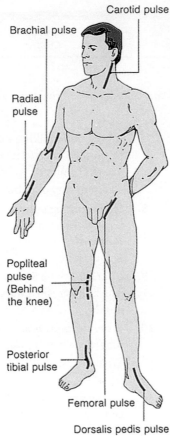

FIGURE 5-13

Pulse sites.

Pulse Site	Location
Radial	Thumb side of the wrist approximately one inch below base of the thumb. This is the most frequently used site for counting pulse rate.
Brachial	Inner (antecubital fossa/space) aspect of the elbow. This is the pulse heard and felt when taking blood pressure.
Carotid	Between larynx and the sternocleidomastoid muscle in the side of the neck. This is the pulse used during cardiopulmonary resuscitation (CPR). It can be felt by pushing the muscle to one side and pressing gently against the larynx.
Temporal	At the side of the head just above the ear.
Femoral	Near the groin where the femoral artery is located.
Popliteal	Behind the knee. This pulse is located deeply behind the knee and can be felt when the knee is slightly bent.
Dorsalis pedis	On the top of the foot slightly lateral to midline. This pulse can be an indication of adequate circulation to the feet.

TABLE 5-6

Location of Common Pulse Sites

PROCEDURE: Measuring Radial Pulse Rate

Terminal Performance
Competency: Student must be able to accurately perform the procedure and provide a radial pulse reading with 100% accuracy, unless otherwise instructed.

Equipment and Supplies
Paper and pen/pencil
Patient's record
Watch with second hand

Procedural Steps

1. Wash hands.

2. Identify patient. *Note:* To avoid error call patient by name and check against the name on the patient's record.

3. Explain procedure.

4. Ask the patient about any recent physical activity or smoking.
   Rationale: Exertion can increase pulse rate. Wait 10 minutes after physical exertion of patient to take pulse.

5. Ask patient to sit down and place arm in a comfortable, supported position. The hand should be at chest level with the palm down.

6. Place finger tips on radial artery on thumb side of wrist. *Note:* Do not use thumb when taking pulse since pulse in thumb may be felt in addition to patient's pulse in wrist.

7. Check quality of pulse.

8. Start counting pulse beats when second hand on watch is at 3, 6, 9, or 12.
   Rationale: One minute is easier to observe at these points.

9. Count the pulse for one full minute. The number will always be an even number.

10. Write the pulse beats per minute immediately on a piece of paper.

11. Wash hands.

12. Record the pulse beats per minute in patient's record, describing any abnormalities in pulse rate.

Charting Example
2/14/XX   4:00 p.m.   pulse = 72 Regular and strong M. King, CMA (AAMA)

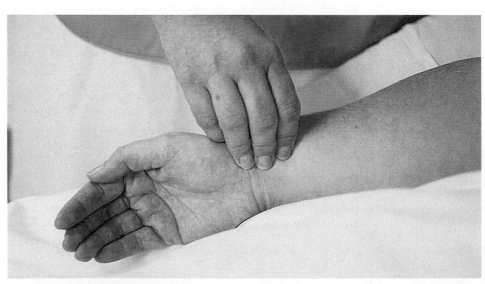

FIGURE 5-14

Measuring a patient's radial pulse.

Med Tip: When taking an apical-radial pulse, have only one person responsible for using the watch. This person will raise one finger when counting begins and lower the finger when a minute has passed. There is better coordination of timing using this method.

▶ RESPIRATION

Respiration, or the act of breathing, is the exchange of oxygen and carbon dioxide (CO_2) between the atmosphere and the body cells. It consists of one expiration or exhalation and one inspiration or inhalation. This is called the respiratory cycle.

PHYSIOLOGY OF RESPIRATION

During the process of inspiration, oxygen, which is necessary for body cells and life, is taken into the lungs. The **diaphragm** moves downward, intercostal muscles move outward, and the lungs expand in order to take oxygen into the lungs. During expiration air containing carbon dioxide is expelled from the lungs as a waste product. The diaphragm moves upward and the lungs deflate.

The respiratory process is both external and internal. The external respiratory process is an exchange of oxygen and carbon dioxide between the **alveoli,** the minute air sacs of the lungs, and the blood. The internal repiratory process takes place when blood in the capillaries comes into contact with the alveoli where it picks up oxygen and carries it to cells throughout the body. Carbon dioxide is thrown off as a waste product, carried back to the lungs where it is exhaled. The process then begins all over again with inhalation.

The **medulla oblongata** located in the base of the brain contains the respiratory, cardiac, and vasomotor centers. When the medulla oblongata receives a message indicating there is a buildup of carbon dioxide, this message is translated by the brain into a need for increased respiration to occur. Breathing is actually controlled by the involuntary nervous system. However, breathing is also under some control of the voluntary nervous system.

Med Tip: Since patients have some control over their respiration it is advisable to take a respiratory count without the patient's awareness. It is recommended that respirations be counted while appearing to count the pulse. This will then be a more accurate indication of the true respiratory rate.

CHARACTERISTICS OF RESPIRATION

When observing a patient's respirations, three characteristics should be noted: rate, rhythm, and depth.

Rate
Rate refers to the number of respirations per minute and can be described as normal, rapid, or slow. The adult normal range of respirations is 14 to 20 cycles per minute. A respiratory rate, below 12

PROCEDURE: Apical-Radial Pulse (Two-person)

**Terminal Performance
Competency:** Student must be able to accurately perform all steps of the procedure and provide an apical heart rate within 1 point difference of the instructor's reading, unless otherwise instructed.

Equipment and Supplies
Stethoscope
Alcohol wipe/cotton balls with Isopropyl alcohol 70%
Paper and pen/pencil
Patient's record
Watch with second hand

Procedural Steps

1. Wash hands.

2. Prepare stethoscope using alcohol wipe or cotton balls with alcohol on ear pieces and diaphragm of scope.
   Rationale: To prevent carrying organisms into ear canal of medical assistant or between patients.

3. Identify patient. *Note:* To avoid error call patient by name and check against the name on the patient's record.

4. Explain procedure. If patient is a child, explain procedure to both parent and child.

5. Uncover left side of patient's chest. Provide privacy with a drape, if necessary.

6. First person places earpieces of stethoscope in ears with opening in tips forward.

7. Locate apex of patient's heart by palpating to left fifth intercostal space (between fifth and sixth ribs) at the midclavicular line. This is found just below the nipple.

8. Warm chestpiece by holding in the palm of hand before placing onto patient's chest.
   Rationale: This is a comfort measure for the patient. A cold stethoscope can be startling to the patient and may cause a faster heart beat.

9. Second person locates radial pulse in the thumb side of wrist one inch below base of thumb.

10. First person places the chestpiece of stethoscope at apex of heart. When heart beat is heard, a nod is made to the second person and counting begins. Ideally, the count should begin when the second hand is at the 3, 6, 9, or 12.

11. Count for one full minute. *Note:* Both systole and diastole (or lubb/dubb) count as one beat.

12. Remove stethoscope and earpieces.

13. Record the rate and quality of heart beats. Include both apical and radial rates using designation "AP." Calculate the pulse deficit by subtracting the radial pulse rate from the apical pulse rate. *Note:* A pulse deficit may indicate that the heart contractions are not strong enough to produce a palpable radial pulse.

14. Assist the patient with replacement of clothing, if necessary. Assist patient from the examining table.

15. Wipe earpieces and chestpiece of stethoscope with alcohol wipes or cotton balls and alcohol. *Rationale:* Prevent cross-contamination.

16. Wash hands.

Charting Example
2/14/XX   4:00 p.m.   82/78 AP
Pulse deficit = 4
Quality of beat strong.   M. King, CMA (AAMA)

(bradypnea) or above 40 (tachypnea) in an adult, should be considered a serious symptom. Rapid respirations are usually shallow in depth.

Children have a much more rapid rate of breathing than adults with an average of 30 to 50 cycles per minute. See Table 5-7 for the ranges of respiratory rates of various age groups.

The respiratory rate is usually at a 1:4 proportion of the pulse rate. Many factors affect the respiratory rate. Some of these include an elevated temperature, age, pain, and medical conditions

Age Group	Average Number Per Minute
Newborn	30–50
1 year old	20–40
2–10 years	20–30
11–18 years	18–24
Adult	14–20

TABLE 5-7

Respiratory Rate Ranges of Various Age Groups

such as asthma. An elevated temperature in both adults and children can result in an elevated respiratory rate. Extreme pain may also cause the respirations to increase.

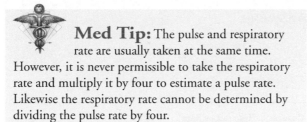

Med Tip: The pulse and respiratory rate are usually taken at the same time. However, it is never permissible to take the respiratory rate and multiply it by four to estimate a pulse rate. Likewise the respiratory rate cannot be determined by dividing the pulse rate by four.

There are several terms relating to rate used to describe the respirations. Each term is specific to a breathing condition and should be used when observing the patient. A description of these terms is in Table 5-8.

The respiratory rate is affected by both emotional and physical conditions. Table 5-9 lists situations which may cause an alteration in the respiratory rate.

Rhythm

Rhythm is the breathing pattern which occurs at either regular or irregular intervals. In a regular rhythm, inspirations and expirations should be the same in rate and depth. In an irregular breathing pattern, the amount of air inhaled and exhaled and the rate of respiration per minute will vary.

Term	Meaning	Example
Apnea	Temporary cessation of breathing	Sleep apnea
Bradypnea	Abnormally slow breathing (an adult below 10 per minute)	Near death
Dyspnea	Difficulty breathing	Asthma, pneumonia
Orthopnea	Difficulty breathing when lying down	Emphysema, congestive heart failure
Tachypnea (or hyperpnea)	Rapid respirations	High fever, pneumonia

TABLE 5-8

Respiratory Terms Relating to Rate

Increased Rate	Decreased Rate
Allergic reactions	Certain drugs (for example, morphine)
Certain drugs (for example, epinephrine)	Decrease of CO_2 in blood
Disease (asthma, heart disease)	Disease (stroke, coma)
Exercise	
Excitement/Anger	
Fever	
Hemorrhage	
High altitudes	
Nervousness	
Obstruction of air passage	
Pain	
Shock	

TABLE 5-9

Situations Causing Changes in Respiratory Rate

If the breathing rhythm appears irregular after one minute of observation then respirations should be observed for several more minutes for comparison purposes. Patients with **emphysema,** an abnormal pulmonary condition, may experience no difficulty with inhalation but may struggle to fully exhale. Asthma may also cause an irregularity in breathing rhythm.

Depth

The depth of respiration refers to the volume of air being inhaled and exhaled. It is described as either shallow or deep. Shallow respirations with a rapid rate occur in some disease conditions such as high fever, shock, and severe pain.

When a patient is unable to take in enough oxygen during inhalation, the skin and nail beds may appear bluish in color. This is called **cyanosis** and is due to the increase of carbon dioxide (CO_2) in the blood. In this situation, both the depth of respiration and cyanosis must be noted in the patient's record.

BREATH SOUNDS

Normal respirations have no noticeable sound. Breath sounds occur in some disease conditions. Terms for describing breath sounds are stridor, stertorous, crackles (rales), rhonchi, and wheezes.

1. *Stridor,* a shrill, harsh sound is heard more clearly during inspiration. This sound may be heard in children with **croup** and patients with laryngeal obstruction.
2. *Stertorous sounds* are noisy breathing sounds such as heard in snoring.
3. *Crackles* or *rales* consist of crackling sounds resembling crushing tissue paper. They are caused by fluid accumulation in the airways and are heard with some types of pneumonia.
4. *Rhonchi,* which are also called gurgles, are rattling, whistling sounds made in the throat. This sound may be heard in a patient with a tracheostomy who requires suctioning of mucous.

5. *Wheezes* are high-pitched, whistling sounds made when airways become obstructed or severely narrowed, as in asthma or chronic obstructive pulmonary disease (COPD).

Med Tip: Chronic obstructive pulmonary disease (COPD) is one of the leading causes of disability and affects approximately 17 million Americans. Cigarette smoking, air pollution, and occupational exposure to dust and fumes are some of the leading causes of this disease. COPD is the result of chronic bronchitis, asthma, emphysema, and heart disease.

Guidelines: Measuring Respirations

1. Do not explain the procedure to the patient. Attempt to keep the patient unaware that respirations are being measured since the patient may alter the breathing pattern. Appear to be taking the pulse.
2. The temperature and pulse may be taken at this same time if desired.
3. Do not take respiration measurements immediately after the patient has experienced exertion, such as climbing stairs, unless so ordered.
4. Count each inhalation and expiration as one respiration (breathing cycle).

▶ BLOOD PRESSURE (BP)

The measurement of blood pressure (BP) is an important vital sign to aid in diagnosis and treatment and is therefore taken routinely. Many medical conditions can be indicated by either a rise or fall in blood pressure. The condition of high blood pressure known as **hypertension** is often **asymptomatic** or without any symptoms. An abnormal blood pressure **reading** can be the first indication of this condition.

Med Tip: Blood pressure measurement is not used solely to determine if hypertension exists. Abnormal blood pressure measurements are found with other conditions including kidney disease and stress.

PHYSIOLOGY OF BLOOD PRESSURE

The blood pressure is actually caused by the action of the blood moving against the walls of the arteries. Blood is pushed out of the heart and into the aorta and pulmonary arteries as the ventricles contract. (See Figure 5-15). This, in turn, exerts continuous pressure on the walls of the arteries.

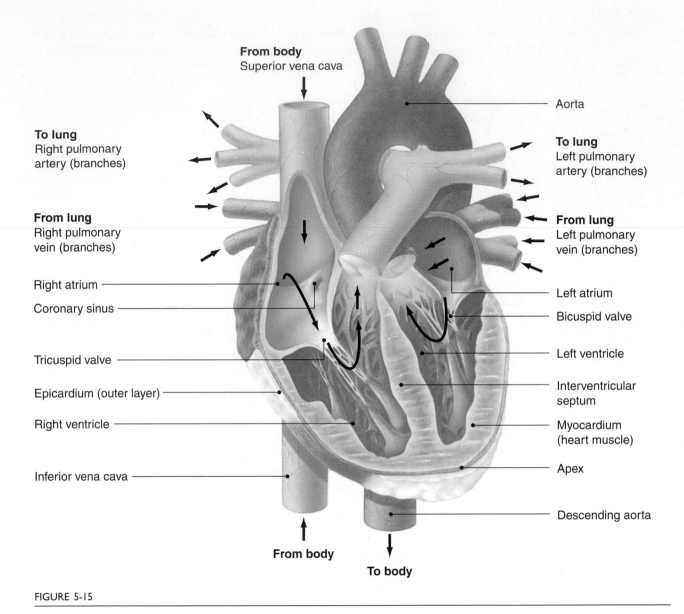

From body
Superior vena cava

Aorta

To lung
Right pulmonary
artery (branches)

To lung
Left pulmonary
artery (branches)

From lung
Right pulmonary
vein (branches)

From lung
Left pulmonary
vein (branches)

Right atrium

Left atrium

Coronary sinus

Bicuspid valve

Tricuspid valve

Left ventricle

Epicardium (outer layer)

Interventricular
septum

Right ventricle

Myocardium
(heart muscle)

Inferior vena cava

Apex

Descending aorta

From body

To body

FIGURE 5-15

Circulation of blood through the heart.

BLOOD PRESSURE READINGS

Blood pressure levels are taken at two different points called "readings." The two blood pressure readings are systolic pressure, or the highest pressure that occurs as the heart is contracting, and diastolic pressure, which is at the lowest pressure level that occurs when the heart is relaxed (the ventricle is at rest). The pulse beat is felt at the systolic pressure level and is absent at the diastolic pressure level.

These two phases of heart activity—contraction and relaxation—are referred to as the **cardiac cycle.** The two **heart sounds** (lubb and dubb) occurring during the cardiac cycle are **systole** at contraction and **diastole** at relaxation.

KOROTKOFF SOUNDS

Korotkoff sounds are the sounds actually heard as the arterial wall distends during the compression of the blood pressure cuff. The sounds were first classified into five different phases by the Russian neurologist, Nicolai Korotkoff.

PROCEDURE: Measuring Respirations

Terminal Performance
Competency: Student must be able to accurately perform all steps of procedure and provide a respiration measurement with 100% accuracy.

Equipment and Supplies
Watch with sweep second hand.

Procedural Steps
1. Wash hands.
2. Identify patient.
3. Assist patient into a comfortable position.
4. Place your hand on the patient's wrist in position to take the pulse.
5. Count each breathing cycle by observing and/or feeling the rise and fall of the chest or upper abdomen.
6. Count for one full minute using a watch with a sweep second hand. If the rate is **atypical**, or unusual, in any way take it for another minute.
7. Record respiratory rate in patient's record noting date, time, any abnormality in rate, rhythm, and depth, and your signature.

Charting Example
2/14/XX   4:00 p.m.   Resp. 20 and regular
                                        M. King, CMA (AAMA)

When the blood pressure cuff is first inflated no sound can be heard since the brachial artery is compressed. As air is slowly removed from the cuff during deflation, the Korotkoff sounds become audible. The deflation of air should be at the rate of 2-3 mm Hg per heart beat. The medical assistant should practice taking blood pressure readings slowly in order to be able to identify each phase. Korotkoff sounds are described in Table 5-10.

Pulse pressure is the difference between the systolic and diastolic readings. This is found by subtracting the diastolic reading from the systolic reading. A pulse pressure which is greater than 50

Phase	Description
Phase I	This is the first faint sound heard as the cuff is deflated. Record this reading as the systolic pressure reading. The cuff must be inflated to a high enough level to hear this first sound during relaxation.
Phase II	The second phase occurs as the cuff continues to be deflated and blood flows through the artery. This sound has a swishing quality. The cuff has to be slowly deflated in order to hear this soft sound. An **auscultatory gap** is said to have occurred if there is a total loss of sound at this stage which then reoccurs later. An auscultatory gap can occur in certain cases of heart disease and hypertension. An auscultatory gap should be reported to the physician.
Phase III	During this phase the sound will become less muffled and develop a crisp tapping sound as the blood flow moves easily through the artery. If the BP cuff was not inflated enough to hear the Phase I sound, then the Phase III sound may be heard and incorrectly stated as the systolic reading.
Phase IV	The sound will now begin to fade and become muffled. The American Heart Association, which believes Phase IV is the best indicator of the diastolic pressure, recommends the reading at this phase be recorded as the diastolic pressure for a child.
Phase V	Sound will disappear at this phase. Some physicians want both phase IV and phase V recorded for the diastolic pressure reading (for example, 120/78/74 rather than 120/74).

TABLE 5-10

Five Phases of Korotkoff Sounds

mm Hg or less than 30 mm Hg is considered to be abnormal. For instance, if the blood pressure is 130/82 the pulse pressure would be 48 which is still within the range considered normal. Extremes of pulse pressure can result in stroke or shock.

Readings of blood pressure are in millimeters (mm) of mercury (Hg). The abbreviations, mm and Hg, are not necessary when recording the blood pressure readings. The actual blood pressure is recorded using just the systolic, or highest pressure reading, over the diastolic, or lowest reading. For example, 120/80 would be considered a normal blood pressure reading for an adult. Generally, a *range of normal* is used for blood pressure readings since slight variations can occur between normal healthy adults. A deviation, either rise or fall, from the patient's baseline measurement of 20-30 mm Hg can be significant for that patient.

Med Tip: Blood pressure readings, as with all vital signs, should be interpreted using the patient's baseline measurement. This means that a previously-taken blood pressure reading, when the patient was not ill, is used as that patient's "normal" measurement. All subsequent readings are then compared to that patient's "normal" baseline reading.

Blood pressure readings should routinely be started at age five as part of the school physical or earlier if medically necessary. Recommendations are that an elevated blood pressure reading should be found on at least two occasions before the patient is placed on medication, unless the diastolic reading is over 120 mm Hg. Patients should have a complete physical to see why their blood pressure is elevated. Patients with a sustained high blood pressure measurement may require further diagnostic evaluation for the presence of other disease conditions, as well as medication to lower the blood pressure. Controlling blood pressure can lower the incidence of stroke and heart attack.

If a patient's blood pressure deviates from the normal range, he or she should be tested again. Ideally, blood pressure is taken while the patient is lying down, sitting, and standing. Average normal blood pressure readings are listed in Table 5-11. While an average blood pressure is listed for a newborn, blood pressure readings are not generally taken on infants. Monitors are used on the very young.

Age Group	Average Blood Pressure (mm Hg)
Newborn	50/25
6–9 years of age	95/65
10–15 years of age	100/65
16 years to adulthood	118/76
Adult	120/80
Older adult	138/86
Normal adult range	90/60 to 140/90

TABLE 5-11

Average Normal Blood Pressure Readings

FACTORS AFFECTING BLOOD PRESSURE

Physiological factors affecting blood pressure include volume or amount of blood in the arteries, peripheral resistance of the vessels, condition of the heart muscle, and the elasticity of vessels. These four factors are discussed in Table 5-12.

Many other factors may affect blood pressure. Two of these are gender and age. Women generally have a lower pressure than men. Blood pressure is lowest at birth and tends to increase as people age. The time of day can also cause blood pressure variations. For example, blood pressure is usually at its lowest point early in the morning just before awakening.

Activities such as standing, sitting, or lying down can affect blood pressure. When blood pressure is measured while the patient is in an erect position it is referred to as an orthostatic blood pressure reading. Orthostatic **hypotension** refers to a lowered blood pressure occurring when a patient moves from a lying down to an erect position. Sudden movement, or a sudden change in position, with a resulting fall in blood pressure is referred to as postural hypotension.

The pressure reading in the right arm is usually 3 to 4 mm Hg higher than in the left arm. Numerous situations that cause changes in blood pressure readings are listed in Table 5-13. Terms relating to abnormal blood pressure readings are described in Table 5-14.

Blood pressure is a routinely taken vital sign. It is especially important for patients with the following characteristics or conditions:

1. Patients on antihypertensive drugs
2. Patient with a history of heart disease, kidney disease, stroke or hypertension
3. Patients receiving a complete physical examination, including children
4. Pregnant women
5. Preoperative and postoperative patients
6. Patients who are bleeding or in shock
7. Patients with symptoms of a neurological disorder
8. Patient experiencing an allergic reaction

EQUIPMENT FOR MEASURING BLOOD PRESSURE

There are two pieces of equipment necessary for measuring blood pressure: a sphygmomanometer and a stethoscope. The sphygmomanometer is the instrument used for measuring the pressure the

Factor	Result
1. **Volume of blood**	Increase of blood volume increases the BP. Decrease of blood volume decreases BP. Example: Polycytopenia increases BP, hemorrhage causes volume and BP to drop.
2. **Peripheral resistance**	Relates to the size of the lumen, the cavity or space, within blood vessels and amount of blood flowing through it. Example: The smaller the size of the lumen, the greater the resistance to blood flow. Fatty cholesterol deposits result in high BP due to narrowing of the lumen.
3. **Condition of heart muscle**	Strength of heart muscle affects volume of blood flow. The pumping action of the heart and how efficiently it does the job affects the BP. Example: A weak heart muscle can cause an increase or decrease in BP.
4. **Elasticity of vessels**	The ability of blood vessels to expand and contract decreases with age. Example: Non-elastic blood vessels, as in arteriosclerosis, cause an elevated BP.

TABLE 5-12

Physiologic Factors Affecting Blood Pressure (BP)

Elevated (Increased) BP	Lowered (Decreased) BP
Anger	Anemia
Certain drug therapies (nicotine, caffeine)	Approaching death
Endocrine disorders, such as hyperthyroidism	Cancer
Exercise	Certain drug therapies (antihypertensives, narcotics, analgesics, diuretics)
Fear, excitement	Decreased arterial blood volume (hemorrhage)
Heart and liver disease	Dehydration
Increased arterial blood volume	Infection and fever
Increased intracranial pressure	Left arm
Late pregnancy	Massive heart attack
Lying down position with legs elevated	Middle pregnancy
Obesity	Pain
Pain	Starvation
Renal disease	Shock
Right arm	Sudden postural changes such as standing
Rigidity of blood vessels (in old age)	Thyroid and adrenal gland disorders: nerve disorders
Smoking	Time of day (during sleep and early morning)
Stress, anxiety	Weak heart
Time of day (late afternoon and early evening)	
Vasoconstriction or narrowing of peripheral blood vessels	

TABLE 5-13

Causes of Blood Pressure (BP) Variations

blood exerts against the walls of the artery (Figure 5-16). The stethoscope is a diagnostic instrument that amplifies sound. It is used to detect sounds produced by blood pressure as well as the heart and other internal organs such as the stomach.

Sphygmomanometers

The components of a sphygmomanometer are: manometer, inflatable rubber bladder, cuff, and bulb. The **manometer** is a scale which registers the actual pressure reading.

The core of the blood pressure cuff is the rubber bladder which, when inflated, distends to temporarily constrict blood circulation in the arm. A soft material cuff covers the bladder and is placed next to the skin of the patient. The pressure bulb has a thumbscrew attached to a control valve which allows for inflation and deflation of the cuff.

The size of the blood pressure cuff is important. There are three additional sizes available: pediatric, large arm adult, and thigh. A small pediatric cuff is available for children. Blood pressure cuffs are not generally used on infants. The pediatric cuff can also be used on small-limbed adults. A

Condition	Description
Hypertension	A condition in which the patient's blood pressure is consistently above the norm for his or her age group. Also called high blood pressure. 140/90 is the baseline.
benign	Slow onset elevated blood pressure without symptoms.
essential	This is a primary hypertension of unknown cause. It may be genetically determined.
secondary	Elevated blood pressure associated with other conditions such as renal disease, pregnancy, arteriosclerosis, atherosclerosis, and obesity.
malignant	Rapidly developing elevated blood pressure which may become fatal if not treated immediately.
renal	Elevated blood pressure as a result of kidney disease.
Hypotension	Condition of abnormally low blood pressure which may be caused by shock, hemorrhage, and central nervous system (CNS) disorders.
orthostatic	A temporary fall in blood pressure that occurs when a patient rapidly moves from a lying to a standing position. Dizziness and blurred vision can also be present.
postural	A temporary fall in blood pressure from standing motionless for extended periods of time.

TABLE 5-14

Abnormal Blood Pressure Readings

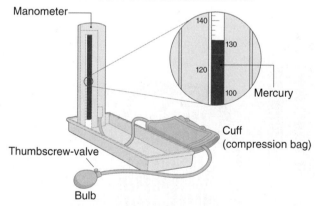

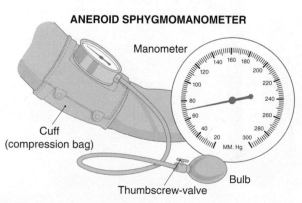

FIGURE 5-16

A sphygmomanometer is the blood pressure instrument.

thigh cuff is available when an adult arm is too large for the large arm cuff. When using a thigh cuff, the popliteal artery is palpated for a pulse.

The two types of sphygmomanometers are mercury and aneroid. A discussion follows with illustrations of portable and wall-mounted versions of each type.

Mercury Sphygmomanometer The mercury sphygmomanometer is considered to be the most accurate and is found on the walls in many physicians offices (Figure 5-17). It contains a column of mercury which will rise as the pressure bulb is pressed and the rubber bladder inflated. A calibrated scale runs down both sides of the mercury column. The reading is taken at eye level at the top of the mercury line next to a calibrated scale. This type of instrument must be placed vertically on the wall or on a flat, level surface so that the mercury will rise in a vertical position. Periodic re-calculation is necessary for accuracy. See Figure 5-18 for an example of a portable mercury sphygmomanometer.

Aneroid Sphygmomanometer The aneroid sphygmomanometer has a round dial that contains a scale calibrated in millimeters (mm) and a needle to register the reading (Figure 5-19). The needle must be at zero before starting the procedure. The aneroid sphygmomanometer should be re-calibrated for accuracy every year by using a mercury manometer as the model. This instrument is easily portable (Figure 5-20).

Diaphragm and Bell Stethoscopes

The stethoscope is used to detect sounds produced by blood pressure. This instrument consists of a chestpiece containing a diaphragm and/or bell, flexible tubing, binaurals, a spring mechanism, and earpieces. The key components of the stethoscope are described in Table 5-15 and shown in Figure 5-21.

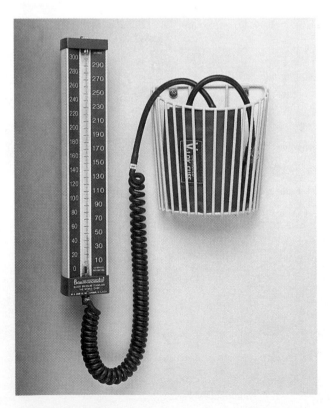

FIGURE 5-17

Wall mounted mercury sphygmomanometer.

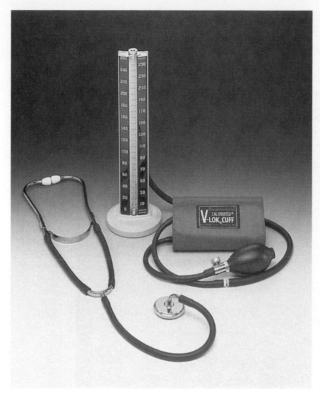

FIGURE 5-18

Portable mercury sphygmomanometer.

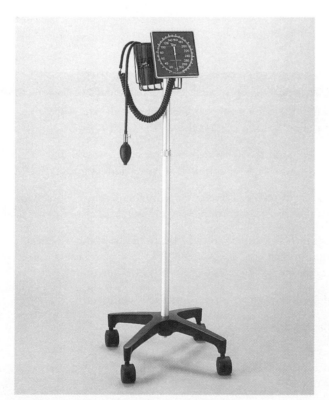

FIGURE 5-19

Aneroid sphygmomanometer.

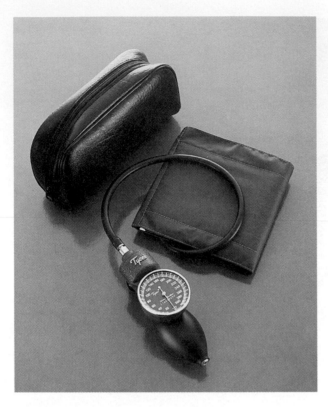

FIGURE 5-20

Portable aneroid sphygmomanometer.

Key Part	Description
Chestpiece	Portion of the instrument that is placed over the site where the sound is to be heard. May consist of a diaphragm or a bell or both.
Diaphragm	A disc-like sound sensor which picks up both low and high-pitched sound frequencies. More useful for high sounds such as bowel and lung sounds.
Bell	A hollow, curved—bell or cup shaped—sound sensor which may have one, two, or three "heads" which are useful in picking up sounds of the cardiovascular system.
Flexible tubing	Rubber or plastic tubing to carry the sound from the patient to the binaurals. The usual length of tubing is 12 to 14 inches. You may prefer using longer tubing up to 22 inches. However, some of the sound clarity is lost as the tubing becomes longer.
Binaurals	Rigid small metal tubes that connect the tubing to the earpieces.
Spring mechanism	Flexible external metal spring that holds the binaural steady so that the earpiece will remain in the ear.
Earpieces	Molded plastic tips which attach to the end of the binaurals and are placed in the medical assistant's ears.

TABLE 5-15

Components of the Stethoscope

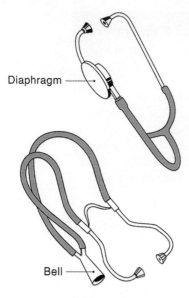

FIGURE 5-21

Diaphragm and bell stethoscopes.

MEASURING BLOOD PRESSURE

After selecting the appropriate equipment, use the following guidelines and the procedure for measuring blood pressure (Figure 5-22).

Estimated Systolic Pressure

The **palpatory method** of feeling the radial pulse while the blood pressure cuff is deflating can be used to determine systolic pressure. This method cannot be used to determine the diastolic pressure or to hear the Korotkoff sounds. However it is useful when a student is learning to take blood pressure readings. The level of inflation necessary to hear the first sound in Phase I can be determined by using the palpatory method. See procedure for using this method.

Note: Follow the general guidelines for taking blood pressure and steps 1 through 10 in the procedure for taking blood pressure. See Figure 5-22 for illustration of measuring blood pressure.

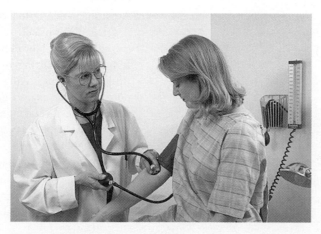

FIGURE 5-22

Measuring a patient's blood pressure.

Guidelines: Measuring Blood Pressure

1. Attempt to relax the patient by explaining in a calm, quiet manner that the procedure is not painful.
2. Ask if the patient knows what his or her last blood pressure reading was and if the patient has any history of high blood pressure.
3. When taking blood pressure for the first time on a new patient, take a reading in both arms. Usually the BP is higher in the right arm than in the left if the patient is right handed.
4. If you hear the systolic beat immediately, then you have not inflated the cuff enough. However, do not add more pressure to the cuff without deflating it first. Always deflate the cuff completely before attempting to do another pressure reading.
5. Give the patient his or her blood pressure results only if the physician has instructed you to do so. Do not make any statement about the blood pressure being high or low. Let the physician explain the results.

PROCEDURE: Taking Blood Pressure

**Terminal Performance
Competency:** Student is expected to obtain a systolic and diastolic reading within 2 mm Hg of the instructor's observance, unless otherwise instructed.

Equipment and Supplies

Sphygmomanometer

Stethoscope

70% Isopropyl alcohol

Alcohol sponges or cotton balls

Paper and pen/pencil

Patient record

Procedural Steps

1. Wash hands
2. Assemble equipment. Thoroughly cleanse the earpieces, bell, and diaphram pieces of the stethoscope. Use an alcohol sponge or cotton ball with 70% Isopropyl alcohol. Allow alcohol to dry.
3. Identify patient verbally and explain the procedure.
4. Assist the patient into a comfortable position. BP is usually taken with patient in sitting position. However, the patient may be lying down, sitting, or standing. If taken while the patient is lying down or standing, note this in the chart. Inform the doctor since the pressure changes in different positions. The patient's arms should not be higher than heart level.
5. Place the mercury sphygmomanometer on a solid surface with the gauge within 3 feet for easy viewing. The sphygmomanometer should be able to be read by the MA but not the patient.

PROCEDURE: Taking Blood Pressure *(Continued)*

6. Uncover the patient's arm by asking patient to roll back sleeve 5 inches above the elbow. If the sleeve becomes constricting when rolled back, ask patient to slip the arm out of the sleeve. Never take a blood pressure reading through clothing.

7. Have patient straighten arm with palms up. Apply the cuff of the sphygmomanometer over the brachial artery (see Figure 5-22) 1 to 2 inches above the antecubital space (bend in the elbow). Many cuffs are marked with arrows or circles to be placed over the artery. Hold the edge of the cuff in place as you wrap the remainder of the cuff tightly around the arm. If the cuff has a Velcro closure, press it into place at the end of the cuff.

8. Palpate with your finger tips to locate the brachial artery in the antecubital space.

9. Place earpieces in your ears and the diaphragm (or bell) of the stethoscope over the area where you feel the brachial artery pulsing. Hold the diaphragm in place with one hand on the chestpiece without placing your thumb over the diaphragm. The stethoscope tubing should hang freely and not touch any object or the patient during the reading.

10. Close the thumbscrew on the hand bulb by turning clockwise with your dominant hand. Close the thumbscrew just enough so that no air can leak out. Do not close so tightly that you will have difficulty re-opening with one hand.

11. Pump air into the cuff quickly and evenly, until the level of mercury is 20-30 mm Hg above the previously measured BP or the approximated method. Some physicians prefer inflating the cuff to 180 mm Hg as a starting point.

12. Slowly turn the thumbscrew counter-clockwise with your dominant hand. Allow the pressure reading to fall only 2-3 mm Hg at a time.

13. Listen for the point at which the first clear sound is heard (Phase I of the Korotkoff sounds). Note where this occurred on the mercury column (or spring gauge scale on an aneroid manometer). This is the systolic pressure.

14. Slowly continue to allow the cuff to deflate. The sounds will change from loud to murmur and then fade away. (Phases I, II, III, IV of Korotkoff sounds). Read the mercury column (or spring gauge scale) at the point where the sound is muffled or dull. This is the diastolic pressure (Phase IV of Korotkoff sounds).

15. Continue to deflate the cuff and read the mercury column (or spring gauge scale on aneroid manometer) until the sound is gone. This is Phase V of the Korotkoff sounds. Many physicians will want both Phase IV and Phase V reported for the diastolic reading.

16. Quickly open the thumbscrew all the way to release the air and deflate the cuff.

17. If you are unsure about the BP reading wait at least a minute or two before taking a second reading. Never take more than two readings in one arm since blood stasis may have occurred resulting in an inaccurate reading.

18. Immediately write the BP as a fraction on paper. You may inform the patient of the reading if this is the policy in your office.

19. Remove the cuff.

20. Clean the earpieces of the stethoscope with an alcohol sponge.

21. Wash hands.

22. Chart the results including the date, time, BP reading and your name.

Charting Example
2/14/XX   9:00 am B/P 134/88 left arm, sitting.   M. King, CMA (AAMA)

CAUSES OF ERRORS IN BLOOD PRESSURE READINGS

Table 5-16 describes causes of errors in taking blood pressure readings.

Source/Cause	Problem
Equipment	Cuff is improper size. The cuff bladder should be 20% wider than the diameter of the extremity where cuff is placed. Large cuffs for obese arms and small cuffs for children should be available in all offices.
	Air leaks around the valve may cause mercury to drop suddenly.
	Air leak in the bladder of cuff delays the inflation rate and could give a false high reading. Air leaks may also occur along the tubing if it is old or worn.
	Mercury column is not calibrated to the zero point.
	Velcro may be worn and does not hold.
Procedure	Patient's arm is not uncovered.
	Medical assistant is too far away from manometer to accurately read gauge.
	Cuff is improperly applied (too loose or too small).
	Cuff is not centered over the brachial artery, 1-2 inches above bend in the elbow.
	End of the cuff is not secured tightly.
	Part of stethoscope tubing or chestpiece touches the blood pressure cuff while taking the pressure reading.
	Failure to locate brachial pulse before placing stethoscope in position.
	The rubber bladder in the cuff was not deflated completely before beginning the procedure.
	Valve on bulb is not completely closed before beginning to pump air into cuff.
	Cuff was not inflated to a level 20–30 mm Hg above the palpated or previously measured systolic pressure or 200 mm Hg.
	Deflation occurs too rapidly to accurately determine the sounds.
	The arm used for the reading is not at the same level as the heart. The arm cannot be held above the level of the heart.
	Failed to wait 1-2 minutes before taking second reading.
	Failed to notice the auscultatory gap.
Patient	Patient is nervous or anxious resulting in a false high reading.
	Patient's arm is too large for accurate reading with available equipment.

TABLE 5-16

Causes of Errors in Blood Pressure Readings

► MEASURING HEIGHT AND WEIGHT

Height and weight are two important measurements even though they are not considered vital signs in the true sense of the term. These measurements are called anthropometric measurements since they relate to **anthropometry,** the science of size, proportion, weight, and height.

Height and weight can provide indications of the general health of the patient. Infants who fail to gain weight or "fail to thrive" need close supervision of weight gains and losses. The diagnosis of hormonal imbalances in children resulting in abnormal growth patterns can be picked up through routine comparisons of the child's height and weight against national growth charts. Diabetic patients, pregnant women, cardiac patients, patients with fluid retention, and patients suffering from eating disorders such as bulimia and obesity need to have frequent weight monitoring. Patients prefer privacy when having their body measurements taken. They can remain fully clothed for this procedure. Indicate on the medical record if measurements were taken with clothes on or off.

Scales may be calibrated in either kilograms (metric weight) or pounds (Figure 5-23). In some cases, a scale will have a ruled panel which can be flipped up to reveal both pounds and kilograms. However, the medical assistant must know how to do conversions from pounds into kilograms and vice versa. Table 5-17 contains conversion charts to be used when converting a weight from pounds to kilograms or from kilograms to pounds.

INFANT HEIGHT AND WEIGHT

Figures 5-24 and 5-25 show baby scales used to measure an infant's weight. See the Procedure for Measuring Infant Height and Weight.

PROCEDURE: Estimating Systolic BP Using Palpatory (Approximated) Method

Terminal Performance
Competency: Student is expected to obtain a systolic reading that is within 2 mm Hg of the instructor's, unless otherwise instructed.

Equipment and Supplies
Sphygmomanometer

Stethoscope

70% Isopropyl alcohol

Alcohol sponges or cotton balls

Paper and pen

Patient record

Note: American Heart Association recommends that approximate systolic BP be determined first by palpatating radial pulse, then pumping up cuff until pulse in no longer felt. This is standard procedure in many cases.

Procedural Steps
1. Place the blood pressure cuff in the usual position on the upper arm.
2. Locate the radial pulse on the thumb side of the wrist.

3. Inflate the blood pressure cuff until the pulse disappears and note the reading on the manometer.
4. Re-inflate the cuff until the pulse once again disappears and inflate another 30 mm Hg to get above the systolic pressure.
5. Slowly deflate the cuff while keeping fingers on the pulse. The point at which the pulse is felt is the systolic pressure.
6. Remember this number if you are going to take a brachial artery blood pressure reading immediately. Write the number on paper if there will be a delay before you can take the complete blood pressure.

Charting Example
Note: This number is not usually charted since it is only used to estimate the systolic BP.

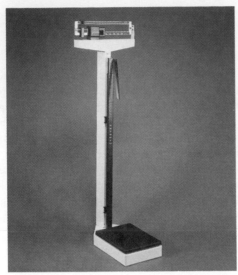

FIGURE 5-23

Upright scale.

To convert kilograms to pounds (kg to lb):
1 kilogram (kg) = 2.2 pounds (lbs)
Multiply the number of kilograms by 2.2
Example: If a patient weighs 64 kilograms, multiply 64 by 2.2.
$64 \times 2.2 = 140.8$ or 141 pounds
To convert pounds to kilograms (lb to kg):
1 pound = 0.45 kilograms
Multiply the number of pounds by 0.45
Example: If a patient weighs 130 pounds, multiply 130 by 0.45.
$130 \times 0.45 = 58.5$ or 59 kilograms

TABLE 5-17

Conversion Chart for Pounds and Kilograms

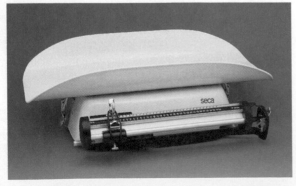

FIGURE 5-24

Baby scale.

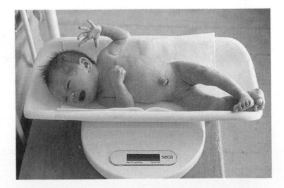

FIGURE 5-25

Electronic baby scale.

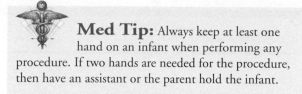

Med Tip: Always keep at least one hand on an infant when performing any procedure. If two hands are needed for the procedure, then have an assistant or the parent hold the infant.

CIRCUMFERENCE OF THE INFANT'S HEAD

Some physicians wish to have a measurement taken of the circumference or area around the infant's head. This is performed periodically during infancy to observe for any abnormal enlargement. This is generally performed during each check-up visit until the age of 36 months.

PROCEDURE: Measuring Adult Height and Weight

**Terminal Performance
Competency:** Student is expected to obtain a height and weight that is equal to the instructor's observance, unless otherwise instructed, and to perform math conversions.

Equipment and Supplies
Balance scale with bar to measure height
Paper towel
Pen
Patient record

Procedural Steps

1. Wash hands
2. Identify the patient.
3. Explain procedure to the patient.
4. For patients who wish to remove shoes, place a paper towel on the scale. Heavy objects such as keys should be removed and female patients should set their purses aside.
5. Set all the weights to zero. Balance the scale by adjusting the small knob at one end until the balance bar pointer floats in the center of the frame. (A coin can be used to make this adjustment.)
6. Assist the patient onto the scale.
7. Ask the patient to stand still.
8. First move the large weight into the groove closest to the weight you estimate for the patient. If the balance bar pointer touches the bottom of the bar then move the large weight back one notch. Move the small weight by tapping it gently until it reaches a point in which the pointer floats in the center of the frame.
9. Leave the weights in place.

Continue with Height:

10. Ask the patient to place his or her back to the scale, stand erect, and look straight ahead.
11. Raise the height bar in a collapsed position making sure the tip is over the patient's head.
12. Open the bar into the horizontal position and bring it down gently to touch the top of the patient's head. Leave this setting in place.
13. Assist the patient in stepping off the scale.
14. Read the weight scale by adding the number at the large weight to the number behind the small weight to the nearest 1/4 pound. For example, 150 pounds at the large weight and 23 1/2 at the small weight = 173 1/2 pounds.
15. Record this measurement on the patient's record.
16. Read the height as marked behind the movable level of the ruled bar. Record this measurement to the nearest 1/4 inch on the patient's record. (Convert inches to feet by dividing by 12. Chart height in feet and inches.)
17. Return the weights to zero and the height bar to the normal position.
18. Discard paper towel.
19. Wash hands.

Charting Example
2/14/XX   wt. = 140 1/4 lbs with shoes;
ht. = 5' 7" (67 inches)   M. King, CMA (AAMA)

PROCEDURE: Measuring Infant Height and Weight

Terminal Performance

Competency: Student is expected to obtain a height and weight that is equal to the instructor's observance, unless otherwise instructed and convert to metric readings.

Equipment and Supplies

Baby scale

Patient record

Pen

Small towel or protector for scale

Tape measure

Procedural Steps

1. Wash hands.

2. Identify infant by stating the infant's name to the parent. Have infant remain with parent while the equipment is being prepared.

3. Place a towel/protector on the baby scale.

4. Balance the scale by placing all the weights to the far left side. Turn the bolt at the right edge of the scale until the balance bar pointer is at the middle of the balance bar.

5. Undress infant (or ask parent to undress infant). Gently lay infant on the scale. Always keep one hand on the infant until the weights are adjusted. Do not leave the infant unattended at any time.

6. Keeping one hand over the infant's body as a safety precaution, move the large pound weight into the groove closest to the weight estimated for the baby. Then move the smaller ounce weight by tapping it gently until it reaches a point in which the pointer floats in the center of the frame.

7. Keep the weights in place while the infant is moved to the examination table for height measurement.

Continue with Height:

8. Holding the tape measure with one hand, place the tape at the top of the side of the infant's head. Stretch the infant out full length as you pull the tape measure down to the bottom of the feet. If you are using a table with a measure bar, place the infant's head at one end of the table with the soles of his or her feet touching the foot board. *Note:* It is preferred to have two people measure the length of an infant. The parent can assist by holding the infant's head still. To measure an active child, make pencil marks at the top of the child's head and at the bottom of the feet on the exam table paper. Then measure the area between the marks.

9. Note the height in inches and fractions of an inch and write it on the paper covering the exam table. Do not take your hands off the infant.

10. Ask the parent to hold the infant while the height and weight are charted in the infant's record.

11. Tell the measurements to the parent.

12. Discard paper towel.

13. Wash hands.

Charting Example

2/14/XX   weight 16 lb. 3 oz., length 30 inches

M. King, CMA (AAMA)

Using a flexible (soft) measuring tape, wrap it once around the baby's head at the forehead level. The circumference is then charted to the nearest 0.1 cm or 1/4 inch along with the height and weight.

The physician may also request to have the infant's chest measurement taken until the age of 12 months. This is used to monitor abnormal growth patterns. A flexible tape measure is held by the medical assistant's thumb at the infant's midsternal level. The tape is wrapped once around the chest above the nipple line and under the axilla. The measurement should be taken while the child is breathing normally and not during crying.

► SKIN-FOLD FAT MEASUREMENT

In some medical practices body fat is calculated using skin-fold calipers. Areas of fat tissue at the under side of the upper arm are measured by gently grasping the skin (but not the muscle) between the calipers. The measurement is read from the scale on the caliper and charted as "taken by skin-fold caliper."

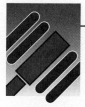

LEGAL AND ETHICAL ISSUES

The medical assistant has an ethical responsibility to use careful, proper technique when performing procedures to measure vital signs since an incorrect reading could lead to misdiagnosis and result in serious consequences for the patient. Proper technique includes: allowing enough time for the temperature to register; using a watch with a second hand when taking pulse and respiration; and never guessing the time when measuring pulse and respirations, just to name a few. Incorrect documentation of vital signs can lead to serious complications for the patient and legal consequences for the physician and the medical assistant.

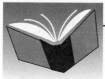

PATIENT EDUCATION

The medical assistant acts as the resource person for instructing the patient on the correct use of equipment, such as the thermometer, to ensure accuracy in reporting temperatures to the physician.

Teaching methods, include verbal instructions, demonstration and return demonstration, educational pamphlets, and drawings, when necessary, depending on what you are teaching and the patient's educational and motivational level.

Patients must be cautioned that an abnormal vital sign, such as an elevated temperature, should not be ignored with a "wait and see" attitude since a prolonged high fever can result in brain damage and even death.

Patient education will vary. For example, patients suffering from cardiovascular disease should be taught to take their own pulse and to detect abnormalities in pulse rate, rhythm, and volume. Hypertensive patients should be taught the symptoms and causes of high blood pressure and how to monitor their own blood pressure. In addition, patient education is needed to alert the patient to risk prevention, dietary control, the role of exercise, lifestyle choices, and compliance with drug therapy.

Summary

Vital signs are an important objective indication of the patient's overall physical condition. One vital measurement taken alone does not necessarily provide a complete picture. The medical assistant must be able to skillfully take all vital measurements and be able to assess what she or he is observing such as the rate, rhythm, and depth of respirations. Other factors such as age, gender, nervousness and physical condition of the patient may effect vital sign readings.

The accuracy of obtaining and recording vital sign measurements is critical for the ultimate diagnosis and treatment of the patient. Communication skills, while important in all aspects of medical assisting work, are essential when obtaining vital measurements. A positive and sincere approach in interacting with the patient may be enough to put the patient at ease and result in obtaining more valid vital sign measurements.

Competency Review

1. Define and spell the glossary terms for this chapter.
2. Take and record 10 oral temperatures using an oral thermometer within 0.2° of instructor's reading.
3. Take and record an axillary temperature using an oral thermometer within 0.2° of instructor's reading.
4. Take and record 5 aural temperatures using a tympanic membrane thermometer within 0.2° of instructor's reading.
5. Take and record 10 patients' pulse rates within 1 pulse beat per minute of instructor.
6. Count and chart 10 patients' respirations within 1 respiration of instructor's count.
7. Take 10 blood pressure readings within 2 mm Hg of instructor's reading.
8. Measure and record height and weight of 5 patients within 1/4 inch and 1/4 pound of instructor's measurement with conversion to metric included in charting.

PREPARING FOR THE CERTIFICATION EXAM

Test Taking Tip — Circle any key word in the question, such as always or never, to focus on that concept when answering a multiple choice question.

Examination Review Questions

1. Dinesha Reynolds has an oral temperature of 100.4°F. The medical term for this is
   - (A) pyuria
   - (B) purulent
   - (C) hyperpyrexia
   - (D) pyrexia
   - (E) none of the above

2. Which of the following is NOT considered a vital sign?
   - (A) body temperature
   - (B) weight
   - (C) blood pressure
   - (D) respiration
   - (E) all of these are vital signs

3. What is considered the least accurate indicator of temperature?
   - (A) axilla
   - (B) oral
   - (C) eardrum
   - (D) rectum
   - (E) all are equally accurate

4. The ratio of pulse to respirations is usually
   - (A) 1:5
   - (B) 4:1
   - (C) 1:3
   - (D) 1:2
   - (E) none of the above

5. During which phase of the Korotkoff sounds will the sound fade and become muffled?
   - (A) Phase I
   - (B) Phase II
   - (C) Phase III
   - (D) Phase IV
   - (E) Phase V

6. Blood pressure that becomes low when a patient assumes an erect position is called
   - (A) postural hypertension
   - (B) orthostatic hypertension
   - (C) essential hypertension
   - (D) orthostatic hypotension
   - (E) none of the above is correct

7. Mr. Daniels weighs 83.92 Kg. How many pounds does he weigh?
   - (A) 185 lb
   - (B) 195 lb
   - (C) 180 lb
   - (D) 200 lb
   - (E) 210 lb

8. The normal pulse rate (beats per minute) for adults is
   - (A) 40–60
   - (B) 60–80
   - (C) 80–100
   - (D) 100–120
   - (E) 120–160

9. When taking an oral temperature, the thermometer should be left in the mouth for at least how many minutes?
   - (A) 3 minutes
   - (B) 5 minutes
   - (C) 10 minutes
   - (D) 12 minutes
   - (E) 15 minutes

10. When taking a rectal temperature, the thermometer should be left in the rectum for how many minutes?
    - (A) 3 minutes
    - (B) 5 minutes
    - (C) 10 minutes
    - (D) 12 minutes
    - (E) 15 minutes

Problem Solving

An established patient of 35 years of age is being seen by Dr. Bean. He is complaining of fever, chest congestion, and difficulty breathing. Joan performs the initial procedures and assists the patient in a comfortable position. The patient has difficulty breathing when he reclines on the exam table. The vital signs were as follows: temperature—102F, blood pressure—140/80, respirations—28 and shallow, pulse—100 and bounding, ht—63≤ and wt—170 pounds.

1. What should Joan do immediately to assist the patient?

2. Are this patient's vital signs abnormal? List the correct range for each vital sign.

3. Should the physician be consulted immediately?

4. Chart your findings according to the correct procedure.

MEDICAL ASSISTANT ROLE DELINEATION CHART

Highlight indicates material covered in this chapter

ADMINISTRATIVE

ADMINISTRATIVE PROCEDURES

- Perform basic clerical functions
- Schedule, coordinate, and monitor appointments
- Schedule inpatient/outpatient admissions and procedures
- Understand and apply third party guidelines
- Obtain reimbursement through accurate claims submission
- Monitor third-party reimbursement
- Perform medical transcription
- Understand and adhere to managed care policies and procedures
- *Negotiate managed care contracts (adv)*

PRACTICE FINANCES

- Perform procedural and diagnostic coding
- Apply bookkeeping principles
- Document and maintain accounting and banking records
- Manage accounts receivable
- Manage accounts payable
- Process payroll
- *Develop and maintain fee schedules (adv)*
- *Manage renewals of business and professional insurance policies (adv)*
- *Manage personal benefits and maintain records (adv)*

CLINICAL

FUNDAMENTAL PRINCIPLES

- Apply principles of aseptic technique and infection control
- Comply with quality assurance practices
- Screen and follow up patient test results

DIAGNOSTIC ORDERS

- Collect and process specimens
- Perform diagnostic tests

PATIENT CARE

- Adhere to established triage procedures
- Obtain patient history and vital signs
- Prepare and maintain examination and treatment areas

- Prepare patient for examinations, procedures, and treatments
- Assist with examinations, procedures, and treatments
- Prepare and administer medications and immunizations
- Maintain medication and immunization records
- Recognize and respond to emergencies
- Coordinate patient care information with other health care providers

GENERAL (TRANSDISCIPLINARY)

PROFESSIONALISM

- Project a professional manner and image
- Adhere to ethical principles
- Demonstrate initiative and responsibility
- Work as a team member
- Manage time efficiently
- Prioritize and perform multiple tasks
- Adapt to change
- Promote the CMA credential
- Enhance skills through continuing education

COMMUNICATION SKILLS

- Treat all patients with compassion and empathy
- Recognize and respect cultural diversity
- Adapt communications to individual's ability to understand
- Use professional telephone technique
- Use effective and correct verbal and written communications
- Recognize and respond to verbal and non-verbal communications
- Use medical terminology appropriately
- Receive, organize, prioritize, and transmit information
- Serve as liaison
  Promote the practice through positive public relations

LEGAL CONCEPTS

- Maintain confidentiality
- Practice within the scope of education, training, and personal capabilities
- Prepare and maintain medical records
- Document accurately
- Use appropriate guidelines when releasing information
- Follow employer's established policies dealing with the health care contract
- Follow federal, state, and local legal guidelines
- Maintain awareness of federal and state health care legislation and regulations
- Maintain and dispose of regulated substances in compliance with government guidelines
- Comply with established risk management and safety procedures
- Recognize professional credentialing criteria
- Participate in the development and maintenance of personnel, policy, and procedure manuals
- *Develop and maintain personnel, policy, and procedure manuals (adv)*

INSTRUCTION

- Instruct individuals according to their needs
- Explain office policies and procedures
- Teach methods of health promotion and disease prevention
- Locate community resources and disseminate information
- *Orient and train personnel (adv)*
- *Develop educational materials (adv)*
- *Conduct continuing education activities (adv)*

OPERATIONAL FUNCTIONS

- Maintain supply inventory
- Evaluate and recommend equipment and supplies
- Apply computer techniques to support office operations
- *Supervise personnel (adv)*
- *Interview and recommend job applicants (adv)*
- *Negotiate leases and prices for equipment and supply contracts (adv)*

SOURCE: Reprinted by permission of the American Association of Medical Assistants from the *AAMA Role Delineation Study: Occupational Analysis of the Medical Assisting Profession*.

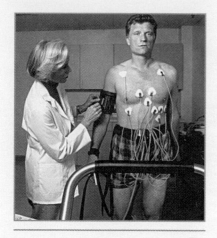

- Heart Structure and Function
- The Electrocardiogram
- Cardiology Specials
- Holter Monitor
- Pulmonary Function
- Pulmonary Volume Tests
- Peak Flowmeter
- Oximeter
- Legal and Ethical Issues
- Patient Education

ELECTROCARDIOGRAPHY AND PULMONARY FUNCTION

OBJECTIVES

After completing this chapter, you should:

- Define and spell the glossary terms for this chapter.
- Practice within the scope of education, training and personal capabilities.
- Conduct oneself in a courteous and diplomatic manner.
- Treat all patients with empathy and impartiality.
- Prepare and maintain examination and treatment area.
- Prepare patients for procedures.
- Assist physician with examinations and treatments.
- Perform selected tests that assist with diagnosis and treatment.
- Document accurately.
- Maintain and operate electrocardiogram and pulmonary function equipment.
- Identify by name and function the controls on an electrocardiograph machine.
- Name the standard 12 leads and the locations of their sensors.
- State the cause and correction of artifacts.
- Name six abnormalities that can be detected in an electrocardiogram.

- Explain Forced Vital Capacity (FVC), Forced Expiratory Volume in 1 second (FEV1) and Maximal Midexpiratory Flow (MMEF).
- Differentiate between obstructive and restrictive pulmonary disease.

CLINICAL PERFORMANCE COMPETENCIES

After completing this chapter, you should perform the following tasks:

- Prepare the patient and obtain a clear and accurate electrocardiograph tracing.
- Obtain a clear and accurate recording of a patient's pulmonary function.
- Correctly attach patient to holter monitor.

Glossary

amplitude   Degree of variation from zero or the baseline, up or down, in recording electrical output of the heart. Also called voltage.

artifact(s)   In reference to EKGs, these are deflections caused by electrical activity other than from the heart; irregular and erratic markings.

baseline   No electrical charge or activity; return to zero; flat on electrocardiogram recording. Also known as isoelectric line.

cardiac cycle   One heartbeat, designated arbitrarily as P, Q, R, S, and T, consisting of contraction and relaxation of both atria and ventricles; one pulse.

cardiac rate   Pulse rate, number of beats or contractions per minute.

channel(s)   On a machine capable of receiving more than one signal at once, a channel is the pathway for one signal.

deflection   Deviation, up or down, from zero or the isoelectric line.

depolarized (depolarization)   Discharge of electrical activity that precedes contraction.

depolarization, atrial   Discharge of electrical activity in the upper heart chambers.

depolarization, ventricular   Discharge of electrical activity in the lower chambers.

electrocardiogram   Record of electrical activity of the heart; voltage with respect to time.

electrocardiograph   Machine used to record electrical activity of the heart.

electrode(s)   Device that detects electrical charges. Also know as sensor.

electrolyte   Material applied to the skin to enhance contact between skin and the sensor.

endocardium   Lining of the heart.

interval   Time between beginning of one phase and beginning of the next phase.

isoelectric line   *See baseline.*

lead(s)   An electrical connection to the body to receive data from a specific combination of sensors.

myocardium   Heart wall composed of muscle and fibrous tissue.

obstructive lung disease   Those diseases that obstruct the flow of air out of the lungs characterized by generally slow expiratory rate and increased residual volume.

pacemaker   The portion of cardiac electrical tissue that establishes the beat; the sinoatrial node; also the artificial equipment used when the natural pacemaker fails.

pericardium   A double-walled sac that encloses the heart.

polarized   State of electrical charge in living cells.

pulmonary volume tests   Under constant conditions, the patient breathes with extreme inhalations and exhalations, and the amount of gas inhaled or exhaled is recorded.

QRS complex   Multiple waves or deflections occurring in a group.

repolarization   Return to polarization from the depolarized state; return to rest.

repolarization, atrial   Return to polarization of the upper heart chambers.

repolarization, ventricular   Return to polarization of the lower chambers.

restrictive lung disease   Those diseases that prevent the expansion of the lungs, diminish the total lung capacity, vital capacity, and inspiratory capacity.

segment   Time from the end of one phase to the beginning of another phase.

sensitivity   Ability of the equipment to detect a change in amplitude; normally a state of one.

sensors   *See electrode.*

standardization   Test performed to document a machine's compliance with the international agreement.

tracing   Recording.

voltage   *See amplitude.*

wave   *See deflection.*

WARNING!

For all patient contact, adhere to Standard Precautions.
Wear protective equipment as indicated.

Within the thorax or chest are the major organs of both respiration and circulation. These two systems work very closely together; both are vital for survival, and a problem with one is likely to cause a problem with the other. Because many patients suffer with disorders of these two systems, both primary care physicians and specialists monitor and treat these patients, and the tests performed to evaluate their status are performed frequently by a medical assistant. Figure 6-1 shows the heart and an electrocardiogram.

Assessment of the heart and lungs begins when any patient visits the physician, whether they are sick or well. A stethoscope is used to evaluate the sounds made as the heart works. These sounds represent the closing of the valves and usually occur close together followed by a pause, as in "lubb-dubb . . . lubb-dubb. . . ." S1 designates the first sound and represents the closing of the tricuspid and bicuspid (mitral) valves. S2 results from the closing of the aortic and pulmonary valves (Figure 6-2). The physician notes on the patient record any abnormalities in heart sounds and rhythm.

When more specific cardiac documentation is needed, an **electrocardiogram** (ECG or EKG) is made. The electrocardiogram is a **tracing,** or recording, of electrical activity as it moves through the heart. Thus, it is a recording with respect to time. The physician orders this painless, non-invasive test when the heart sounds are unusual, the rhythm is irregular, the patient has any heart related complaints or has a condition that might affect the heart or be due to the heart. A recording will also be made to serve as a reference with which to compare future recordings in evaluating any changes. This may be called a baseline electrocardiogram, not to be confused with the baseline in the recording itself.

▶ HEART STRUCTURE AND FUNCTION

Located between the lungs behind the sternum, the heart is a hollow triangular organ enclosed within a double-walled sac called the **pericardium.** The middle layer or **myocardium** makes up most of the heart wall and is composed of interconnected muscle and fibrous tissue. The **endocardium** lines the upper chambers, or atria, and lower chamber, or ventricles, of the heart.

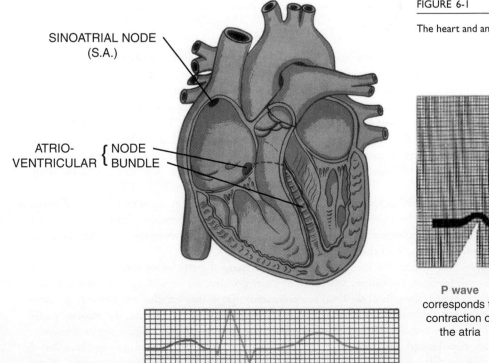

SINOATRIAL NODE
(S.A.)

ATRIO-
VENTRICULAR { NODE
{ BUNDLE

FIGURE 6-1

The heart and an electrocardiogram tracing.

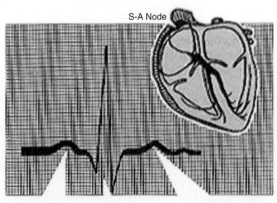

S-A Node

P wave
corresponds to
contraction of
the atria

QRS complex
correlates to
ventricles
contracting

T wave
represents
preparation for
next series of
complexes

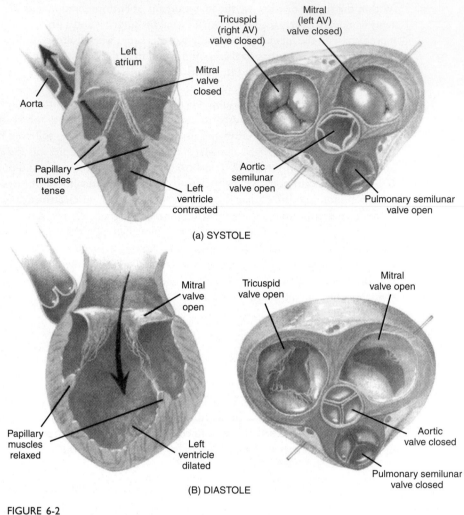

FIGURE 6-2

Heart valves.

Blood circulates throughout the body and returns from the general circulation by way of the superior and inferior vena cava, to the right atrium, moving in one direction through the heart. When the right atrium is full, the atrium contracts and blood is pumped into the right ventricle through the tricuspid valve. Upon filling, blood is pumped by contraction of the right ventricle through the semilunar valves into the pulmonary artery going to the lungs. There, blood is oxygenated and returned to the left atrium through the four pulmonary veins. When that chamber is full, it contracts and blood is squeezed into the left ventricle through the mitral (bicuspid) valve. In the left ventricle, blood will enter the aortic semilunar valve and move into all parts of the body except the lungs.

Heart valves act as gates to prevent the backward flow of blood. They open and shut in response to the changing pressure brought about by cardiac contraction and relaxation. The contraction and relaxation of the chambers occurs in sequence because electrical impulses move smoothly along the electrical conduction system of the heart.

This conduction system involves the movement of charged particles or ions during different phases. Minerals (sodium, potassium, and calcium) are responsible for smooth contractions and consistent rhythm. At rest, the cells of the heart are **polarized**; that is, they are charged with energy (negative inside the cell and positive outside). As the cells are stimulated to contract, the mineral particles move like a wave and the charge within the cells changes to positive inside and negative outside. The cells are **depolarized** and contraction occurs. The cells then return to a resting state, called **repolarization**, as their electrical charge returns to the original negative inside and positive outside.

The four major components of this conduction system are the sinoatrial (SA) node, atrioventricular (AV) node, the bundle of His with the right and left bundle branches, and the Purkinje fibers. The heartbeat is controlled by rhythmic impulses that arise in the SA node and move through the conduction system. The SA node, located in the right atrium, is made of modified myocardial cells and acts like a battery. It is known as the **pacemaker** of the heart because it establishes the pace. It may accelerate or slow the rate under the influence of the autonomic nervous system.

The conduction system carries the impulse from the SA node and spreads it through the atria, causing them to contract. Contraction of the atria is called **atrial depolarization**. The impulses reach the atrioventricular or AV node (also made of modified myocardial cells) where they are momentarily delayed. During this delay, the atria rest and recover. This is known as atrial recovery, atrial rest, or **atrial repolarization**. The impulse passes from the AV node down the bundle of His as it divides into 2 bundle branches, carrying the impulse along both sides of the interventricular septum. The bundle branches spread to form a network, the Purkinje system, that distributes the impulse to all parts of the ventricular muscle, resulting in ventricular contraction or **ventricular depolarization**. Ventricular depolarization follows atrial repolarization, and is followed by a period of ventricular recovery known as **ventricular repolarization** or rest. There is a brief pause, and the cycle begins again. Atrial and ventricular depolarization plus atrial and ventricular repolarization comprise the **cardiac cycle**, one pulse and one heart beat.

A unique property of cardiac muscle is that all conductive tissue has the potential to serve in the role of pacemaker; that is, any area can set the **cardiac rate** if the SA node fails. Under abnormal circumstances, such as when damage has occurred, other areas may assume the role of pacemaker. Slower rhythms will be generated by the AV node (40 to 60 beats per minute), by the bundle of His (less than 40 beats per minute), and by the Purkinje system. But normally the SA node generates the controlling impulses at a resting rate of 60 to 80 beats per minute.

► THE ELECTROCARDIOGRAM

As the electrical changes are passed through the cardiac conduction system, they also spread throughout the body and can be detected by **sensors**, or **electrodes**, placed on the skin. These sensors will be placed on arms, legs, and specific places across the chest. Wires from sensors on the skin transmit these minute changes via a patient cable to the **electrocardiograph** machine; the machine amplifies them and converts electrical energy to mechanical action, causing movement of a writing instrument, the stylus. When there is no energy being recorded, there is no movement of the stylus, and a **baseline** or **isoelectric line** or straight flat line appears. Movement away from the baseline is called a **deflection** or **wave**. The waves or deflections may go up (positive) or down (negative) from the baseline and represent **amplitude** or **voltage**. An increase in voltage will cause a larger deflection. Smaller deflections mean only a small amount of voltage is being detected and recorded. The deflections are arbitrarily labeled P, Q, R, S, and T. (Sometimes a small U wave follows the T wave. This is considered normal and is most probably due to a potassium deficiency.) A normal cardiac cycle is one series of PQRST waves. The P represents atrial depolarization, the QRS complex represents ventricular depolarization, and the T is repolarization.

On an ECG, the horizontal axis (line) represents time; a slower heart rate will have more space between the PQRST complexes. On a patient with a faster heart rate, the cardiac cycles will be closer together. When a heart skips a beat, there is a long flat line between PQRSTs. Additionally, the amount of space between the P wave and the QRS complex indicates the time required for the conduction system to carry the inpulse from the SA node to the Purkinje fibers.

Recordings are made from a variety of perspectives or angles known as **leads**. Each lead will record from a specific combination of sensors. When completed, the 12 lead electrocardiograph produces a three dimensional record of cardiac impulses. The pattern of deflections will appear quite different on each lead. The pattern of deflections recorded, voltage or amplitude and time, assists the physician in evaluating the status of the patient's heart.

In some instances, it may be necessary to enlarge or shrink the recording. Under ordinary circumstances, a recording is made in **sensitivity** 1 (This represents a 10 mm deflection per 1 millivolt of electricity). The size is doubled in sensitivity 2 or halved in sensitivity 1/2.

TIME AND THE CARDIAC CYCLE

The P wave represents the impulse that originated in the sinoatrial node and spread throughout the atria. It is atrial depolarization. If the P wave is present in normal size and shape, it can be assumed that the stimulus originated in the SA node.

Normally, the P-R **interval** (time from the beginning of P to the beginning of QRS) is between 0.12 and 0.20 seconds (3 to 5 small boxes on the EKG graph paper). A deviation from these times could represent pathology. This interval represents the time it takes for the impulse to cross the atria and the atrioventricular node and reach the ventricles. A P-R interval that is too short means the impulse has reached the ventricles through a shorter than normal pathway. If the interval is too long, a conduction delay in the AV node might be assumed.

The **QRS complex** represents the time necessary for the impulse to travel through the bundle of His, the bundle branches, and the Purkinje fibers to complete ventricular activation or contraction, known as ventricular depolarization. This usually takes less than 0.12 seconds (3 small boxes).

Repolarization of the ventricles is represented by the ST segment and the T wave. The ST **segment** is normally flat (on the isoelectric line or baseline) or is only slightly elevated.

The T wave represents a part of recovery of the ventricles after contraction. Usually the QRS complex and the T wave point in the same direction. T waves that are opposite in direction from the QRS may indicate pathology. While the medical assistant should not try to interpret the electrocardiogram, a knowledge of what is normal in the cardiac cycle is helpful.

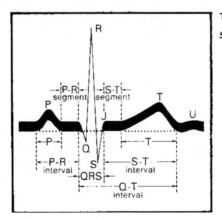

The cardiac cycle.

Source: The Burdick Corporation, Milton, Wisconsin

ECG MACHINES

There are a great variety of machines in use, but all should be calibrated to align with the international standard. This means that the paper moves at the same speed of 25 mm per second and, given the same amount of electrical energy, the recording stylus will move the same distance (1 mv of electricity input will cause the stylus to deflect 10 mm), thus giving uniform recordings worldwide. **Standardization** is a means of verifying that each machine deflects 10 mm in response to 1 mv of electricity in sensitivity 1.

Older models are manual; you must tell the machine what to do. You may record from arms and legs in fairly rapid succession, but you must move the chest sensor and record from each lead, then move the sensor again. Computerized models have automatic features so you may only need to push a button. You place all sensors on the patient at the beginning of the procedure and the computer switches from lead to lead in rapid succession. These automated machines can be overridden by the operator if there is a need for manual controls. Many computerized models can record from more than one lead at once, to save time. Each is recorded in a separate channel or pathway for the signal, and typically these machines record 3 channels at once. Some other machines have a built-in interpretive feature as in Figure 6-3 and will print out a statement as to the status of the heart. Others can connect directly via fax with a regional office that will carry out the interpretation function and fax results to your office. Many automated machines require that you type in pertinent patient data such as height, weight, age, blood pressure, and prescription drugs being taken.

It is your responsibility to produce a clear and accurate tracing from each patient, so you must be familiar with the machines in your office. Read the manufacturer's instructions for the machine before using. Knowledge of the control panel will help you produce a tracing that is clear, accurate, and easily read.

- *Main power switch (off/on).* Allow for a warm-up of 2 minutes (or whatever is specified by the manufacturer) before using.
- *Record switch.* This switch moves the paper at the standard "run 25" speed (25 mm/sec). EKGs are usually recorded at this speed. Another option is "run 50" (50 mm/sec or twice as fast). This is used when the heart rate is so rapid that interpretation requires that it be stretched out.
- *Lead selector.* This determines from which sensors the machine will record. Standard (limb) leads: Record from 2 sensors placed on all extremities. Augmented leads: Record from the midpoint between 2 limb sensors to a third limb sensor. Chest leads (also called precordial leads): Record from various positions on the thorax.
- *Standard adjustment screw.* Increases or decreases the size of the deflection in response to 1 mv electricity.
- *Sensitivity control.* Allows the operator to increase or decrease the recording size in order to enlarge or shrink the deflections to fit on the paper. When changing from the international standard of sensitivity 1 to sensitivity of 1/2 or 2, the operator needs to include a standard for the interpreter's information.
- *Standard button.* Allows verification of calibration to the international standard.
- *Stylus control.* Centers the recording in the middle of the page or the center of each channel by moving the stylus.
- *Stylus heat control.* Increases or decreases heat and adjusts for the sharpest tracing.
- *Marker.* Indicates, by a code, which lead is being recorded.

ELECTROCARDIOGRAM PAPER

There are "time" markers printed on all electrocardiogram paper, referred to as 3 second markers. Look for them at the top of single channel paper and between **channels** in multichannel paper.

A heated stylus melts the light colored coating and reveals the black base of this special electrocardiogram paper. The stylus temperature is adjustable with a screwdriver; if it becomes too hot, a hole will be burned in the paper. If it is not hot enough, insufficient coating is removed and the line revealed is very faint. The paper is also pressure sensitive and must be handled carefully. Note that it is marked in small squares with a light line and in larger squares with a darker line. The small squares are 1 mm square and represent 0.1 mv of voltage in the height, and .04 seconds time in the width. The larger squares are 5 mm square and represent 0.5 mv of voltage in the height, and 0.20 seconds time in the width. Thus the paper records both time (horizontally) and voltage (vertically).

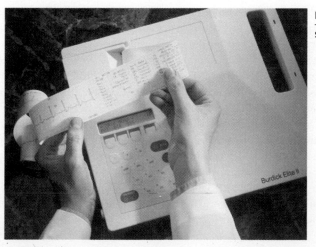

FIGURE 6-3

Single channel electrocardiograph.

HEART RATE

It is possible to estimate the heart rate from an electrocardiogram. Some offices have a protocol that states you should record some additional cycles if the heart rate is above or below certain numbers. Many cardiologists also expect you to perform an exact calculation of the heart rate before you place the recording in the patient record or on the doctor's desk. Here are two methods for estimation of the heart rate and one for exact calculation.

Note the "3 second markers" that are printed by the manufacturer on the paper. To estimate the cardiac rate (beats per minute) from the tracing use the "6 second method." Begin at one 3 second marker and go to the right for two additional markers, a total of 6 seconds. Count the number of QRS complexes between the first and third markers and add a zero. This is your estimated ventricular rate per minute. A similar atrial estimate can be made by counting the P waves between these markers. This estimate is accurate even if the rhythm is irregular (arrhythmia).

The heart rate can also be estimated by locating a QRS complex close to a 5 mm line, the darker line on the paper. Move to the next deflection at the right or the left, counting how many 5 mm lines intersect the tracing before the next QRS complex. Count off at each 5 mm line, beginning at the deflection near the 5 mm line and saying "zero, 300, 150, 100, 75, 60, 50." Stop counting when you reach the next QRS complex. This "count-off method" is an estimate of the ventricular rate. This estimate is accurate only for the complexes where it was done.

To get the exact calculation of the heart rate, recall that the paper moves at a standard speed of 25 mm/second, so it will move at 1500 mm/minute (25 mm × 60 seconds = 1500). An exact calculation of ventricular heart rate is achieved by counting the mm boxes between two QRS complexes and dividing that number into 1500. For instance, if there are 20 mm between two QRS complexes, 1500 divided by 20 equals 75 beats per minute. An exact calculation of atrial heart rate is achieved by counting the mm boxes between two P waves and by dividing that number into 1500. These calculations are accurate only for the complexes where they were done.

Rate is the same as beats per minute. Rhythm is the regularity of the occurrence of those beats. Ventricular rhythm is determined by measuring the distance between QRS complexes. There should be a fairly consistent space between complexes. Atrial rhythm is determined by measuring the distance between P waves. There should be a fairly consistent space between waves. Again, train yourself to look at the rhythm while you are recording. Some offices have protocols about what extra tracings to record in the event the rhythm appears irregular to you.

SENSOR PLACEMENT

The EKG machine records the cardiac cycle through sensors placed on the patient's bare skin. Sensors are placed over the fleshy part of the inner aspect of both lower legs and both upper arms or forearms, avoiding the bony prominences. These locations are abbreviated LA for left arm, RA for right arm, LL for left leg and RL for right leg. The RL sensor serves as an electrical reference point and is not actually used in the recording. If you have a patient on whom you cannot place the sensor as planned, you must place the sensors on both extremities symmetrically. For example, a patient in a cast up to the knee requires that both sensors be placed above the knee. If a hand and forearm are amputated, both arm sensors are placed on the upper arm. The chest sensor, abbreviated with V, is used in six locations, with a number following the V, as in V1, V2, and so forth. Placement of chest sensors must be anatomically correct. Figure 6-4 A-H shows the 12-lead ECG.

By recording from different combinations of sensors, the electrical activity of the heart is seen from different angles. A lead selector switch or lead indicator selects the combination of sensors for that lead. One sensor is used for chest (unipolar) leads. A combination may be two sensors, as with standard limb (bipolar) leads, or 3 sensors, as with augmented limb leads.

With many sensors and many views possible, you will need to indicate on the tracing from which lead you are recording. An international marking system has been devised using dashes and dots. Some machines automatically mark the code just above the cardiac tracing. Others require manual marking with the international code. Table 6-1 lists *limb*, *augmented*, and *chest* leads indicating proper placement and marking codes.

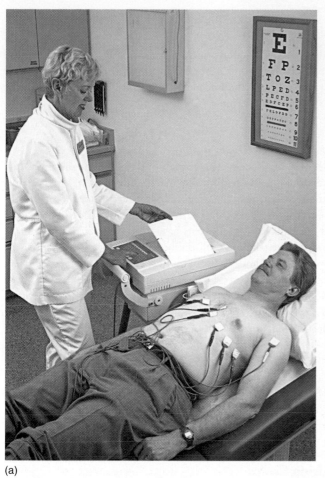

(a)

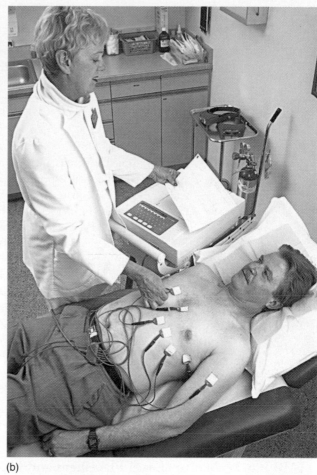

(b)

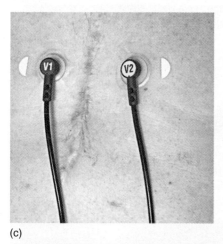

(c)

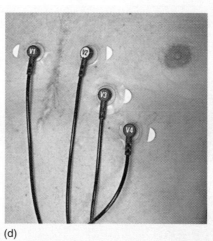

(d)

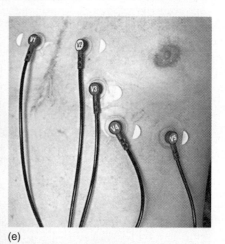

(e)

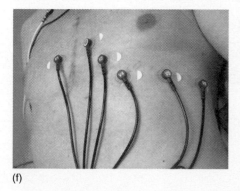

(f)

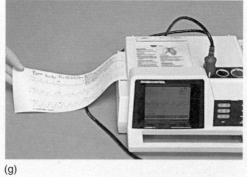

(g)

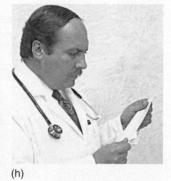

(h)

FIGURE 6-4 A-H

Sensors of a 12-lead ECG.

It is beneficial to memorize the sensors used in the limb and augmented leads. Then, if you have difficulty getting a clear recording from one lead, you do not have to look at all the sensors, only those involved. Some find it easier to remember all the leads and the sensors being recorded using Table 6-1 or by picturing Einthoven's triangle, as in Figure 6-5.

PATIENT PREPARATION

A well informed patient is more cooperative and less anxious. Explain the equipment and procedure as well as what you will expect the patient to do. The surroundings should be pleasant and the table wide enough for adequate support. Patients will need to be bare to the waist so privacy should be provided for disrobing. Offer female patients a gown, to be worn with the opening at the front. In addition, you will need access to bare skin on the lower legs. Patients have to remove socks or stockings. Roll long pant legs out of the way. Position the patient comfortably supine with a pillow under the head, and another under the knees, if needed, to eliminate back strain. Jewelry usually does not interfere with sensor placement. Prepare the skin where the sensors will be applied. Any area that has been treated with talcum powder or skin lotion must be rubbed with alcohol to remove the residue. Some shower gels leave sufficient moisturizer as a residue that interfere with sensor contact and this must be removed with alcohol. Then the electrolyte sensors may be applied.

THE PROCEDURE

If you are to obtain a clear recording of the patient's cardiac cycle, you will need a machine, calibrated and in good working order with a supply of special paper. You may also need a screwdriver for adjustment of stylus temperature and the standard control screw. A patient gown should be available for female patients. You will also need the sensors to place on the skin and a supply of **electrolyte** or con-

TABLE 6-1   Sensor (Lead) Placement and Marking Codes

Limb Leads	Placement	Abbreviation	Marking Code
Lead I	Right arm to left arm	RA - LA	•
Lead II	Right arm to left leg	RA - LL	••
Lead III	Left arm to left leg	LA - LL	•••
Augmented Leads			
aVR	RA-midpoint (LA-LL)	(LA-LL) RA	-
aVL	LA-midpoint (RA-LL)	(RA-LL) LA	- -
aVF	LL-midpoint (RA-LA)	(RA-LA) LL	- - -
Chest Leads	Placement		Marking Code
V1	4th intercostal space, right sternal border	- •	
V2	4th intercostal space, left sternal border	- ••	
V3	Midway between V2 and V4		- •••
V4	5th intercostal space, mid-clavicular left	- ••••	
V5	Left anterior axillary fold horizontal to V4	- •••••	
V6	Left mid-axillary horizontal to V4 and V5	- ••••••	

Note: The right leg is never used for the tracings, but is an electrical ground.

duction cream, gel, or pads to improve the contact between the skin and electrodes. The sensors may be metal plates that attach with rubber straps or they may be small suction cups called Welch electrodes. These will need to be cleaned between patients to prevent the accumulation of electrolyte. Adhesive disposable sensors that contain electrolyte are also available.

To begin, assemble the necessary supplies, plug the machine into a properly grounded outlet, allow for it to warm-up, and verify that the machine is operational and in compliance with the international standard. Using manual controls, run the machine at "run 25" and push the standard button briefly to release 1 millivolt of electricity. Stop the machine and count the small boxes covered by the deflection of the stylus. The 1 mv of electricity should have caused a positive deflection of 10 mm. If not, adjust the standard screw with a screwdriver until the deflection is precisely 10 mm, or call your service representative.

Identify, interview, and instruct the patient. Following skin preparation, the electrolyte and sensors may be applied. There are many forms of electrolyte, including gel, lotion and paste. Each office selects one that is compatible with the type of sensors they are using and their machines. The most recent development is a disposable gummy sensor containing electrolyte. It requires that small alligator clamps be added to the sensor wires. These clip onto the edge of the sensor.

The procedure to attach the sensors will vary slightly, depending on the machine you are using. Some sensors are secured with a rubber strap. One electrolyte saturated pad is placed on the skin

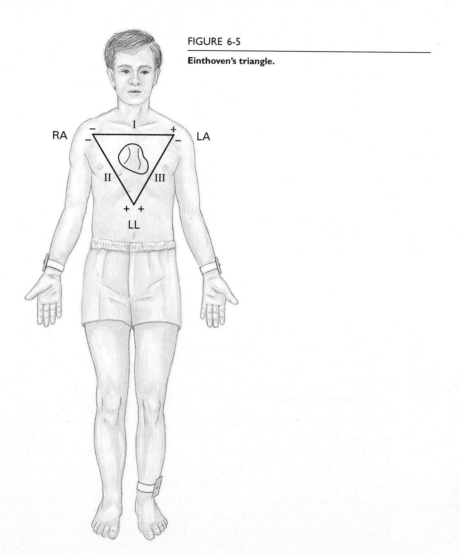

FIGURE 6-5

Einthoven's triangle.

Med Tip: Know what format you will use for mounting the ECG before you begin recording so that there is minimal waste.

and the sensor plate strapped over it. The limb sensors are attached and the first six leads are recorded, one at a time. Then the one chest sensor is moved from position to position as each lead is recorded. Newer machines use a small amount of electrolyte lotion and suction cup sensors, referred to as Welch electrodes. Electrolyte and all sensors are placed on the skin at once. All 12 leads are run in rapid succession because the computerized machines can switch from one lead to another quickly.

The placement of chest sensors must be precise. It is possible to complete this task without unnecessary exposure for female patients. The landmarks you will need to palpate or view are the sternum, the fourth intercostal space, both clavicles, and the left axilla. Stand on the left side of the patient and expose the sternum. Locate the right clavicle and the space immediately inferior to it. This is a supracostal space; that is, it is above the first rib and does not count as an intercostal space. Proceed toward the feet at the right edge of the sternum and, using the tips of your fingers, palpate the first rib and first intercostal space, second rib and intercostal space, and so forth until you feel the fourth intercostal space. This space at the right sternal margin is the location of V 1. V 2 is at the same level on the left side of the sternum. Next, you will need to locate V 4 to find V 3. From the middle of the left clavicle, draw an imaginary line towards the feet, stopping one intercostal space below the level of V 2. This is V 4 (5th intercostal space, mid-clavicular left). Lift a female patient's gown up from the hemline in respect of patient privacy. V4 must be at the base of the breast and, in some patients, under the breast. In males, it should be about nipple level. Now you can locate V 3 midway between V 2 and V 4. It is on a rib. V 5 is at a point where 2 imaginary lines intersect. Continue to work under the patient's gown. Draw a line from the front of the left axillary fold toward the feet, parallel to the table on which the patient is lying. Draw another line toward the table from V 4. Where these lines intersect is V 5. V 6 is at the mid-axilla, in line with V4 and V5. You will need to practice locating the landmarks and sensor sites on different body sizes and shapes. Remember to keep your female patients covered.

Arrange the patient cable to follow body contours, avoiding coils. Connect the patient cable and begin to record by performing a standard. For manual machines, select the STD lead, "run 25", and push the standard button. Stop the machine and count the boxes included in the deflection. You should have 10 mm. If more or less, adjust the standard control as needed with a screwdriver. Then use the lead selector knob and select the leads in sequence, running a six inch strip, marking the lead code, if necessary. The length of the tracing you will need depends on how your office mounts single channel cardiograms. Have information about your mounting format before you begin to record. Adjust the stylus to the center of the paper. For automatic machines, depress "auto run" and adjust the stylus to the center of each channel. Record the tracing, using problem-solving skills. When the cardiogram is completed, remove the sensors and wipe the electrolyte from the patient's skin. Dismiss the patient.

Med Tip: The medical assistant is responsible for adhering to the international agreement for sensor placement, recording and coding for leads.

Clean the machine. Mount the electrocardiogram, if necessary, and transfer the patient information. Sign or initial your work.

MAKING ADJUSTMENTS

A satisfactory tracing is one that is accurate, readable, clear, travels down the center of the page, and has a baseline that is consistently horizontal. If the baseline begins to drift upward or downward, use the position control knob to return it to the center of the page. Observe whether the tracing remains within the graph portion of the paper. If the deflections are so large that they exceed the upper and lower limits of the graph, you will have to reduce the sensitivity from 1 to 1/2. This will make the tracing half as large, and you will need to include a standard to let the interpreter know what you have done. 1 mv of electricity will cause a deflection of 5 mm in sensitivity 1/2. However, if your tracing in sensitivity 1 is so tiny that it is not readable, increase the size by changing the sensitivity from 1 to

PROCEDURE: Recording A 12 Lead Electrocardiogram

Terminal Performance
Competency: Will be able to perform an ECG, obtaining a satisfactory tracing with 100% accuracy, without assistance.

Equipment and Supplies
ECG machine with sensors, patient cable, power cord
ECG Paper
Electrolyte
Alcohol
Screwdriver for adjustments, if needed
Patient gown, if needed

Procedural Steps
1. Wash hands.
2. Assemble necessary supplies.
3. Attach and plug in the power cord.
4. Verify that the machine is operational and positioned properly.
5. Identify, interview, and instruct the patient. Offer female patients a gown, to be worn with the opening down the front.
6. Position the patient flat on a table with a pillow under the head and one under the knees if needed.
7. Prepare the electrode sites and attach the electrodes:
   - Limb electrodes should be applied over the fleshy part of the inner aspect of lower legs and forearms.
   - Chest leads should be applied as illustrated in Figure 6-6 A and B.
8. Connect the patient cable.
9. Instruct the patient to relax, breathe normally, and refrain from speaking.
10. Standardize the machine.
11. Adjust the stylus to the center of the paper or the center of each channel.
12. Record—For automatic machines, depress AUTO-RUN; for manual machines, select the leads in sequence and use RUN 25. Use your problem-solving skills if you encounter any artifacts.
13. Mark the leads, if necessary.
14. Remove the sensors; wipe electrolyte from the patient's skin.
15. Dismiss the patient.
16. Wash hands.
17. Clean the machine, straps, and sensors.
18. Mount the electrocardiogram and transfer the patient information.
19. Chart the procedure in the patient's record. Sign or initial your work.

Charting Example
3/11/XX   2:10 PM   12-lead ECG performed.
M. King, CMA (AAMA)

2. Again, place a standard on the page to let the physician know that you have made a change. 1 mv of electricity will cause a deflection of 20 mm in sensitivity two.

Since the paper moves through the machine at the rate of 25 mm per second, an option available in recording is to move the paper twice as fast, or at 50 mm per second. This would only be necessary if the cardiac cycles were compacted by a very rapid heart rate. In this case, a better quality cardiogram would be produced if the cycles were stretched out. Mark the tracing to indicate you have changed the speed. In machines that mark the lead with an international code, the code marks are stretched out; the dots appear as dashes, and the dashes are long ones.

The multi-channel machines produce an EKG very quickly, on a single sheet of paper about 8 inches by 11 inches. You will have to center three baselines. A sensitivity or speed change affects all three channels.

Knowledge of the leads and their sensor locations will help the medical assistant to trace back to the source any irregular or erratic markings, known as **artifacts**. You can also perform other trouble-shooting techniques during the recording process. Failure to make the necessary corrections will result in an unsatisfactory or no tracing. The physician will not be able to read and interpret such a recording.

ARTIFACTS

Occasionally, the sensors will detect electrical activity from a source other than the heart. These deflections or artifacts impair accurate interpretation of the tracing. The medical assistant needs to find the cause of the artifact and correct it. The different causes of artifacts and how to correct them include:

1. *Somatic tremor.* A tense muscle or a muscle contraction, even one that you cannot see, is called somatic tremor. It may result from patient discomfort, tension, chills, and talking or moving. Calm and reassure the patient. Suggest that the patient relax, breathe normally, and not talk. If necessary, place the patient's hands palm-side down under the hips. This is especially helpful if the patient is not relaxed on the narrow table. This position is also best for patients with a tremor disorder. They will display the least artifacts in this position.
2. *Wandering baseline, baseline shift.* This artifact is caused by poor sensor contact with the skin, such as when sensors are dirty or applied too tightly or too loosely, when lotion or talcum prevents good contact with the skin, or when the patient cable slips toward the floor, pulling on the lead wires. You need to readjust, reapply, or clean the sensors, and place the patient cable securely on the table.
3. *AC (alternating current) interference.* The current in wires and equipment may leak into the room and be picked up by the patient's body and the recording machine. This appears in the recording as small regular spikes or static, and is due to improper grounding, nearby electrical equipment in use, or twisted and coiled lead wires. Ground the machine properly. Unplug other electrical equipment in the area. Move the machine to the patient's feet and away from walls containing cables. You may have to wait until a procedure in an adjacent room, such as an x-ray, is completed.
4. *Erratic stylus.* Loose or broken lead wires cause the stylus to thrash erratically, and go off the page. Repair the wires, replace them or call for service on the equipment.

MOUNTING AN ELECTROCARDIOGRAM

Machines that record one lead at a time produce a tracing that is 6 or 12 feet long. To have a document that will fit into the patient record, use a mounting device. Manufacturers make heavy paper folders with pockets or self-stick areas labeled for each of the leads. There are many different forms available. Knowing the form you will use for mounting will help avoid the waste in obtaining a longer tracing than you need. Select the best part of the recording for that lead. It must have a straight baseline and no artifacts. Cut and trim it, and place it in the appropriate area of the folder. Double check your work to make certain you have read the international code for leads correctly. Repeat the process until all 12 leads have been properly mounted. Employer preference will determine where to place the standardization. Machines that record from 3 leads at once do not require mounting. The final product fits nicely into a patient record.

WHAT IS NORMAL?

A normal sinus rhythm means that each heartbeat has 3 distinct waves, a P wave, a T wave, and between the two, a QRS complex where the Q is a downward deflection, the R is an upward deflection, and the S is a downward deflection following an R. The beats come at regular intervals, indicating the impulse originates in the SA node. Within the lead being recorded, each cardiac cycle appears the same as previous cycles.

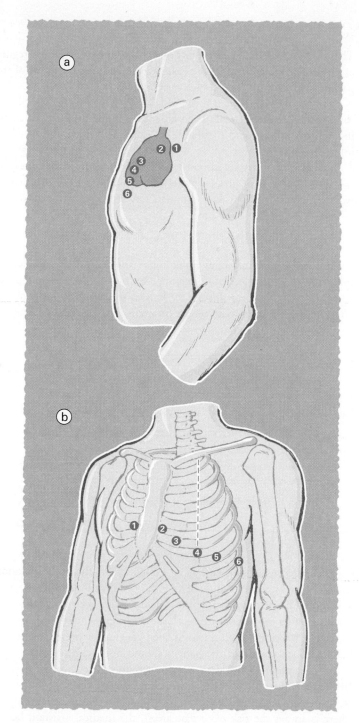

FIGURE 6-6 A AND B

Placement of chest leads.

ABNORMALITIES

Occasionally a tracing will reveal an abnormality caused by cardiac pathology in the patient. An observant medical assistant will recognize the more common abnormalities and draw them to the attention of the physician or follow office protocol, which often calls for an additional recording in a particular lead. A few examples are listed in Table 6-2. Figures 6-7 A-D illustrate varying paper runs of EKGs.

► CARDIOLOGY SPECIALS

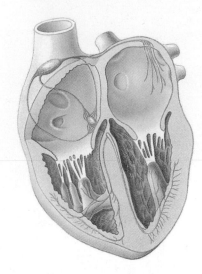

There are a few EKG-related diagnostic procedures performed regularly in the primary care office or in cardiology. The first two are additional lengths of tracings, and may be part of written office protocol for cardiograms.

A rhythm strip will be run in Lead II for 20 seconds on the physician's request or, in some instances, if the medical assistant sees anything that appears abnormal on the tracing. This is not cut and mounted, but carefully folded and given to the physician for interpretation.

An inspiration strip is run on Lead II for 10 seconds with the patient holding his or her breath. This is of greatest value when, as the patient breathes, your tracing shows wandering baseline. This will eliminate any respiratory impact on the tracing.

EXERCISE TOLERANCE TESTING

A stress test or treadmill is an evaluation of the heart's response during moderate exercise following a 12 lead electrocardiogram. This may be used to evaluate patients with a high risk for developing heart disease, or known to have early heart disease, and for patients about to begin a strenuous exercise program. This test is also done on patients who have

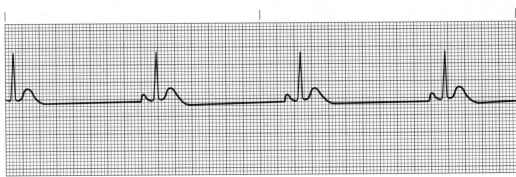

FIGURES 6-7 A

Sinus bradycardia.

cardiac complaints when exercising and as an evaluation of their rehabilitation following cardiac surgery. Figure 6-8 shows a technician discussing the EKG read-out with the patient.

The patient should be prepared before the scheduled day with instructions to wear comfortable exercise or walking shoes and loose fitting clothes. The patient should know that ECGs will be recorded as he or she walks at a carefully prescribed pace in the presence of the physician. Increases in rate or incline will be made but the patient should not feel discomfort or shortness of breath. The medical assistant prepares the patient, connects the patient to the recording devices (ECG, heart rate, BP) and frequently checks blood pressure during the test. The physician evaluates the effect of exercise on the heart rate, blood pressure, and the electrocardiogram.

Because there is always the risk of cardiac arrest, the medical assistant becomes responsible for maintaining emergency equipment that might be needed and having it in the room at the time of the test. Oxygen equipment, a defibrillator, an airway, intravenous solutions, and medications should be periodically checked and replaced, if outdated or not functioning. Figure 6-9 shows the patient being closely observed during a stress test.

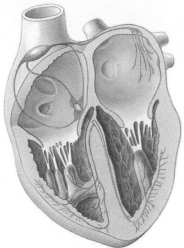

FIGURES 6-7 B

Sinus tachycardia.

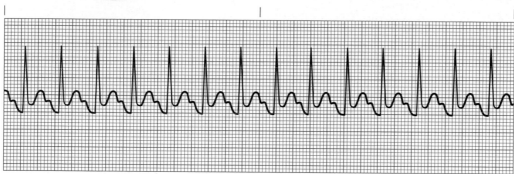

FIGURES 6-7 C

Premature ventricular contractions.

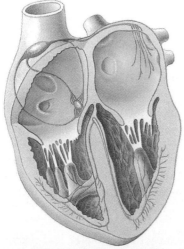

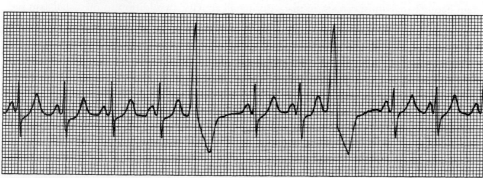

FIGURES 6-7 D

Premature artrial contractions.

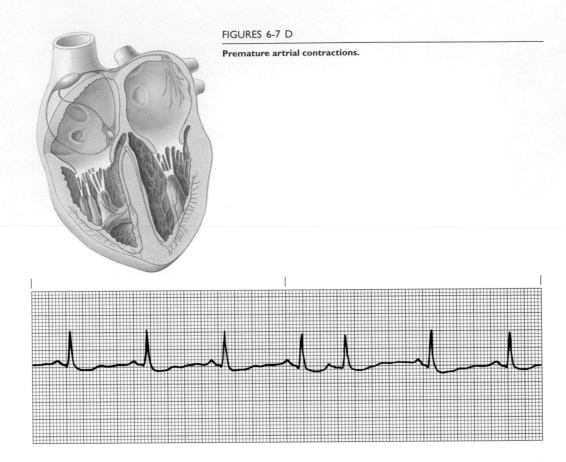

► HOLTER MONITOR

The Holter monitor is performed when the ECG is not conclusive or the cardiac irregularity was not captured on the tracing. The Holter monitor records cardiac activity while the patient is ambulatory for at least a 24 hour period. A small tape recorder and a patient diary are used to detect heart irregularities that are infrequent and not detected on the standard 12-lead cardiogram. It may be set to record continuously and/or to record when the patient presses an "event" button at the onset of symptoms. A medical assistant may instruct the patient and apply the chest sensors.

Patient preparation should stress the importance of the diary. Patients carry out all routine daily activities except showering or bathing. They must also avoid areas of high voltage as the tape will be affected. Patients use the diary to record their activities during the day. They also indicate in the diary or by depressing an "event button" when they experience any cardiac symptoms, such as chest pain, shortness of breath, or palpitations. See Figure 6-10 A and B for an example of the Holter monitor with and without the patient.

The five special disposable chest sensors are attached more securely than in the 12 lead electrocardiogram because they must remain in place during all activity. In addition to the usual skin preparation to remove oils, areas for attachment may have to be shaved and an abrasive skin cleaner used. Peel off the cover on the adhesive backing and attach one sensor to each of the following locations:

- 3rd intercostal space 2 or 3 inches to the right of the sternum
- 3rd intercostal space 2 or 3 inches to the left of the sternum
- 5th intercostal space at the left sternum margin
- 6th intercostal space at the right anterior axillary line
- 6th intercostal space at the left anterior axillary line

TABLE 6-2 Abnormalities Caused by Cardiac Pathology

Abnormality	Description
Sinus tachycardia	There are over 100 beats per minute; cycles are normal.
Sinus bradycardia	There are less than 60 beats per minute; cycles are normal.
Sinus arrhythmia	Normally seen in children and young adults, all aspects of the EKG are normal except the irregularity. The space between QRS complexes is not equal. The heart rate increases on inspiration and decreases on expiration.
Premature atrial contractions or PACs	There is an early P wave occurring before expected, usually from a source outside the sinus node. Therefore P waves are distorted.
Paroxysmal atrial tachycardia or PAT	This is a common arrhythmia, usually seen in young adults with normal hearts. There are no visible P waves because they are hidden by the T wave of the previous cycle. The atrial rate is between 140-250/minute. In many ways it looks on the ECG like repeated PACs.
Atrial flutter	This rapid fluttering of the upper chambers appears on the electrocardiogram like the pattern of teeth on a saw. The atrial rate is 250-350/minute. Not all the impulses are conducted through the AV node because they are coming too fast. There is some "blockage" at the AV node. This is one type of heart block.
Atrial fibrillation	There are as many as 350 irregular P waves and 130-150 irregular QRS complexes per minute.
AV heart block	The node is diseased and does not conduct the impulse well. There are three types. First degree where the PR interval is prolonged, second degree where some waves do not pass through to the ventricles, and third degree or complete AV block where the atria and ventricles beat independently.
Premature ventricular contractions or PVCs	The wide QRS complexes occur without preceding P waves. They may be caused by electrolyte imbalance, stress, smoking, alcohol or toxic reactions to drugs and in a majority of patients who have had a heart attack.
Ventricular tachycardia	Three or more consecutive PVCs. Usually originating below the SA node, the complexes are wide and bizarre in appearance.
Ventricular fibrillation	The waves are irregular and rounded, the contractions uncoordinated. Death may occur in as little as 4 minutes.
MI or myocardial infarction	There are broad and deep Q waves. Old injury: The ST segment is usually depressed below the baseline. New Injury: The ST segment is usually elevated above the baseline. Angina pectoris is the name for the syndrome of pain and oppression in the anterior chest due to heart tissue being deprived of oxygen. If this pain lasts 20-30 minutes, suspect a myocardial infarction in which the heart tissue is actually dying.

▶ PULMONARY FUNCTION

Pulmonary function tests are performed to evaluate lung volume and capacity, to assist in the differential diagnosis of patients with suspected pulmonary dysfunction (obstructive or restrictive disease processes), and to assess the effectiveness of drug therapies. These tests may be done by physicians devoted to primary care or allergy, or by a specialist in lung diseases (pulmonologist).

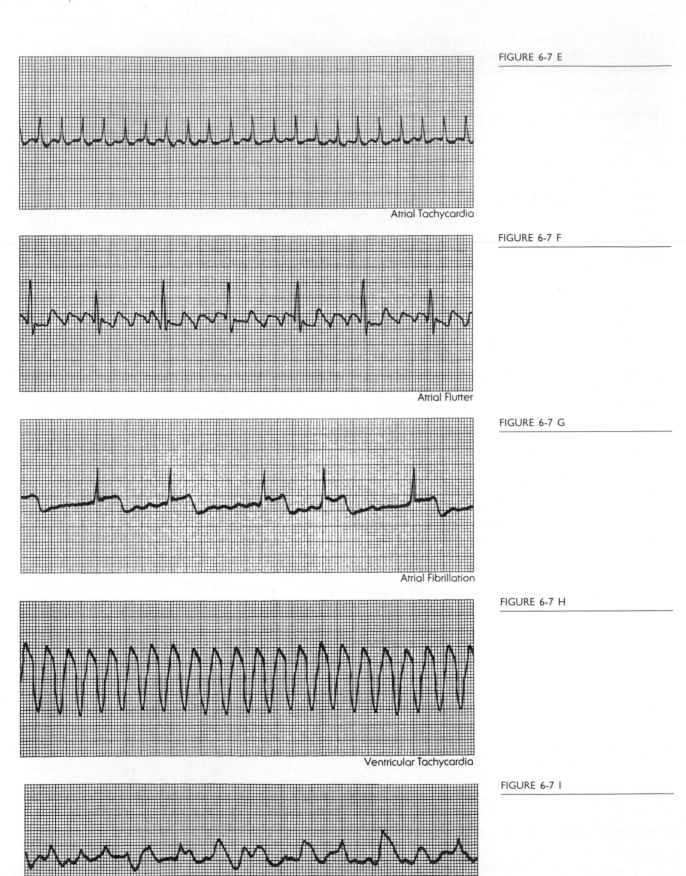

FIGURE 6-7 E

Atrial Tachycardia

FIGURE 6-7 F

Atrial Flutter

FIGURE 6-7 G

Atrial Fibrillation

FIGURE 6-7 H

Ventricular Tachycardia

FIGURE 6-7 I

Ventricular Fibrillation

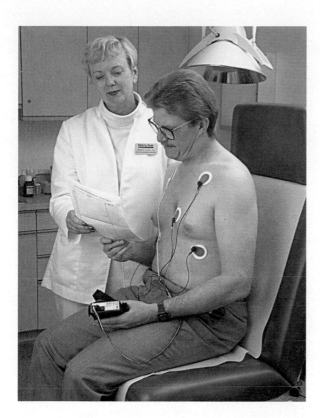

FIGURE 6-8

Technician with EKG read-out.

Sometimes patients complain of difficulty breathing after minimal exertion, or shortness of breath. Other patients have no symptoms or may have been diagnosed with asthma, chronic bronchitis, emphysema, cystic fibrosis or a combination of these. An awareness of the long-term effects of smoking and exposure to occupational or environmental toxins has increased the frequency with which this assessment is performed. Because lung disease tends to worsen with age, it is important to make a diagnosis early and, thereby, slow the rapid loss of function that occurs without treatment. Allergic patients may undergo a status change quite suddenly. Pulmonary patients can expect to have pulmonary function tests performed quite frequently.

▶ PULMONARY VOLUME TESTS

The first part of the procedure is to discover the amount of air the lungs move normally, and how much lung space is available after a normal inhale and a normal exhale. These are called **pulmonary volume tests** and there are four of them:

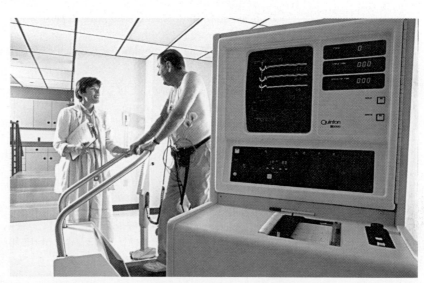

FIGURE 6-9

The patient must be observed very closely during a stress test.

PROCEDURE: Treadmill Stress Test

**Terminal Performance
Competency:** Will be able to apply monitors, instruct the patient, monitor and record ECG, BP, and heart rate periodically and make adjustments to the treadmill as requested with 100% accuracy, without assistance.

Equipment and Supplies
Treadmill
Sensors
Blood pressure monitor

Procedural Steps
1. Assemble necessary supplies.
2. Plug in the power cord and turn on the machine.
3. Verify that the treadmill is operational.
4. Identify, interview, and instruct the patient. Offer female patients a gown, to be worn to open down the front.
5. Perform a baseline ECG.
6. Disconnect the patient cable from the ECG machine.
7. Attach a sphygmomanometer to the patient's arm.
8. Permit the patient to walk about the room or on the slow moving treadmill to see what it feels like.
9. Connect the patient to all recording devices.
10. The physician will determine the pace and incline of the treadmill.
11. Record BP, ECG, and heart and respiratory rate periodically as you observe the patient's face for redness, difficulty breathing, chest pain, and so on.
12. When the test is completed, clean the patient's skin and assist with dressing as needed.
13. Organize the documentation into the patient record.

Charting Example
3/11/XX   2:10 PM   Stress test performed and tolerated well.   M. King, CMA (AAMA)

- Tidal Volume is abbreviated VT. It is the amount of air inhaled or exhaled during normal breathing (about 500 ml).
- Expiratory Reserve Volume is abbreviated ERV. This is the amount of air that can be forcibly exhaled after a normal exhale.
- Inspiratory Reserve Volume is abbreviated IRV. It is the amount of air that can be forcibly inspired after a normal inhale.
- Residual Volume is abbreviated RV. It is the volume of air left in the lungs at the end of an exhale (around 1200 ml).

From these volume tests, pulmonary capacity can be calculated, based on two or more volumes. Capacities include:

- Total Lung Capacity, or TLC, is the volume of the lungs at peak inspiration, and is equal to the sum of the four volumes above.
- Vital Capacity, or VC, is the amount of air that can be exhaled following forced inspiration and includes maximum expiration.
- Inspiratory Capacity, or IC, is the amount of air that can be inhaled after normal expiration.
- Functional Residual Capacity, or FRC, is the amount of air remaining in the lungs after a normal expiration.

Total Lung Capacity and Functional Residual Capacity will increase in **obstructive lung disease** (those diseases that obstruct the flow of air out of the lungs and generally slow expiratory rate and

PROCEDURE: Applying a Holter Monitor

Terminal Performance

Competency: Will be able to apply a Holter monitor, instruct the patient and obtain a satisfactory recording with 100% accuracy, without assistance.

Equipment and Supplies

Holter monitor with sensors, patient cable

Patient activity diary

Fresh batteries

Blank recording tape

Adhesive tape

Razor

Alcohol

Procedural Steps

1. Assemble necessary supplies.
2. Install new batteries and a blank tape.
3. Verify that the machine is operational.
4. Identify, interview, and instruct the patient.
5. Have the patient remove clothing to the waist (female patients may wear a gown opened down the front) and sit on an examination table.
6. Prepare the electrode sites and attach the electrodes.
7. Attach the wires so that they point toward the feet and connect the patient cable.
8. Secure each sensor with adhesive tape.
9. Connect the patient cable to the ECG machine and record a baseline cardiogram.
10. Assist the patient with replacing his or her shirt. Extend the cable between the buttons or under the hem.
11. Place the recorder in the carrying case and either attach to the patient's belt or to the shoulder strap. Check that there is no tension on the wires.
12. Plug the cable into the recorder.
13. Record the starting time in the diary.
14. Confirm an understanding of what the patient is to do.
15. Confirm the time for return to the clinic for removal of the Holter monitor.
16. Dismiss the patient.
17. Chart the procedure in the patient's record. Sign or initial your work.

Charting Example

3/11/XX   2:10 PM Holter monitor applied and instruction given. Will return in 24 hours. M. King, CMA (AAMA)

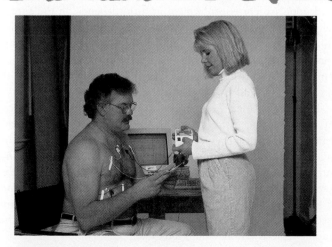

FIGURE 6-10 A

Holter monitor with patient.

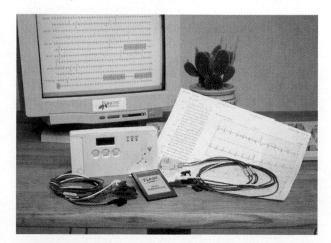

FIGURE 6-10 B

Holter monitor equipment.

increase residual volume). Patients with asthma have a decreased ability of the lungs to deflate during expiration. In **restrictive lung disease** the volumes are decreased because expansion of the lungs is prevented, thereby diminishing total lung capacity, vital capacity, and inspiratory capacity.

These tests are performed by a Respiratory Care Specialist, usually in a hospital setting, as ordered by the Pulmonologist. The capacities are included here because, in working with the specialist and pulmonary patient, you encounter the terms and volumes. It is helpful to know what they describe. To continue monitoring the effects of respiratory disease, an evaluation can be carried out by the medical assistant in an office or clinic.

VOLUME CAPACITY SPIROMETRY

A diagnostic spirometer is employed to evaluate the patient's ability to ventilate during a maximum forced exhale. This device measures and records the volume exhaled and the time required to do so. This air movement is recorded on special paper with vertical second marks and horizontal liter marks in one of three ways:

- Forced Vital Capacity (FVC)—Amount of air exhaled after maximum inspiration or one of the two timed FVCs
- Forced Expiratory Volume in 1 second (FEV1)—Amount of air exhaled on 1st second of FVC maneuver
- Maximal Midexpiratory Flow (MMEF)—Average flow rate during middle half of FVC

Figure 6-11 shows one type of spirometer.

PATIENT PREPARATION

The patient must have accurate instructions and reassurance with questions answered. Generally, preparation begins when the patient schedules the appointment. Patients should eat lightly and not smoke prior to the test, and should avoid using analgesics or bronchodilators for 24 hours prior to the test, if the physician so orders.

SPIROMETRY PROCEDURE

When the patient arrives for the procedure, obtain his or her height, weight, and vital signs. Reassure patients that they will be given time to rest if dyspnea or fatigue occur during the test. The test will be stopped if the patient experiences any chest pain, palpitations, nausea, or wheezing. After a basic test, some patients are asked to breathe an aerosolized bronchodilator, and the physician evaluates the value of the drug in causing an increase in capacity. The graphic test results become part of the patient's permanent record.

Spirometric measurements depend upon patient effort, which, in turn, depends on the coaching of the medical assistant. Generally, 3 good measurements are performed and the best is considered for evaluation. Patients usually need some practice with wrapping their lips around the disposable mouthpiece and forcibly exhaling. Next, the patient may wish to experiment with a standing versus sitting position. Since it makes no difference with the results, the choice depends on patient comfort.

There are a variety of spirometers available in the marketplace, but they must meet minimum standards for acceptable performance. When using automated computerized machines, the spirometry procedure is complicated by the necessity of dealing with the computer program. You must enter patient data into the computer, such as age, height, weight, vital signs, medication, and so forth, depending on the machine and the computer program used. The machine usually makes predictions about what the graphic representation should look like.

The basic spirometry procedure is as follows: Plug in and turn

Med Tip: Remind the patient that it is important to blow hard and fast from the very beginning, as if all the candles on the birthday cake were not extinguished. The patient should avoid doubling over at the waist. Demonstrate the maneuver and have the patient practice. Then begin, reminding the patient to take as deep a breath as possible, blast the air out hard and fast, and keep blowing, blowing, blowing until told to stop.

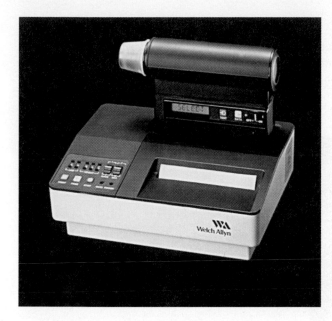

FIGURE 6-11

One type of spirometer.

on the machine, allowing it to warm up. Verify that the equipment is operational. Explain the procedure to the patient. The patient will breathe in and out through a mouthpiece. The quantity of this air is measured and the nose is kept shut with a nose clip. Apply the nose clip to the patient's nose and allow the patient to adjust it for comfort. Set the machine according to the manufacturer's guidelines. Have the patient take a big breath in. Have the patient place the mouthpiece in his or her mouth and seal the lips around the mouthpiece. Push the start button at the same time as you instruct the patient to "blow". Have the patient exhale as hard, fast, and long as possible, while you coach to "blow, blow, blow. . . ." Most machines will have you stop at this point—you have recorded the forced vital capacity, forced expiratory volume at 1 second, and the mean expiration flow rate. With a few other machines, the patient must record an inhale. Keeping the tube in his or her mouth, have the patient take a big breath in. Have the patient exhale normally. Remove the noseclip and mouthpiece, permitting the patient to rest. Repeat this procedure as often as needed, up to eight attempts. Submit the best of three acceptable trials to the physician.

There are changes anticipated with lung disease. Note that in obstructive disease, more time is required for a complete exhale, and in a restrictive pattern, maximum exhale is reached quickly but the volume is small.

With the test results, the patient's pulmonary measurement is compared to the predicted values for the patient's height, weight, age, race and sex by the physician who takes into account the patient's clinical status at the same time. Clinical status refers to the patient's physical condition at the time of the test. A fever, asthma attack, poor night's sleep, scoliosis, or any of a number of other variables could affect the pulmonary function results. A prediction indicator result of 85% to 100% would indicate no impairment; 75-85% would be slight impairment, and so on.

▶ PEAK FLOWMETER

A patient may use a flowmeter at home to monitor breathing and assist the physician with determining the medication regimen that is most effective. On a "good" day, the patient blows as hard as possible into the device to establish a goal or baseline against which to compare other expiratory attempts.

▶ OXIMETER

For patients suffering from cardiac and pulmonary disorders it may be necessary to determine the oxygen content of the blood. An electronic device called an oximeter, which can be clipped on the bridge of the nose, the forehead, earlobe, or to the tip of a finger, determines the oxygen concentration in arterial blood. A pulse oximeter is illustrated in Figure 6-12.

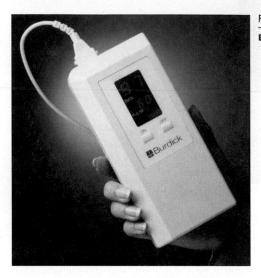

FIGURE 6-12

Burdick 100 Pulse Oximeter.

PROCEDURE: Performing Spirometry

Terminal Performance
Competency: Will be able to obtain spirometric results (instruct the patient and obtain a satisfactory recording) with 100% accuracy, without assistance.

Equipment and Supplies
Functioning spirometry machine
Nose clip
Mouthpiece

Procedural Steps
1. Plug in and turn on the machine; verify that the equipment is operational.
2. Explain the procedure to the patient.
3. Apply the noseclip to the patient's nose.
4. Set the machine according to the manufacturer's guidelines. All spirometers will be different even though they operate on the same principle. Some require movement of parts.
5. Have the patient take a big breath in.
6. Have the patient place the mouthpiece in his or her mouth and seal his or her lips around the mouthpiece.

7. Push the start button at the same time as you give instructions to the patient.
8. Have the patient blast breath out as hard, fast, and long as possible.
9. Repeat the procedure to get three good trials, up to eight attempts.
10. Submit to the physician the best of three trials. Some computerized machines will select the best attempt and print it.

Note: All equipment, including tubing and disposable mouthpieces should be properly cleaned or disposed of after use, using Standard Precautions.

Charting Example
3/11/XX   2:10 PM   Spirometry performed
with 3 good results.   M. King, CMA(AAMA)

LEGAL AND ETHICAL ISSUES

Provide an appropriate explanation to reinforce the physician's explanation of the necessary procedure. Accurate understanding assists the patient in giving expressed or written consent and in being cooperative.

Perform your cardiac and pulmonary diagnostic tasks quickly and accurately. Improper technique or error could affect the patient's diagnosis and treatment. However, if an error is made, admit it and seek to put things right, even if it is embarrassing to you.

The patient's right to privacy and dignity must be considered at all times. Many procedures performed by the internist and specialist are uncomfortable for the patient. The medical assistant must respect the patient's need for privacy during these tests.

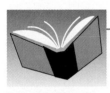

PATIENT EDUCATION

Patients with pulmonary disease may need some educational materials on breathing exercises, a moderate exercise program, the avoidance of inhaled irritants, and the use of an inhaler. As you work in these areas you will pick up some interesting tips from other patients that you can pass along.

Many patients need dietary guidance, especially regarding the reduction of salt and cholesterol, and some will need information about weight loss and moderate exercise programs. Never give out materials or educational information without the specific direction of the physician.

Summary

The use of electrocardiography and spirometry for the early diagnosis and treatment of heart and lung disease has contributed to the lengthened life expectancy of many patients and has improved their quality of life. Accuracy in carrying out your duties during these tests will provide the physician with the best possible data to make that diagnosis and institute the correct treatment.

Competency Review

1. Define and spell the glossary terms for this chapter.
2. Describe how to maintain and operate electrocardiograph equipment; pulmonary function equipment.
3. Identify by name and the location of their sensors the standard 12 leads on an electrocardiograph machine.
4. Name and describe six abnormalities that can be detected in an electrocardiogram.
5. Explain Forced Vital Capacity (FVC), Forced Expiratory Volume in 1 second (FEV1), and Maximal Mixexpiratory Flow (MMEF).
6. Explain the difference(s) between *obstructive* and *restrictive* pulmonary disease.

PREPARING FOR THE CERTIFICATION EXAM

Test Taking Tip — When studying a textbook in preparation for an examination, write in the margin of the book the important word or concept covered in each paragraph. Then do a final quick study for the examination by just reviewing the notes in the margin.

Examination Review Questions

1. An artifact in leads 1, 2, and AVR would cause you to recheck the sensors attached to which body part?
   - (A) chest
   - (B) left arm
   - (C) left leg
   - (D) right arm
   - (E) right leg

2. When performing an EKG on a patient with a right lower leg cast, the leg sensors are placed
   - (A) on the left leg
   - (B) on both upper legs
   - (C) on both upper arms
   - (D) on the bottom of the feet
   - (E) they are eliminated

3. An electrocardiogram is a
   - (A) recording of the voltage with respect to time
   - (B) recording of the mechanical action of the heart
   - (C) technique for making recordings of heart activity
   - (D) machine used to make cardiac tracings
   - (E) recording of the size of the heart

4. Normally, a complete EKG consists of ___sensors and ___leads
   - (A) 10, 10
   - (B) 8, 10
   - (C) 6, 12
   - (D) 12, 10
   - (E) 10, 12

5. The SA node is located in or on the
   - (A) right atrium
   - (B) right ventricle
   - (C) apex
   - (D) valve between the right atrium and right ventricle
   - (E) septum between the atria

6. The portion of the EKG that relates to ventricular depolarization is the
   - (A) P wave
   - (B) QRS complex
   - (C) T wave
   - (D) U wave
   - (E) P-R interval

7. A standard limb lead monitors voltage from
   - (A) any limb sensor
   - (B) any two limb sensors
   - (C) the chest sensor
   - (D) two of the following: RA, LL, RL
   - (E) two of the following: RA, LA, LL

8. The little "spark" that begins or starts the heart beat originates in the
   - (A) Purkinje fibers
   - (B) Vagus nerve
   - (C) SA node
   - (D) AV node
   - (E) artificial pacemaker

9. The correct order of stimulation in the electrical conduction system of the heart is
   - (A) AV node, SA node, bundle of His, bundle branches, Purkinje network
   - (B) SA node, AV node, bundle of His, bundle branches, Purkinje network
   - (C) Bundle of His, AV node, SA node, bundle branches, Purkinje network
   - (D) Purkinje network, Purkinje fibers, SA node, AV node
   - (E) bundle of His, SA node, AV node, bundle branches, Purkinje network

10. Leads 1, 2, and 3 (I, II, III) are called
    - (A) standard limb or bipolar leads
    - (B) Welch sensors
    - (C) augmented leads
    - (D) chest leads
    - (E) precordial leads

Section Three

CERTIFICATION
EXAM PREPARATION

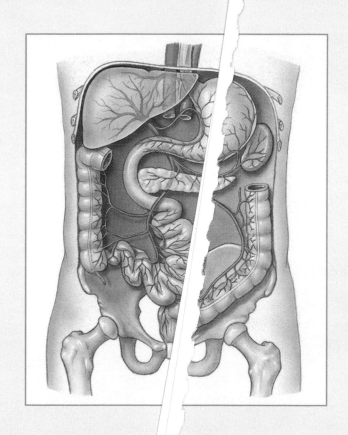

► CHAPTER 7, PART ONE: ELECTROCARDIOGRAPHY REVIEW

1. The heart is located

   (A) on the right side of the chest
   (B) entirely on the left side of the chest
   (C) behind the scapula
   (D) between the lungs
   (E) just to the right of the liver

   (D) is correct. The heart is located between the lungs and slightly to the left side of the body.

2. The serous inner membrane lining of the heart is the

   (A) myocardium   (D) pacemaker
   (B) endocardium   (E) cardiac cycle
   (C) pericardium

   (B) is correct. The endocardium is the serous inner membrane lining of the heart.
   (A) The myocardium is the muscular middle layer of the heart.
   (C) The pericardium is the double-walled sac surrounding the heart.
   (D) The pacemaker is the portion of cardiac electrical tissue that establishes the beat. This is also known as the sinoatrial (SA) node.
   (E) The cardiac cycle is one heartbeat, designed arbitrarily as P, Q, R, S, and T. It consists of contraction and relaxation of both atria and ventricles. It is one pulse.

3. The primary purpose of the heart valves is to

   (A) force blood through the chambers of the heart
   (B) prevent blood from rushing through the heart too fast
   (C) separate the chambers of the heart
   (D) prevent the backward flow of blood
   (E) none of the above

   (D) is correct. The primary purpose of the heart valves is to prevent the backward flow of blood.

4. When listening to the heart with a stethoscope, the sound heard is actually the

   (A) epicardium   (D) myocardium
   (B) the closing of the heart valves   (E) pericardium
   (C) pacemaker

   (B) is correct. The sound heard through the stethoscope is actually the closing of the heart valves.
   (A) The epicardium is the outer layer of the heart.
   (C) The pacemaker of the heart is located in the sinoatrial node and is silent.
   (D) The myocardium of the heart is the muscular middle layer of the heart.
   (E) The pericardium of the heart is the double-walled sac surrounding the heart.

5. The SA node, located in the right atrium of the heart, is known as the

   (A) sensor   (D) pacemaker of the heart
   (B) electrode   (E) C and D
   (C) sinoatrial node

   (E) is correct. The sinoatrial (SA) node is known as the pacemaker of the heart.
   (A) A sensor is a device that detects electrical charges, also called an electrode.
   (B) An electrode and sensor are the same.

6. The SA node is located in or on the

   (A) right atrium
   (B) right ventricle
   (C) apex
   (D) valve between right atrium and right ventricle
   (E) septum between atria

      (A) is correct. The SA node is located in or on the right atrium.

7. The "little spark" that begins or starts the heartbeat originates in the

   (A) Purkinje fibers
   (B) vagus nerve
   (C) SA node
   (D) AV node
   (E) artificial pacemaker

      (C) is correct. The SA node produces the "little spark" that begins or starts the heartbeat and sets its pace. The SA node has a rate between 60 and 80 impulses per minute.
      (A) The Purkinje fibers extend from the right and left bundle branches of the heart to the ventricular walls and cause the ventricles to contract.
      (B) The vagus nerve is the 10th cranial nerve. It affects the actions of the heart, pharynx, larynx, lungs, bronchi, esophagus, stomach, small intestines, and gallbladder.
      (D) The atrioventricular (AV) node is a cardiac muscle located in the lower right atrial septum.
      (E) An artificial pacemaker is one that is surgically implanted into a patient's chest, which will automatically control the rate of the heart.

8. The correct order of stimulation in the electrical conduction system of the heart is

   (A) bundle of HIS, AV node, SA node, bundle branches, Purkinje network
   (B) AV node, SA node, bundle of HIS, bundle branches, Purkinje network
   (C) SA node, AV node, bundle of HIS, bundle branches, Purkinje network
   (D) Purkinje network, Purkinje fibers, SA node, AV node
   (E) bundle of HIS, SA node, AV node, bundle branches, Purkinje network

      (C) is correct. The order of stimulation in the electrical conduction of the heart originates in the SA node and moves through the AV node, bundle of HIS, bundle branches, and Purkinje network.

9. The portion of the EKG that relates to ventricular depolarization is the

   (A) P wave
   (B) QRS complex
   (C) T wave
   (D) U wave
   (E) P-R interval

      (B) is correct. The QRS complex is the portion of the EKG that relates to ventricular depolarization.
      (A) The P wave is the first upward deflection and represents atrial depolarization (contraction).
      (C) The T wave represents the electrical repolarization (recovery), which gives the cells time to recharge in preparation for ventricular depolarization (contraction).
      (D) The U wave, when present, is a small upward deflection, which occurs after the T wave.
      (E) The P-R interval occurs at the beginning of the P wave and ends at the onset of the QRS wave. It represents the conduction of the electrical impulse through the atria from the SA node to the AV node.

10. The contraction and relaxation of both atria and ventricles equal

   (A) one cardiac cycle
   (B) two cardiac cycles
   (C) three cardiac cycles
   (D) four cardiac cycles
   (E) none of the above

   (A) is correct. One cardiac cycle consists of the contraction and relaxation of both atria and ventricles.

11. The electrical state of the heart in which the cardiac cells are in a state of resting is

   (A) depolarization
   (B) polarization
   (C) negatively charged
   (D) A and C
   (E) B and C

   (E) is correct. During the state of polarization, the cardiac cells are in a state of rest and are negatively charged.

12. When the cardiac cells are discharging a positively charged electrical impulse, which creates a contraction, they are said to be in a state of

   (A) repolarization
   (B) depolarization
   (C) polarization
   (D) rest
   (E) none of the above

   (B) is correct. The cardiac cells are in a state of depolarization when they are discharging a positive electrical impulse and in a state of contraction.
   (A) Repolarization or recovery occurs when cardiac cells are transformed from a state of depolarization (active) to a state of polarization (rest).
   (C) Polarization occurs when the cardiac cells are negatively charged and in a state of rest.

13. What wave on an EKG reflects the repolarization of the ventricles?

   (A) P wave
   (B) QRS wave
   (C) T wave
   (D) U wave
   (E) none of the above

   (C) is correct. The T wave reflects the repolarization of the ventricles.
   (A) The P wave reflects the electrical impulse coming from the atria.
   (B) The QRS wave represents the electrical impulse as it passes through the ventricles.
   (D) The U wave, when present, is the small upward deflection that follows a T wave.

14. An electrocardiogram is a

   (A) recording of the mechanical action of the heart
   (B) recording of the voltage with respect to time
   (C) technique for making recordings of heart activity
   (D) machine used to make cardiac tracings
   (E) recording of the size of the heart

   (B) is correct. An electrocardiogram is a recording of the voltage with respect to time.

15. An electrocardiogram is also referred to as an

   (A) ECG
   (B) EKG
   (C) EEG
   (D) A and B only
   (E) A, B, and C

   (D) is correct. The abbreviations ECG and EKG both mean electrocardiogram.
   (C) EEG stands for electroencephalogram, which is a study of the electrical impulses of the brain.

16. Another name for an electrode is a/an

(A) lead

(B) tracing

(C) sensor

(D) channel

(E) artifact

(C) is correct. An electrode is also called a sensor.

(A) A lead is an electrical connection to the body to receive data from a specific combination of sensors.

(B) A tracing is a recording of data.

(D) On an EKG machine capable of receiving more than one signal at once, a channel is the pathway for one signal.

(E) An artifact is a deflection caused by electrical activity other than from the heart. This is an irregular and erratic marking.

17. Normally, a complete ECG/EKG consists of how many sensors and how many leads?

(A) 8, 10

(B) 10, 10

(C) 6, 12

(D) 12, 10

(E) 10, 12

(E) is correct. A complete ECG/EKG consists of 10 sensors and 12 leads.

18. The type of EKG sensors that appear to be small suction cups are called

(A) styluses

(B) electrolytes

(C) Welch electrodes

(D) leads

(E) none of the above

(C) is correct. The small suction cup sensors are known as Welch electrodes.

(A) A stylus is the penlike apparatus on an EKG machine that records the electrical impulses onto the EKG paper.

(B) Electrolytes are the gel materials applied to the skin to enhance contact between the skin and the sensor.

(D) Leads are the electrical connections to the body to receive data from a combination of sensors.

19. The only cardiac sensor that is NOT actually used in the recording of an EKG is the

(A) LL

(B) RL

(C) RA

(D) LA

(E) all of the above are used

(B) is correct. The right leg (RL) is used to ground the system. The left arm (LA), right arm (RA), and left leg (LL) are all used in recording the EKG.

20. A lead is

(A) one negative pole

(B) one positive pole

(C) one ground

(D) all of the above

(E) none of the above

(D) is correct. A lead consists of one negative pole, one positive pole, and a ground (the right leg).

21. Remembering all of the EKG leads and sensors can be facilitated by visualizing the

(A) Einthoven's triangle

(B) chambers of the heart

(C) polarization and repolarization of the heart

(D) alphabet

(E) none of the above

(A) is correct. Einthoven's triangle is a method for picturing where the leads should be placed.

22. The landmarks for the chest leads for an EKG are the sternum, both clavicles, the left axilla, and the

   (A) right axilla
   (B) supracostal space
   (C) fourth intercostal space
   (D) third intercostal space
   (E) second intercostal space

   (C) is correct. The fourth intercostal space is used as a landmark for the chest leads.

23. The time markers printed on all EKG paper are referred to as

   (A) 1-second markers
   (B) 2-second markers
   (C) 3-second markers
   (D) 4-second markers
   (E) 5-second markers

   (C) is correct. The time markers on the EKG paper are referred to as 3-second markers. They are found at the top of single-channel paper and between channels in multichannel paper.

24. The small squares on EKG paper are

   (A) 1 mm square and represent 0.0 mv of voltage
   (B) 1 mm square and represent 0.1 mv of voltage
   (C) 5 mm square and represent 0.5 mv of voltage
   (D) 5 mm square and represent 0.1 mv of voltage
   (E) none of the above

   (B) is correct. The small squares on EKG paper are 1 mm square and represent 0.1 mv of voltage.

25. To use the EKG to estimate heart rate, you would

   (A) use the "six-second method"
   (B) begin at one 3-second marker and go to the right for 2 additional markers
   (C) count the number of QRS complexes between the first and third markers and add a zero
   (D) all of the above
   (E) none of the above

   (D) is correct. The "six-second method" can be used to estimate the heart rate by beginning at one 3-second marker and moving to the right for 2 additional markers (6 seconds). Then count the number of QRS complexes between the first and third markers and add a zero to get the heart rate.

26. A normal P wave is how many squares/blocks on the EKG paper?

   (A) 2.5
   (B) 3
   (C) 3–5
   (D) can be all of the above
   (E) none of the above

   (B) is correct. A normal P wave is 3 squares or blocks on the EKG paper.
   (A) The duration of the QRS complex is normally 2.5 squares wide.
   (C) The PR interval is normally 3 to 5 small blocks wide.

27. The paper on an EKG machine, as part of an international standard, moves at the rate of

   (A) 10 mm per second
   (B) 15 mm per second
   (C) 20 mm per second
   (D) 25 mm per second
   (E) 30 mm per second

   (D) is correct. The paper on an EKG machine moves at the rate of 25 mm per second.

28. When performing an EKG, if the baseline begins to drift to such a degree that it exceeds the parameters of the graph

   (A) stop the procedure, standardize, and begin again
   (B) reduce the sensitivity from 1 to ½
   (C) decrease the speed with which the paper moves through the machine
   (D) all of the above
   (E) none of the above

   (B) is correct. If the baseline begins to drift to such a degree that it exceeds the parameters of the graph, reduce the sensitivity from 1 to ½.

29. A deflection on an EKG tracing caused by electrical activity other than from the heart is known as a/an

   (A) isoelectric line   (D) artifact
   (B) wave   (E) interval
   (C) segment

   (D) is correct. An artifact is a deflection on an EKG tracing caused by electrical activity other than from the heart.
   (A) The isoelectric line, or baseline, is the point on an EKG line in which there is no electrical charge or activity. This is a flat line on the EKG recording.
   (B) A wave, or deflection, is any upward or downward deviation from zero or the isoelectric (baseline) line.
   (C) A segment on an EKG tracing is the time from the end of one phase to the beginning of another phase. This is the distance between selected wave marks but not including them.
   (E) An interval is the time between the beginning of one phase and the beginning of the next phase.

30. The degree of variation from zero, up or down, in recording the electrical output of the heart is known as the

   (A) isoelectric line   (D) amplitude
   (B) baseline   (E) none of the above
   (C) deflection

   (C) is correct. The degree of variation from zero, up or down, in recording the electrical output of the heart is known as the deflection.

31. During an EKG, a tense muscle or a muscular contraction may produce an artifact called a/an

   (A) erratic stylus defect   (D) baseline shift
   (B) somatic tremor   (E) none of the above
   (C) AC interference

   (B) is correct. A somatic tremor artifact is produced by a tense muscle or muscular contraction during the process of taking an EKG.

32. An artifact in leads 1, 2, and AVR would cause you to recheck the sensors attached to which body part?

   (A) chest   (D) right arm
   (B) left arm   (E) right leg
   (C) left leg

   (D) is correct.

33. A standard limb lead monitors voltage from

   (A) any limb sensor   (D) two of the following: RA, LL, RL
   (B) any two limb sensors   (E) two of the following: RA, LA, LL
   (C) the chest sensor

   (E) is correct. A standard limb lead monitors voltage from two of the following: RA, LA, LL.

34. Lead V1 of the precordial chest leads is placed at the

   (A) fourth intercostal space just to the left of the sternum
   (B) fourth intercostal space just to the right of the sternum
   (C) line midway between leads V2 and V4
   (D) left midaxillary line at the same level as V4
   (E) left midclavicular line in the fifth intercostal space

      (B) is correct. Lead V1 is placed at the fourth intercostal space just to the right of the sternum.
      (A) Lead V2 is placed at the fourth intercostal space just to the left of the sternum.
      (C) Lead V3 is placed at the line midway between leads V2 and V4.
      (D) Lead V6 is placed at the left midaxillary line at the same level as lead V4.
      (E) Lead V4 is placed at the left midclavicular line in the fifth intercostal space.

35. Lead I of the limb leads measures electrical activity from the

   (A) left arm to left leg (LA to LL)   (D) augmented vector right side
   (B) right arm to left leg (RA to LL)   (E) augmented vector left side
   (C) right arm to left arm (RA to LA)

      (C) is correct. Lead I of the limb leads measures electrical activity from the right arm to the left arm (RA to LA).
      (A) Lead III of the limb leads measures electrical activity from the left arm to the left leg (LA to LL).
      (B) Lead II of the limb leads measures electrical activity from the right arm to the left leg (RA to LL).
      (D) The augmented vector for the right side is indicated by aVR.
      (E) The augmented vector for the left side is indicated by aVL.

36. The marking codes used on the older models of EKG machines indicate lead III as

   (A) .   (D) ---
   (B) ..   (E) -.
   (C) ...

      (C) is correct. Three dots (...) mark lead III on the EKG paper.
      (A) One dot (.) indicates lead I.
      (B) Two dots (..) indicate lead II.
      (D) Three dashes (---) indicate AVF lead.
      (E) A dash and dot (-.) indicate V1 lead.

37. When performing an EKG on a patient with a right lower leg cast, the leg sensors are

   (A) on the left leg   (D) on the bottom of the feet
   (B) on both upper legs   (E) eliminated
   (C) on both upper arms

      (B) is correct. The leg sensors are placed on both upper legs when performing an EKG on a patient with a right lower leg cast.

38. A majority of patients who have had a heart attack have an EKG tracing that exhibits

   (A) PACs   (D) a ventricular fibrillation
   (B) PVCs   (E) AV heart block
   (C) a PAT

      (B) is correct. Premature ventricular contractions (PVCs) appear in the heart tracings of a majority of patients who have had a heart attack.
      (A) Premature atrial contractions (PACs) occur when an early P wave appears before expected, usually from a source outside the sinus node.
      (C) A paroxysmal atrial tachycardia (PAT) is a common arrhythmia, seen in young adults with normal hearts. There are no visible P waves. The atrial rate is between 140 and 250/minute.

(D) Ventricular fibrillation appears on the EKG tracing as irregular and rounded waves in which the contractions are uncoordinated. Death may occur in as little as 4 minutes with ventricular fibrillation.

(E) An AV heart block occurs when the node is diseased and does not conduct the impulse well. There are three types: first-degree, second-degree, and third-degree heart blocks.

39. An elevated T wave may be present on a patient's EKG when the patient

(A) is suffering an acute myocardial infarction
(B) is suffering from ischemia
(C) is taking digitalis
(D) has enlarged ventricles
(E) has an elevated serum potassium

(E) is correct. An elevated T wave may be present if the patient has an elevated serum potassium blood level.
(A) An acute myocardial infarction may be apparent on an EKG with an ST elevation.
(B) Ischemia may be evidenced by a flat, inverted T wave on the EKG.
(C) The drug digitalis may cause an ST depression on the EKG tracing.
(D) Enlarged ventricles may be indicated by a tall R wave on the EKG.

40. One of the dangers of performing a stress test in the medical office is the risk of a

(A) tachycardia
(B) bradycardia
(C) heart attack
(D) all of the above
(E) none of the above

(C) is correct. One of the dangers of performing a stress test in the medical office is the risk of the patient suffering a heart attack. This is the reason that emergency equipment and a physician should always be in the medical office when a stress test is administered.

41. A device used to record cardiac activity while the patient is ambulatory for at least 24 hours is called a/an

(A) ECG
(B) portable EKG
(C) cardiac stress monitor
(D) Holter monitor
(E) none of the above

(D) is correct. A Holter monitor is a device used to record cardiac activity while the patient is ambulatory for at least 24 hours.

42. The test performed to evaluate lung volume and capacity in a patient is called a

(A) spirometry procedure
(B) pulmonary function test
(C) pulmonary volume test
(D) total lung capacity
(E) none of the above

(B) is correct. A pulmonary function test is performed to evaluate lung volume and capacity in a patient.

► CHAPTER 7, PART TWO: VITAL SIGNS AND MEASUREMENTS REVIEW

1. What part of the brain controls body temperature?

    (A) medulla oblongata   **(D)** hypothalamus
    (B) midbrain   **(E)** cerebrum
    (C) thalamus

    (D) is correct. The hypothalamus is a portion of the brain located just below the thalamus. It controls autonomic nervous system functions, and it is able to adjust the body temperature, appetite, sleep, sexual desire, and emotions such as fear.

    (A) The medulla oblongata, located in the base of the brain, contains the respiratory, cardiac, and vasomotor centers.

    (B) The midbrain is located in the base of the brain in what is commonly referred to as the brain stem. It serves as a two-way conduction pathway, and a relay for visual and auditory impulses.

    (C) The thalamus is located just above the hypothalamus. It acts as a center for relaying impulses from the eyes, ears, and skin to the cerebrum. Perception of pain is controlled by the thalamus.

    (E) The cerebrum is the largest section of the brain. It is located in the upper portion of the brain and is the area that processes thoughts, judgment, memory, association skills, and the ability to discriminate between items.

2. The part of the brain that controls respiratory, cardiac, and vasomotor functions is the

    (A) medulla oblongata   **(D)** hypothalamus
    (B) midbrain   **(E)** cerebrum
    (C) thalamus

    (A) is correct. The medulla oblongata, located in the base of the brain, contains the respiratory, cardiac, and vasomotor centers.

3. Which of the following statements is FALSE?

    (A) the highest body temperature usually occurs in the evening between 5:00 PM and 8:00 PM
    (B) infants and children normally have a lower body temperature than adults
    (C) pregnancy may cause body temperature to rise
    (D) pyrexia is a body temperature above 100.4°F
    (E) hyperpyrexia develops when the body temperature exceeds 105.8°F

    (B) is false. Infants and children normally have a higher body temperature, due to immature heat regulation.

4. Which of the following temperatures is considered normal?

    (A) oral, 98.6°F/37°C   **(D)** aural, 98.6°F/37°C
    (B) rectal, 99.6°F/37.6°C   **(E)** all of the above.
    (C) axillary, 97.6°F/36.4°C

    (E) is correct. All are normal temperatures.

5. Which of the following statements is FALSE?

    (A) the oral method of temperature measurement is the most commonly used
    (B) one of the newest technologies for temperature measurement involves the aural site
    (C) the axillary method has proven to be the most accurate method for temperature measurement
    (D) the rectal route is more reliable than the oral method
    (E) patients who have just eaten, smoked, drunk liquids, or come in from the cold or hot outdoors should not have their temperature taken for a period of at least 10 minutes

    (C) is correct.

6. A temperature of 101 degrees F is equal to how many degrees Celsius?

   (A) 38.3°C   (D) 39.0°C
   (B) 24.1°C   (E) 37.6°C
   (C) 88.1°C

   (A) is correct. To convert Fahrenheit (F) to Celsius (C), subtract 32, then multiply by 5/9. To convert Celsius (C) to Fahrenheit (F), multiply by 9/5 and then add 32.

7. A temperature of 37 degrees Celsius is equal to how many degrees Fahrenheit?

   (A) 70.3°F   (D) 98.6°F
   (B) 98.0°F   (E) 101.2°F
   (C) 99.0°F

   (D) is correct. (See question 6 for the rationale.)

8. When reading a mercury thermometer, each short line represents

   (A) a degree   (D) two-tenths of a degree
   (B) two degrees   (E) three-tenths of a degree
   (C) one-tenth of a degree

   (D) is correct. Each short line represents two-tenths of a degree (0.2). A whole degree is marked with a long line. The even numbered degrees are printed on the thermometer.

9. When taking a rectal temperature on a pediatric patient, insert the thermometer into the anal canal approximately

   (A) 2 to 2½ inches   (D) 1 to 1½ inches
   (B) ¼ of an inch   (E) no more than 3 inches
   (C) ½ to 1 inch

   (C) is correct. For an adult, you may insert the thermometer approximately 1 to 1½ inches into the anal canal.

10. An accurate axillary temperature registers approximately how many degrees lower than a rectal temperature?

   (A) one degree   (D) four degrees
   (B) two degrees   (E) it registers the same as a rectal temperature
   (C) three degrees

   (A) is correct. The average normal temperature orally is 98.6 degrees F, and the average normal rectal temperature is 99.6 degrees F, which equals one degree difference.

11. The average normal rectal temperature is

   (A) 99°F   (D) 101°F
   (B) 97.6°F   (E) 99.6°F
   (C) 98.6°F

   (E) is correct. (See question 10 for the rationale.)

12. The gradual drop of a fever is termed

   (A) lysis   (D) remittent
   (B) crisis   (E) continuous
   (C) intermittent

   (A) is correct.
   (B) Crisis is a sudden drop of a high body temperature to or below a normal level.
   (C) Intermittent describes a fever that is elevated at certain times within a 24-hour period but that falls to normal or subnormal levels during the same period of time.
   (D) Remittent describes a fever that fluctuates frequently but does not fall to normal.
   (E) Continuous describes a fever that remains elevated and does not fluctuate.

13. Which of the following statements is FALSE?

    (A) when taking an aural temperature on an adult, the MA must gently pull upward on the patient's outer ear
    (B) when taking an aural temperature on a pediatric patient, the MA must not pull the child's ear in any direction
    (C) an electronic thermometer has probes for both oral and rectal temperature measurements
    (D) the term afebrile means without fever
    (E) the term sublingual means under the tongue

    (B) is correct. The MA must gently pull downward on an infant's or child's ear when taking an aural temperature.

14. Which of the following statements is TRUE?

    (A) keep a glass/mercury thermometer in place orally for at least 3 minutes
    (B) keep a glass/mercury thermometer under the axilla for at least 10 minutes
    (C) keep a glass/mercury thermometer within the anal opening for 5 minutes
    (D) keep a tympanic thermometer in the aural till it beeps
    (E) all of the above are true

    (E) is correct. It is critical for accuracy to allow the thermometer enough time to register the patient's true temperature. Not keeping a glass/mercury thermometer in place for the appropriate time can lead to inaccurate readings that are below the patient's actual temperature.

15. Which of the following statements is FALSE?

    (A) activity may increase a pulse rate by 20 to 30 beats per minute
    (B) as age increases, pulse rate increases
    (C) female pulse rate is about 10 BPM higher than a male of the same age
    (D) athletes and people in good physical condition tend to have a slower pulse rate
    (E) increased pulse rate in thyroid disease, fever, and shock is due to an increased metabolism

    (B) is correct. As age increases, pulse rate decreases. Remember, infants and children have a faster pulse rate than adults. Pulse rate is proportionate to the size of the body. Heat loss is greater in a small body, resulting in the heart pumping faster to compensate.

16. A child less than 1 year old may have a pulse rate that ranges between

    (A) 50 and 65   (D) 80 and 120
    (B) 60 and 80   (E) 120 and 160
    (C) 70 and 90

    (E) is correct.
       2–6 yrs. = 80–120
       6–10 yrs. = 80–100
       11–16 yrs. = 70–90
       Adult = 60–80
       Older adult = 50–65

17. The force or strength of the pulse is commonly referred to as the

    (A) condition of the arterial wall   (D) pulse pressure
    (B) rhythm   (E) pulse deficit
    (C) volume

    (C) is correct. Volume is noted as full, normal, bounding, weak, feeble, or thready (barely perceptible). Volume is influenced by the forcefulness of the heartbeat, the condition of the arterial walls, and dehydration. A variance in intensity of the pulse may indicate heart disease.
    (A) The condition of the arterial wall should be felt as elastic and soft. A pulse taken in a blood vessel that feels hard and rope-like is considered abnormal and may indicate heart disease, such as arteriosclerosis (narrowing of the artery with loss of elasticity), whereas atherosclerosis refers to hardening of the arteries (note the h when discriminating between arteriosclerosis and atherosclerosis).

(B) Rhythm refers to the regularity, or equal spacing of all the beats, of the pulse. It is not considered abnormal for the heart to occasionally skip a beat. This is referred to as an intermittent pulse. Exercise or caffeine may cause this to occur. An arrhythmia is a pulse lacking in regularity and should be brought to the physician's attention.

(D) Pulse pressure is the difference between the systolic and diastolic readings. This is found by subtracting the diastolic reading from the systolic reading. A p.p. that is greater than 50 mm Hg or less than 30 mm Hg is considered to be abnormal. Extremes of pulse pressure can result in stroke or shock.

(E) Pulse deficit is the difference between the apical and radial pulse rate, taken at the same time by two MAs (or by taking the apical first and then taking the radial immediately after if only one MA is available). A pulse deficit is said to be present if the radial pulse beat is less than the apical. This condition is seen in patients with atrial fibrillation.

18. Hardening of the arteries is referred to as

(A) arteriosclerosis
(B) atherosclerosis
(C) arthrosclerosis

(D) pulse deficit
(E) pulse pressure

(A) is correct.
(B) Atherosclerosis is a form of arteriosclerosis in which yellowish plaques of cholesterol form in the arteries.
(C) Arthrosclerosis is hardening of a joint.
(D) A pulse deficit is the difference between the apical and the radial pulse.
(E) Pulse pressure is the difference between the systolic and diastolic blood pressure.

19. The most common site for taking a pulse on infants and young children is

(A) brachial
(B) pedis
(C) radial

(D) apical
(E) carotid

(D) is correct. The apical pulse is found at the apex of the heart, which is located on the left side of the chest at the fifth intercostal space.
(A) The brachial site is only used on an infant in an emergency and is more typically used when taking blood pressure. It is located on the inner antecubital space of the arm.
(B) Pedis, as in dorsal pedis, refers to the foot (specifically, the top of the foot slightly lateral to the midline). This site should always be checked on patients with diabetes in order to detect adequate circulation in the feet.
(C) A radial pulse on the thumb is the most frequently used site for counting pulse rate in adults.
(E) The carotid site is located between the larynx and the sternocleidomastoid muscle in the side of the neck. This site is used during CPR.

20. When taking a pulse, the medical assistant should count the pulse for at least

(A) 10 seconds
(B) 15 seconds
(C) 20 seconds

(D) 30 seconds
(E) 60 seconds

(E) is correct. Although one may take a pulse for 15 seconds and multiply it by 4, or take a pulse for 30 seconds and multiply it by 2, to get an estimate of BPM, neither allows enough time to adequately evaluate for arrhythmias.

21. What term describes a pulse rate above 100 BPM?

(A) tachycardia
(B) pulse deficit
(C) pulse pressure

(D) thready
(E) bradycardia

(A) is correct. See question 18 for the rationale to (B) and (C). Thready (D) indicates that a pulse rate is barely perceptible. Bradycardia (E) is a term that describes a pulse rate below 60 BPM.

22. Which of the following statements is FALSE?

   (A) fear, anxiety, and anger may cause the pulse rate to rise
   (B) depression, hypothyroidism, or brain injuries that cause intracranial pressure may lower the pulse rate
   (C) it is normal if the heart occasionally skips a beat
   (D) a fever may lower the pulse rate
   (E) shock may increase the pulse rate

   (D) is correct. A fever will cause the pulse rate to increase, due to an increased metabolism.

23. During the process of inspiration, the diaphragm

   (A) moves downward   (D) moves outward
   (B) moves upward   (E) does not move
   (C) moves inward

   (A) is correct. The diaphragm moves downward, the intercostal muscles move outward, and the lungs expand in order to take oxygen into the lungs.

24. The minute air sacs of the lungs are termed

   (A) alveoli   (D) aural
   (B) diaphragm   (E) croup
   (C) medulla oblongata

   (A) is correct. Alveoli are minute air sacs in the lungs.
   (B) The diaphragm is a musculofibrous partition that separates the thoracic and abdominal cavities.
   (C) The medulla oblongata is a vital part of the brain that controls the respiratory, cardiac, and vasomotor centers.
   (D) Aural pertains to the ear or hearing.
   (E) Croup is an acute viral infection of the upper and lower respiratory tract in children that may result in difficult, noisy breathing.

25. The average respiratory rate in adults ranges between

   (A) 30 and 50   (D) 18 and 24
   (B) 20 and 40   (E) 14 and 20
   (C) 20 and 30

   (E) is correct. The adult range for respiratory rate is 14 to 20.
   (A) 30 to 50 is the average range for newborns.
   (B) 20 to 40 is the average range for 1-year-olds.
   (C) 20 to 30 is the average range for 2- to 10-year-olds.
   (D) 18 to 24 is the average range for 11- to 18-year-olds.

26. The average respiratory rate in newborns ranges between

   (A) 120 and 160   (D) 30 and 50
   (B) 80 and 120   (E) 50 and 65
   (C) 60 and 80

   (D) is correct. The average respiratory rate for newborns ranges between 30 and 50.

27. Difficult breathing when lying down is termed

   (A) tachypnea   (D) bradypnea
   (B) orthopnea   (E) apnea
   (C) dyspnea

   (B) is correct. Orthopnea is seen in patients suffering from emphysema or congestive heart failure.
   (A) Tachypnea is characterized by rapid breathing (above 40 RPMs), as seen in patients suffering from high fever or pneumonia.
   (C) Dyspnea is difficulty breathing, as seen in patients suffering with asthma or pneumonia.
   (D) Bradypnea is slow breathing (an adult below 10 RPMs), as seen in patients who are near death.
   (E) Apnea is temporary cessation of breathing, as seen in sleep apnea patients.

28. Which of the following ratios is accurate for the proportion of respiratory rate to pulse rate?

    (A) 10:1   (D) 5:1
    (B) 20:1   (E) 1:5
    (C) 1:4

      (C) is correct. The proportion 1:4 means that for each respiration the heart will generally beat 4 times. (Example: if a patient's respiration rate is 20, the pulse rate will be 4 times greater [20 × 4 = 80 BPM].) This method for estimating a pulse rate is not an acceptable practice for determining a patient's pulse rate. It is simply a general gauge. Since there is a definite correlation between respirations and pulse rates, it is safe to say that the situations that cause the pulse rate to rise or fall will typically cause the respiration rate to rise or fall.

29. Which of the following will cause a decreased respiratory rate?

    (A) allergic reactions   (D) asthma
    (B) epinephrine   (E) fever
    (C) morphine

      (C) is correct. All of the other situations will cause an increase in respiratory rate. In addition, heart disease, exercise, excitement, anger, hemorrhage, high altitudes, shock, and pain will also increase the respiratory rate. However, a decrease of carbon dioxide, a stroke, coma, sleep, and injuries that cause pressure on the brain will decrease the respiratory rate.

30. Cyanosis is due to a/an

    (A) increase in carbon dioxide   (D) rich oxygen levels
    (B) decrease in carbon dioxide   (E) poor carbon dioxide levels
    (C) increase in oxygen

      (A) is correct. Typically when this occurs there is a decrease in oxygen and the patient's skin and/or nail beds may appear bluish in color.

31. Which breath sound resembles the crackling sound of crushing tissue paper and is caused by fluid accumulated in the airways?

    (A) stridor   (D) rhonchi
    (B) rales   (E) wheezes
    (C) stertorous sounds

      (B) is correct. Rales occur with some types of pneumonia.
      (A) Stridor is a shrill, harsh sound that is heard more clearly during inspiration. It may be heard in children with croup and in patients with laryngeal obstruction.
      (C) Stertorous sounds are noisy breathing sounds, such as snoring.
      (D) Rhonchi, or gurgles, are rattling, whistling sounds made in the throat. It is heard in patients with tracheostomies or those requiring suctioning of mucous.
      (E) Wheezes are high-pitched, whistling sounds made when airways become obstructed or severely narrowed, as in asthma or chronic obstructive pulmonary disease (COPD).

32. Which of the following statements is FALSE?

    (A) prior to measuring a patient's respirations, explain the procedure to him or her
    (B) don't take respiration measurements immediately after the patient has experienced exertion
    (C) count each inhalation and expiration as one respiration
    (D) Cheyne-Stokes respiration is a breathing pattern characterized by a period of apnea for 10 to 60 seconds, followed by increased depth and frequency of respirations
    (E) the depth of respiration refers to the volume of air being inhaled and exhaled; it may be described as either shallow or deep

      (A) is correct. One should attempt to keep the patient unaware that respirations are being measured since the patient may alter the breathing pattern. Therefore, the MA should appear to be taking the pulse while he or she is actually taking respirations.

33. The pressure against the walls of the arteries when the heart contracts is considered to be

    (A) hypertension   **(D)** cardiac cycle
    (B) diastolic pressure   **(E)** systolic pressure
    (C) pulse pressure

    (E) is correct. Systolic pressure is the highest pressure that occurs as the heart is contracting.

    (A) Hypertension is simply defined as high blood pressure.

    (B) Diastolic pressure is the lowest pressure level that occurs when the heart is relaxed (the ventricle is at rest).

    (C) Pulse pressure is the difference between the systolic and diastolic readings.

    (D) Cardiac cycle is considered to be the two phases of heart activity—contraction and relaxation. It is identified by two heart sounds (lubb and dubb) occurring during the cardiac cycle.

34. During which of the Korotkoff phases might an auscultatory gap occur?

    (A) I   **(D)** IV
    (B) II   **(E)** V
    (C) III

    (B) is correct. During this phase, the sound has a swishing quality. An auscultatory gap is said to have occurred if there is a total loss of sound at this stage, which then reoccurs later. It may be an indication of heart disease and/or hypertension. Due to this phenomenon, it is advisable to get an estimated systolic reading prior to taking a patient's blood pressure.

    (A) Phase I is the first faint sound heard as the cuff is deflated.

    (C) Phase III sound will become less muffled and develop a crisp tapping sound.

    (D) Phase IV sound will now begin to fade and become muffled. The American Heart Association, which believes Phase IV is the best indicator of the diastolic pressure, recommends the reading at this phase be recorded as the diastolic pressure for a child.

    (E) Phase V sound will disappear at this phase. Some physicians want both Phase IV and Phase V recorded for the diastolic pressure reading (for example, 120/78/74).

35. The average blood pressure reading in children between the ages of 6 and 9 is

    (A) 138/86   **(D)** 100/65
    (B) 120/80   **(E)** 95/65
    (C) 118/76

    (E) is correct.

    (A) 138/86 is the average normal reading for older adults.

    (B) 120/80 is the average normal reading for adults.

    (C) 118/76 is the average normal reading for age 16 to adulthood.

    (D) 100/65 is the average normal reading for 10- to 15-year-olds.

    Newborns tend to have an average normal reading of 50/25. However, blood pressure readings are not generally taken on infants.

36. Which of the following physiological factors may affect blood pressure?

    (A) volume of blood   **(D)** elasticity of vessels
    (B) peripheral resistance   **(E)** all of the above
    (C) condition of the heart

    (E) is correct. All may affect blood pressure.

    (A) An increase of blood volume increases the BP, and a decrease of blood volume decreases BP. For example, polycytopenia increases BP; hemorrhage causes blood volume and BP to drop.

    (B) Peripheral resistance relates to the size of the lumen within blood vessels and amount of blood flowing through them. For example, the smaller the lumen, the greater is the resistance to blood flow, and thus, a high BP.

(C) The condition of the heart, the strength of heart muscle, affects the volume of blood flow. For example, a weak heart muscle can cause an abnormal increase or decrease in BP.

(D) Elasticity of vessels allows them to expand and contract easily. Elasticity decreases with age, and with this an increase in BP is seen.

37. Which is a primary hypertension of unknown cause?

(A) renal
(B) essential
(C) benign

(D) malignant
(E) secondary

(B) is correct.

(A) Renal hypertension is seen with an elevated blood pressure as a result of kidney disease.

(C) Benign hypertension is characterized by a slow onset of elevated blood pressure without symptoms.

(D) Malignant hypertension is a rapidly developing hypertension that may become fatal if not treated immediately.

(E) Secondary hypertension is elevated blood pressure associated with other conditions, such as renal disease, pregnancy, arteriosclerosis, and obesity. Essentially, if you correct the primary condition, such as renal disease, the hypertension will dissipate.

38. Which is a temporary fall in blood pressure that occurs when a patient rapidly moves from a lying to a standing position?

(A) hypotension
(B) postural hypotension
(C) orthostatic

(D) Korotkoff
(E) none of the above

(C) is correct.

(A) Hypotension is abnormally low blood pressure, which may or may not be caused by shock, hemorrhage, and/or central nervous system disorders.

(B) Postural hypotension is a temporary fall in blood pressure from standing motionless for extended periods of time.

(D) Korotkoff refers to the Korotkoff sounds heard in auscultation of blood pressure.

39. Which of the following statements is FALSE?

(A) hypertension has many noticeable symptoms
(B) blood pressure is measured in millimeters of Hg
(C) a patient's BPs are usually tested at least twice before being placed on medication
(D) women generally have lower blood pressure than men
(E) blood pressure tends to increase with age

(A) is correct. Hypertension is often called the silent killer because it is usually asymptomatic, or without any symptoms.

40. Which of the following conditions will cause an increased BP?

(A) anemia
(B) approaching death
(C) exercise

(D) hypothyroidism
(E) infection and fever

(C) is correct. Exercise will cause an increase in BP. Anger, nicotine, caffeine, hyperthyroidism, fear, excitement, liver disease, renal disease, late pregnancy, smoking, and rigidity of blood vessels can also cause an increase in BP. The other conditions can cause a decrease in BP.

41.   Which artery is most commonly used for taking a patient's BP?

    (A)   carotid   **(D)**   dorsalis pedis

    (B)   brachial   **(E)**   apical

    (C)   popliteal

      (B)   is correct. The brachial artery, located at the inner aspect of the antecubital space of the elbow, is the most common artery used in taking BPs.

      (A)   The carotid artery, located between the larynx and the sternocleidomastoid muscle in the side of the neck, is most commonly used to detect a pulse during cardiopulmonary resuscitation.

      (C)   The popliteal artery is located behind the knee.

      (D)   Dorsalis pedis, located on top of the foot slightly lateral to midline, is used to determine adequate circulation to the feet (especially in diabetics).

      (E)   The apical artery, located on the left side of the chest by the fifth intercostal space at the midclavicular line, is found just below the nipple.

42.   Which of the following statements is FALSE?

    (A)   the mercury sphygmomanometer is considered to be the most accurate

    (B)   BP is usually higher in the right arm than the left if the patient is right-handed

    (C)   when taking a blood pressure, the patient's arm should be just below the level of the heart

    (D)   the BP cuff should be placed 1 to 2 inches above the antecubital space

    (E)   BP is measured in mm Hg

      (C)   is correct. The patient's arm should be level with his or her heart.

43.   Which of the following statements is FALSE?

    (A)   when getting an estimated systolic pressure, one should feel the radial pulse while the blood pressure cuff is being inflated

    (B)   when taking a BP, one should inflate the cuff 30 mm Hg above the estimated systolic pressure reading

    (C)   the mercury column should be calibrated to 1

    (D)   a BP that is too small for a patient may give an abnormally high reading

    (E)   if you are unsure about the BP reading, wait at least 1 minute before taking a second reading

      (C)   is correct. The mercury column should be calibrated to zero.

44.   Which of the following will NOT cause an error in blood pressure readings?

    (A)   improper cuff size

    (B)   a loosely applied cuff

    (C)   rapid deflation

    (D)   nervous patient

    (E)   inflating the cuff 30 mm Hg above the previous BP

      (E)   is correct. Inflating the cuff 30 mm Hg above the previous BP will generally not cause an error in BP reading.

45.   One kilogram (kg) is equal to how many pounds?

    (A)   0.45 lb.   **(D)**   4.2 lbs.

    (B)   2.2 lbs.   **(E)**   5.4 lbs.

    (C)   3 lbs.

      (B)   is correct. One kilogram is equal to 2.2 pounds.

46. One pound (lb.) is equal to how many kilograms?

    (A) 0.45 kg.   **(D)** 4.5 kg.
    (B) 0.4 kg.   **(E)** 5.4 kg.
    (C) 3.0 kg.

        (A) is correct. One pound is equal to 0.45 kilogram.

47. Mr. Duffy weighs 220 lbs. How many kilograms does he weigh?

    (A) 48.40 kg.   **(D)** 99.00 kg.
    (B) 26.40 kg.   **(E)** 136.08 kg.
    (C) 102 kg.

        (D) is correct. 220 lbs. $\times$ 0.45 kg. = 99.00 kg.

48. Ms. DeBeir weighs 52.00 kg. How many pounds does she weigh?

    (A) 114 lbs.   **(D)** 195 lbs.
    (B) 144 lbs.   **(E)** 123 lbs.
    (C) 23.40 lbs.

        (A) is correct. 52.00 kg. $\times$ 2.2 lbs. = 114 lbs.

49. Which decimal is equal to ¼ of a pound?

    (A) 0.25   **(D)** 1.25
    (B) 0.75   **(E)** 1.50
    (C) 0.50

        (A) is correct. 0.25 is ¼ of a pound.
        (B) 0.75 is ¾ of a pound.
        (C) 0.50 is ½ of a pound.
        (D) 1.25 is 1¼ of a pound.
        (E) 1.50 is 1½ of a pound.

50. Which of the following statements is FALSE?

    (A) set all weights to zero and check if the scale is calibrated before weighing a patient
    (B) a scale must be calibrated by a trained scale technologist
    (C) ″ is the symbol for inch
    (D) there are 12 inches to 1 foot
    (E) when measuring height, the patient's back should face the scale

        (B) is correct. A medical assistant can calibrate a scale. Set all weights to zero and balance the scale by adjusting the small screw-like knob at one end until the balance bar pointer floats in the center of the frame. (A coin or paper clip can be used if a screw driver is not available to make this adjustment.)

51. Which of the following statements is FALSE?

    (A) an infant's head circumference is usually measured during each checkup until the age of 36 months
    (B) there are 12 ounces to 1 pound
    (C) a small child may be weighed by weighing the mother and then weighing the mother holding the child; subtracting the two weights will give you the weight of the small child
    (D) when weighing an infant, keep one hand over the infant's body as a safety precaution
    (E) never raise the height bar in an opened position

        (B) is correct. There are 16 ounces in 1 pound.

Section Four
APPENDICES

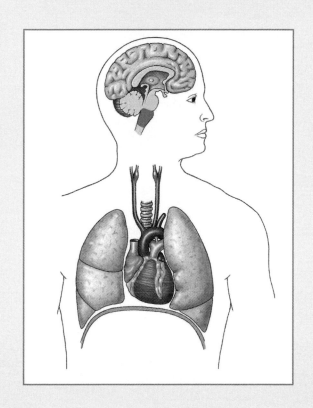

Appendix A

UPDATED SYLLABUS AND PROCEDURE COMPETENCY CHECKLISTS

Contained within this section are updated sheets for your book. Please use these and discard the ones in your books. These sheets were created in an effort to update your course material and assure it meets all requirements by the accrediting bodies.

In accomplishing the tasks required as a medical assistant, it is necessary to be able to incorporate cognitive knowledge (theory) in the performance of psychomotor skills (hands on procedures) and affective skills (behaviors). The new materials provide the procedures that give students the opportunity to demonstrate their ability to take the theory and put it into practice while at the same time exhibiting professional behaviors such

1) Applying critical thinking skills
2) Using language skills that enable patient understanding
3) Demonstrating respect for diversity
4) Displaying sensitivity to patient rights, and
5) Recognizing local, state, and federal legislation that affect the medical assistant's legal scope of practice.

For a more thorough explanation of cognitive, psychomotor, and affective skills, students can visit the Commission on Accreditation of Allied Health Education Programs at http://www.caahep.org/

EVEREST
Medical Assistant Diploma Program

MODULE D—CARDIOPULMONARY AND ELECTROCARDIOGRAPHY

Syllabus and Topic Outline

Prerequisite: None   **Module Length: 20 days**

Date: **Instructor:**

Time:

Module Description:

Module D examines the circulatory and respiratory systems, including the structure and function of the heart and lungs, and diseases, disorders, and diagnostic tests associated with these systems. Students learn about the electrical pathways of the heart muscle in preparation for applying electrocardiography (ECG or EKG) leads and recording a 12-lead electrocardiogram. A cardiopulmonary resuscitation (CPR) course is taught which enables students to respond to cardiac emergencies. Students check vital signs and differentiate between normal values for pediatric and adult patients. They obtain blood samples and prepare syringes and medications for administration. Students learn essential medical terminology, build on their keyboarding and word processing skills, and develop the self-directed job search process by identifying and demonstrating what a successful job interview contains and how to answer common interview questions accurately.

Students attend classes as follows:

Theory Lecture Classroom: 20 hours / module
Computer Classroom: 20 hours / module
Clinical Lab Classroom: 40 hours / module

Quarter Credits

Lecture:	40 Clock Hours /4 Quarter Credits
Lab:	40 Clock Hours / 2 Quarter Credits
Total:	80 Clock Hours / 6 Quarter Credits

The grade scale is as follows: A = 100-90   B = 89-80   C = 79-70   F = 69-0

Student must receive a grade of 70% or above to pass the module.

Module D Textbooks:

Medical Assisting: Module D— Cardiopulmonary and Electrocardiography, Corinthian Colleges, Inc., 2007
Medical Assisting Student Handbook, Corinthian Colleges, Inc., 2007
Insurance Handbook for the Medical Office, 10th edition, Marilyn T. Fordney, W. B. Saunders, 2008
Student Workbook for the Insurance Handbook for the Medical Office, 10th edition, Marilyn T. Fordney, W.B. Saunders, 2008
Medical Transcribing: Techniques and Procedures, 6th edition, Diehl and Fordney, W.B. Saunders, 2007
Introductory Concepts and Techniques: Microsoft Office Word 2003, Shelly, Cashman, Vermaat, Course Technology, Thomson, 2006 and
Introductory Concepts and Techniques: Microsoft Office Excel 2003, Shelly, Cashman, Vermaat, Course Technology, Thomson, 2006
Or (depending on campus software)
Introductory Concepts and Techniques: Microsoft Office Word 2007, Shelly, Cashman, Vermaat, Course Technology, Thomson, 2008 and
Introductory Concepts and Techniques: Microsoft Office Excel 2007, Shelly, Cashman, Vermaat, Course Technology, Thomson, 2008

Dorland's Pocket Medical Dictionary, 28th edition, Elsevier, 2009
Current ICD-9, CPT-4, HCPCS package, Elsevier, 2009
Computers in the Medical Office, 6th edition, Sanderson, McGraw-Hill, 2009

Additional Reference Material: Medical management software, video series, medical dictionary, ICD-9 and CPT coding, and *Physicians' Desk Reference*

Instructional Methods:
Instructors for Module D will use lectures, classroom discussions, hands-on experiences, laboratory exercises, role-playing, presentations, demonstrations, research, and student assignments (depending on section requirements) to facilitate students' achievement of course objectives.

Grading:
The Clinical/Laboratory section grade will be determined as follows:

Hands-on practice and experiences	50%
Tests/quizzes	50%

The grade distribution for Module A is as follows:

Theory	30%
Clinical/Laboratory	40%
Computer/Keyboarding	30%
Total Module D Grade	100%

Attendance:
Students are expected to attend every class session. Make-up work will be allowed only with instructor's approval. Refer to catalog for explanation of attendance policy.

Date of last review: July 2009

Objectives and Topic Outline:

Upon successful completion of this course the student will be able to:

1. Identify and define terms related to basic medical terminology, including prefixes, suffixes, word parts, abbreviations, and symbols. Define and spell the glossary terms for each chapter.
2. Recognize, define, spell, and pronounce the terms related to the diagnosis, pathology, and treatment of the cardiovascular system.
3. Describe the location and general features of the heart.
4. Trace the flow of blood through the heart, identifying the major blood vessels, chambers, and heart valves.
5. Identify the layers of the heart wall.
6. Describe the events of a typical heartbeat, or cardiac cycle.
7. Describe the components and functions of the conducting system of the heart.
8. Describe the structure and function of arteries, capillaries, and veins.
9. Describe how tissues and various organ systems interact to regulate blood flow and pressure in tissues.
10. Distinguish among the types of blood vessels on the basis of their structure and function.
11. Identify the major arteries and veins and the areas they serve.
12. Describe the age-related changes that occur in the cardiovascular system.
13. Identify the diagnostic tests used for cardiovascular conditions.
14. Describe the diseases and disorders of the circulatory and cardiovascular system.
15. Recognize, define, spell, and pronounce the terms related to the diagnosis, pathology, and treatment of the respiratory system.
16. Describe the primary function of the respiratory system.
17. Explain how the delicate respiratory exchange surfaces are protected from pathogens, debris, and other hazards.
18. Relate respiratory functions to the structural specialization of the tissues and organs in the system.
19. Describe the process of breathing.
20. Describe the actions of respiratory muscles in the respiratory movements.
21. Describe how oxygen and carbon dioxide are transported in the blood.
22. Describe the major factors that influence the rate of respiration.
23. Describe the changes that occur in the respiratory system with aging.
24. Identify common diagnostic examinations used in the respiratory assessment
25. Describe the common diseases and disorders of the respiratory system.
26. Identify the four vital signs and the body functions they measure.
27. Explain how the body controls temperature.
28. Describe the different designs of glass clinical thermometers and their appropriate uses.
29. Demonstrate proper techniques for cleaning and storage of non-mercury thermometers.
30. Accurately measure oral, rectal, and axillary temperatures with disposable, electronic, and infrared thermometers, identifying the normal temperature value and relative accuracy of each.
31. Identify situations in which oral measurement of temperature is contraindicated.
32. Define the purpose of taking a pulse, identify how a pulse feels, and locate the pulse points.
33. Identify normal pulse rates and factors, which might affect pulse rate.
34. Accurately measure radial and apical pulse and describe the quality characteristics to be observed.
35. Define pulse deficit, explain its significance, and describe how it is measured.
36. Accurately measure respiration and identify four abnormal breathing patterns.
37. List the five circulatory factors reflected in the measurement of blood pressure.
38. Identify the phases of blood pressure and compare them to the action of the heart.
39. Accurately measure blood pressure by palpation and auscultation, explaining pulse pressure and normal findings.
40. Define and explain auscultatory gap.
41. Practice within the scope of education, training, and personal capabilities while conducting oneself in a courteous and diplomatic manner.
42. Prepare and maintain examination and treatment area.
43. Prepare patients for procedures and demonstrate the medical assistant's responsibilities for these procedures.
44. Explain the electrical conduction system of the heart.

MA (DIP) v1-2 Syllabus Mod D 2009-0717.doc

45. Maintain and operate the electrocardiogram (ECG) and pulmonary function equipment.
46. Demonstrate the correct placement of limb and chest electrodes for an ECG.
47. Perform a routine 12-lead ECG.
48. State the cause and correction of artifacts.
49. Demonstrate the mounting of an ECG tracing and identify the reason for doing so.
50. Identify the purpose of Holter Monitoring and demonstrate the procedure for proper hookup of a Holter Monitor.
51. Identify the purpose of defibrillation.
52. Identify how to perform various pulmonary function tests with patient education and demonstrate how to perform the Peak Flow Meter.
53. Identify legal and ethical responsibilities of the medical assistant when it comes to performing an electrocardiograph and pulmonary function tests.
54. Obtain and provide documentation for certification in basic cardiac life support (BLS Health Care Provider).
55. Identify and demonstrate techniques used for mouth-to-mouth resuscitation (rescue breathing).
56. Identify and demonstrate techniques used for cardiopulmonary resuscitation (CPR) for adults and infants.
57. Identify the various types of interviews that might be experienced by the job applicant.
58. Identify strategies to be used in preparing for an interview.
59. Identify the steps the candidate can take to make the best first impression at a job interview.
60. Identify characteristics employers look for in the ideal candidate.
61. Identify successful strategies for professional conduct during an interview.
62. Demonstrate how to handle typical and tough interview questions.
63. Identify the actions to be taken following an interview.
64. Demonstrate increasing speed and accuracy on the computer keyboard, medical transcription, and acceptable progress through the identified text(s).
65. Demonstrate knowledge and skill in medical terminology and anatomy and physiology by using software to enhance learning and assist in research material for essay assignments.
66. Demonstrate progressive skill acquisition related to word processing, computerized medical office application, and processing of insurance claim forms with acceptable progress through the identified text(s).
67. Conduct (12 lead) resting EKG procedure (5)
68. Mount EKG strip (5)
69. Perform one rescuer CPR
    a. Adult
    b. Infant
70. Perform two rescuer CPR
71. Clear airway of obstruction
    a. Conscious/unconscious Adult
    b. Conscious/unconscious Infant
72. Correctly apply resuscitation mask
73. Identify AED
74. Obtain/document Peak Flow Meter results (3)
75. Conduct appropriate records charting
76. Engage in Career Development
77. Exhibit professionalism
78. Correctly utilize PDR
79. Correctly code for CPT/ICD-9
80. Accurately measure and record TPR (5)
81. Accurately measure and record BP (5)
82. Perform venipuncture to collect blood specimens (2 Vac., 1 Butterfly, 1 Syringe)
83. Administer intradermal injections (3) 18. Administer subcutaneous injections (3)
84. Administer deltoid injections (3)
85. Administer Z-track injections (3)
86. Demonstrate aseptic handwashing (3)
87. Maintain HIPAA and OSHA Guidelines

TOPIC OUTLINE

I. Terminology Associated with the Cardiovascular and Respiratory Systems
   A. Three types of word parts
      1. Prefixes
      2. Suffixes
      3. Root terms
   B. Prefixes
      1 Numbers
      2. Colors
      3. Opposites
      4. Negative
      5. Size/Comparison
      6. Position
   C. Suffixes
      1. Condition
      2. Surgical
      3. Diagnostic
      4. Clinical
      5. Miscellaneous
   D. Root Terms
   E. Anatomical Terms
   F. Medical Abbreviations
   G. The Medical Record
   H. Prescription and Delivery
   I. Using the Medical Dictionary
   J. Anatomy and Physiology of the Cardiovascular System
   K. Anatomy and Physiology of the Respiratory System

II. Anatomy and Physiology of the Circulatory System
   A. The heart and circulation—The circulatory system is a transportation system.
      1. Transports oxygen and nutrients
      2. Transports carbon dioxide and waste material
      3. Blood is the transportation vehicle.
   B. Circulatory system is composed of four main parts
      1. Heart
      2. Blood Vessels
      3. Blood
      4. Lymphatic System
   C. Three different circulatory systems
      1. Pulmonary Circulation
      2. Systemic Circulation
      3. Portal Circulation
   D. Structure of the heart
      1. Each day the heart pumps 4,000 gallons of blood.
      2. Size of fist weighs 1 pound
      3. Located behind sternum
      4. Acts as a pump for the body
   E. Internal anatomy of the heart
      1. Pericardium—a two-layered sac surrounding heart
         a. Visceral Layer—closest to heart
         b. Parietal Layer—outer layer of the sac
         c. Pericardial Fluid—prevents friction during heart activity
      2. Septum—wall in the center of the heart

3. Atria—(2)
    a. Upper chambers collect blood returning to the heart
    b. Right receives blood from the vena cava
    c. Left receives blood from the pulmonary veins
4. Ventricles
F. Heart Valves
    1. Tricuspid Valve
    2. Bicuspid Valve (Mitral Valve)
    3. Semilunar Valves (2)
G. Heart Wall—Three layers
    1. Epicardium—outer layer
    2. Myocardium—middle layer
    3. Endocardium—inner layer
H. Cardiac Muscle Cells
I. Blood Supply to the Heart
J. Heartbeat—Cardiac Cycle
K. Heart Sounds
    1. Lubb-Dubb Sound
    2. Lubb Sound or S1
    3. Dubb Sound or S2
    4. Ventricular Gallop or S3
    5. Atrial Gallop or S4
L. Conducting System of the Heart
    1. Nodal Cells
    2. Conducting Cells
    3. Electrocardiogram
    4. Explain P, Q, R, S, T.
    5. P Wave
    6. QRS Complex
    7. T Wave
    8. Arrhythmias
    9. Control of Heart Rate
M. Blood Vessels—Arteries, Capillaries, and Veins
    1. Arteries
    2. Capillaries
    3. Veins
N. Blood Pressure—pressure of blood being forced against the walls of the arteries
    1. Pressure and resistance affect blood pressure.
    2. Blood is five times thicker than water.
    3. Normal blood pressure is 120/80 mmHg.
    4. Normal range 90–140 mmHg over 60–90 mmHg
    5. Pulse pressure
    6. Radial pulse range 70–75 beats per minute
O. Regulation of blood flow
    1. Short-term responses
    2. Long-term responses
P. Blood vessels of the body
    1. Pulmonary Circulation Pathway
    2. Systemic Circulation Pathway
    3. Hepatic Portal System
    4. Fetal Circulation
        a. Circulatory Changes at Birth

Q. Aging and the Cardiovascular System
   1. Blood
   2. Heart
   3. Blood Vessels
III. Common Diagnostic Tests
   A. Angiogram
   B. Angiography
   C. Cardiac Catheterization
   D. Cardiac Enzymes
   E. Cholesterol
   F. Triglycerides
   G. Ultrasonography
IV. Common Diseases and Disorders
   A. Hypertension
   B. Hypotension
   C. Ischemia
   D. Myocarditis
   E. Mitral Stenosis
   F. Phlebolith
   G. Tachycardia
   H. Thrombosis
   I. Bradycardia
   J. Cardiomegaly
   K. Arrhythmia
V. Anatomy and Physiology of the Respiratory System
   A. Respiration
      1. Pulmonary Ventilation
      2. Gas Exchange
      3. Gas Pickup and Transport
      4. Cellular Respiration
      5. Major Function of the Respiratory System
      6. Provides a defense against pathogenic invasion
   B. Structure of the Respiratory System
      1. Nose
      2. Pharynx
      3. Larynx
      4. Trachea
      5. Bronchi
      6. Bronchioles
      7. Alveoli
      8. Lungs
   C. Physiology of Respiration—Process of Respiration
      1. Pulmonary Ventilation
      2. Inhalation
      3. Exhalation
      4. Movement of Air
         a. Tidal volume
         b. Dead Space
         c. Inspiratory Reserve Volume
         d. Expiratory Reserve Volume
         e. Vital Capacity
   D. Control of Breathing
   E. Aging and the Respiratory System

VI.   Common Diseases and Disorders
  A. Apnea
  B. Anosmia
  C. Influenza
  D. Dyspnea
  E. Hemoptysis
  F. Bronchitis
  G. Cyanosis
  H. Diaphragmatocele
  I. Rhinorrhagia
  J. Asphyxia
  K. Coryza
  L. Emphysema

VII. Common Diagnostic and Laboratory Tests
  A. Acid-Fast Bacilli (AFB)
  B. Antistreptolysisn (ASO)
  C. Arterial Blood Gases (ABGs)
  D. Bronchoscopy
  E. Culture, Sputum
  F. Culture, Throat
  G. Laryngoscopy
  H. Nasopharyngography
  I. Pulmonary Function Test
  J. Rhinoscopy

VIII. Vital Signs
  A. Cardinal Signs
    1. Heat
    2. Rate, Volume, Rhythm of Heart
    3. Rate and Quality of Breathing
    4. Force
  B. Four Indicators Referred to as T, P, R, and BP
    1. Temperature
    2. Pulse
    3. Respiration
    4. Blood Pressure
  C. Temperature
    1. Balance between heat and heat loss
    2. Conditions affecting body temperature
    3. Average normal body temperature
      a. Oral—98.6 F
      b. Axillary—97.6 F
      c. Rectal—99.6 F
    4. Febrile
    5. Afebrile
    6. Controlling Body Temperature
    7. Thermometer Types and Designs
      a. Non-mercury Glass—most accurate
      b. Plastic Disposable
      c. Digital
      d. Electronic Probe
      e. Tympanic Infrared
    8. Reading a Non-mercury Thermometer and Recording
    9. Care of Thermometers
    10. Measuring Oral Temperature

11. Taking Rectal Temperature
12. Taking Axillary Temperature

D. Pulse—throbbing caused by the alternating contractions and expansion of an artery
1. Pulse Points
   a. Radial
   b. Brachial
   c. Carotid
   d. Femoral
   e. Dorsalis Pedis
   f. Popliteal
2. Pulse Rate
3. Pulse Characteristics
   a. Volume
   b. Rhythm
   c. Affected by caffeine and nicotine
4. Measuring Pulse
5. Measuring Apical Pulse
6. Measuring Apical-Radial Pulse

E. Respiration—One respiration is the combination of total inspiration and total expiration.
1. Quality of Respiration
2. Respiration Rate
3. Measuring and Recording Respiration

F. Blood Pressure—Fluctuating pressure that the blood exerts against the arterial walls as the heart alternately contracts and relaxes
1. Measured in brachial artery of arm at antecubital space
2. Maintaining blood pressure depends on two factors.
   a. Strong effective heart
   b. Correctly functioning brain and autonomic nervous system
   c. Both needed for maintaining homeostasis
3. Blood Pressure Phases
4. Normal Blood Pressure
   a. Measured in millimeters of mercury, with a sphygmomanometer and stethoscope
   b. Expressed as a fraction
   c. Normal reading for adults—systolic pressure 100–140 mm Hg and diastolic pressure 60–90 mm Hg
   d. Hypertension
   e. Hypotension
   f. Equipment to be used
   g. Measuring blood pressure
   h. Factors affecting accuracy
   i. Auscultatory Gap
   j. Record blood pressure
   k. Blood pressure in children
   l. Korotkoff sounds
   m. Phase I through V

IX. Electrocardiography and Pulmonary Function
A. Electrocardiogram
B. Mounting the ECG
C. Medical Assistant's Responsibilities
D. Pathway of Electrical Impulses in the Heart
E. ECG or EKG—Procedure
F. Patient Preparation for ECG / EKG
G. Artifacts—unwanted interference on ECG
1. Somatic Tremor
2. Wandering Baseline

3. Alternating Current (AC)
4. Erratic Stylus

H. Holter Monitor—Procedure
I. Patient Instructions
J. Defibrillator
K. Pulmonary Function Tests
   1. Performed to evaluate lung volume capacity
   2. Pulmonary Volume Test
   3. Volume Capacity Spirometry
   4. Patient Preparation
   5. Peak Flow Meter
   6. Oximeter
L. Legal and Ethical Responsibilities
M. General Patient Education

X. Cardiopulmonary Resuscitation (CPR)
   1. Mouth-to-mouth Resuscitation
   2. Airway Obstruction
      a. Conscious / Unconscious Adult
      b. Conscious / Unconscious Infant or Child
   3. Perform cardiopulmonary resuscitation on an adult
      a. One rescuer
      b. Two rescuer
   4. Perform cardiopulmonary resuscitation on an infant or child
   5. AED

XI. Career Development—Success and the Interview Process
   A. The Interview—Definition
      1. Results of a successful interview
   B. Types of Interviews
      1. In-person Interview (Traditional)
      2. Informational Interview
      3. Telephone Interview
      4. Job Search Interview (Prospective)
   C. Preparing for an Interview
      1. Part of the preparation is researching.
      2. Anticipate what types of questions might be asked.
      3. Your turn to ask questions
      4. Be prepared.
   D. Make the Best First Impression
      1. Personal Appearance
      2. Dressing for the Interview
         a. Guidelines for Women
         b. Guidelines for Men
   E. Characteristics of an Ideal Candidate
   F. What to Take to the Interview
   G. During the Interview
      1. How to conduct yourself during the interview
      2. Behaviors to avoid
      3. Listening
      4. Mirroring
   H. Handling typical and tough interview questions
   I. Inappropriate Interview Questions
      1. Illegal or Inappropriate Questions
   J. After the interview
      1. Leaving graciously

      2. Show respect for the interviewer's time
      3. Send a brief follow-up letter
      4. Analyze and evaluate the interview
   K. Key Ideas

XII. Technical Communication and Professional Development
   A. Medical Terminology
   B. Anatomy and Physiology
   C. Keyboarding
   D. Word Processing
   E. Medical Operations Software
   F. Medical Insurance
   G. Medical Transcribing
   H. Disease Short Essays

_____   _____   _____
Student Name (Print)   **Instructor's Name (Print & Sign)**   **Date**

PROCEDURE COMPETENCY CHECKLIST
PHYSICIANS' DESK REFERENCE (PDR)
ALL MODULES

Terminal Performance Objectives

Given evaluation criteria, procedure sheet, drug list and PDR, student will be able to utilize the Physicians' Desk Reference to identify one indication for use, one contraindication for use, one dosage administration and side effects for each listed drug.

Minimum Practice Requirements (as directed)

Read the procedure on the Physicians' Desk Reference; then complete the exercises. Give completed exercises to your instructor for final evaluation.

Evaluation Criteria	Satisfactory	Unsatisfactory
1. Student demonstrated an ability to identify indications for assigned medications from the PDR.		
2. Student demonstrated an ability to identify contraindications for assigned medications from the PDR.		
3. Student demonstrated an ability to identify dosage and administration of assigned medications from the PDR.		
4. Student demonstrated an ability to identify side effects of assigned medications from the PDR.		
5. Student demonstrated an ability to write a prescription based on instructions given by a physician.		
6. Student's penmanship was legible.		
7. Area cleaned once exercises were finished.		
8. Student demonstrated professionalism throughout procedure and accepted constructive feedback with a problem-solving attitude.		
9. Demonstrate awareness of the consequences of not working within the legal scope of practice.		
10. Recognize the importance of local, state and federal legislation and regulations in the practice setting.		
Comments:	**Score:**	**10 = excellent (all correct)** **8 = good (-1)** **7 = fair (-2)** **0 = failed (-3)**

Student Name (Print)   Instructor's Name (Print & Sign)   Date

PROCEDURE COMPETENCY CHECKLIST
CODING EXERCISES
ALL MODULES

Terminal Performance Objectives

Given evaluation criteria, procedure sheet, CPT/ICD-9-CM codebooks, coding exercises and a pen, student will be able to correctly code the exercises presented.

Minimum Practice Requirements (2)

Read the procedure on CPT and ICD-9-CM codes; then complete the exercises presented. Turn the completed exercises in to your instructor for evaluation.

Evaluation Criteria	Satisfactory	Unsatisfactory
1. Student equipped coding area with appropriate items.		
2. Student demonstrated an understanding of CPT insurance coding system.		
3. Student demonstrated an understanding of ICD-9-CM insurance coding system.		
4. Student demonstrated practical application of CPT coding.		
5. Student demonstrated practical application of ICD-9-CM coding.		
6. Student completed the exercises correctly.		
7. Student's penmanship was legible.		
8. Area cleaned once exercises were finished.		
9. Student demonstrated professionalism throughout procedure and accepted constructive feedback with a problem-solving attitude.		
10. Work with the physician to achieve maximum reimbursement.		
Comments:	**Score:**	**10 = excellent (all correct)** **8 = good (-1)** **7 = fair (-2)** **0 = failed (-3)**

Student Name (Print) _____   Instructor's Name (Print & Sign) _____   Date _____

PROCEDURE COMPETENCY CHECKLIST
VITAL SIGNS I
TEMPERATURE, PULSE AND RESPIRATION
ALL MODULES

Terminal Performance Objectives

Given evaluation criteria, procedure sheet, a classmate, thermometer and watch with second hand, student will be able to accurately measure and document temperature, pulse and respiration within 5 minutes.

Minimum Practice Requirements (5)

Read the procedure on vital signs and complete minimum practice requirements. Document each MPR using appropriate charting format.

Sample Documentation: 4/8/XX   10:00 am, T/O 98.0   P 72   R 24 SOB. (Your Signature)

Evaluation Criteria	Satisfactory	Unsatisfactory
1. Hands washed.		
2. Appropriate communication conducted with patient.		
3. Patient positioned correctly.		
4. Thermometer disinfected and inserted correctly.		
5. Procedures timed correctly		
6. Temperature reading obtained within 2 degrees accuracy.		
7. Pulse obtained within 2 beats accuracy.		
8. Respiration obtained within 2 breaths accuracy.		
9. Equipment cleaned and stored appropriately		
10. Documentation completed correctly.		
11. OSHA guidelines followed.		
12. Student demonstrated professionalism throughout procedure and accepted constructive feedback with a problem-solving attitude.		
13. Apply critical thinking skills in performing patient assessment and care.		
14. Use language/verbal skills that enable patients' understanding.		
15. Demonstrate respect for diversity in approaching patients and families.		
Procedure documentation:	**Score:**	**10 = excellent (all correct)** **8 = good** **7 = fail** **0 = failed**

Student Name (Print)   Instructor's Name (Print & Sign)   Date

PROCEDURE COMPETENCY CHECKLIST
VITAL SIGNS II
BLOOD PRESSURE
ALL MODULES

Terminal Performance Objectives

Given evaluation criteria, procedure sheet, a classmate, stethoscope and sphygmomanometer, students will be able to accurately measure and document blood pressure within 5 minutes.

Minimum Practice Requirements (5)

Read the procedure on vital signs and complete minimum practice requirements. Document each MPR using appropriate charting format.

Sample Documentation: 4/8/XX   10:00 am, 130/100/96 R, MEDS: HydroDIURIL 50 mg qd, Lopressor 50 mg bid. (Your Signature)

Evaluation Criteria	Satisfactory	Unsatisfactory
1. Hands washed.		
2. Appropriate communication conducted with patient.		
3. Patient positioned correctly.		
4. Supplies selected and prepared appropriately.		
5. Palpated BP obtained and utilized accurately.		
6. Stethoscope placed and held correctly.		
7. Cuff inflated and deflated correctly.		
8. BP reading obtained within 2 mm Hg accuracy.		
9. Equipment cleaned and stored appropriately.		
10. Documentation completed correctly.		
11. OSHA guidelines followed.		
12. Student demonstrated professionalism throughout procedure and accepted constructive feedback with a problem-solving attitude.		
13. Apply critical thinking skills in performing patient assessment and care.		
14. Use language/verbal skills that enable patients' understanding.		
15. Demonstrate respect for diversity in approaching patients and families.		
Procedure documentation:	Score:	10 = excellent (all correct) 8 = good (-1) 7 = fair (-2) 0 = failed (-3)

Student Name (Print)   Instructor's Name (Print & Sign)   Date

PROCEDURE COMPETENCY CHECKLIST
VENIPUNCTURE

Terminal Performance Objectives

Given evaluation criteria, procedure sheet, a classmate, and correct supplies, students will be able, using correct aseptic technique, to perform a venipuncture using vacutainer, butterfly or syringe technique within 5 minutes.

Minimum Practice Requirements (4)

Read the procedure on venipuncture and complete minimum practice requirements. Document each MPR using appropriate charting format.

Sample Documentation: 4/8/XX 10:00 am, Venipuncture for FBS R basilic vein, pt NPO 12 hr, no adverse reactions. (Your Signature)

Evaluation Criteria	Satisfactory	Unsatisfactory
1. Hands washed.		
2. Appropriate communication conducted with patient.		
3. Patient chart checked for signed orders and required tests.		
4. Supplies selected and prepared appropriately.		
5. Site chosen, disinfected, and tourniquet applied correctly.		
6. Needle stabilized throughout procedure.		
7. Tubes drawn in correct order.		
8. Tourniquet, tube, needle removed in stated order.		
9. Pressure/elevation applied.		
10. Tubes labeled and mixed appropriately.		
11. Patient observed for adverse reactions.		
12. Documentation completed correctly.		
13. OSHA guidelines followed.		
14. Student demonstrated professionalism throughout procedure and accepted constructive feedback with a problem-solving attitude.		
15. Apply critical thinking skills in performing patient assessment and care.		
16. Use language/verbal skills that enable patients' understanding.		
17. Demonstrate respect for diversity in approaching patients and families.		
18. Display sensitivity to patient rights and feelings in collecting specimens.		

Evaluation Criteria	Satisfactory	Unsatisfactory
19. Explain the rationale for performance of a procedure to the patient.		
20. Show awareness of patient's concerns regarding their perceptions related to the procedure being performed.		
Procedure documentation:	**Score:**	**10 = excellent (all correct)** **8 = good** **7 = fair** **0 = failed**

Student Name (Print)   **Instructor's Name (Print & Sign)**   **Date**

PROCEDURE COMPETENCY CHECKLIST
INTRADERMAL INJECTION

Terminal Performance Objectives   Given evaluation criteria, procedure sheet, a classmate, and correct supplies, students will be able, using correct aseptic technique, to administer an intradermal injection within 5 minutes.

Minimum Practice Requirements (3)   Read the procedure on syringe preparation and practice intradermal injections, and complete minimum practice requirements. Document each MPR using appropriate charting format.

Sample Documentation: 4/8/XX 10:00 am, TB, 0.1 cc ID R ant forearm, wheal card given, request CB 48-72 hr, no erythema observed. (Your Signature)

Evaluation Criteria	Satisfactory	Unsatisfactory
1. Hands washed.		
2. Appropriate communication conducted with patient, including allergy verification.		
3. Patient chart checked for signed orders.		
4. Supplies selected and prepared appropriately.		
5. Medication label checked 3 times.		
6. Site chosen, prepared correctly.		
7. Injection delivered at correct angle.		
8. Adequate wheal obtained.		
9. Needle stabilized and removed at correct angle.		
10. Patient observed for adverse reactions.		
11. Documentation completed correctly.		
12. OSHA guidelines followed.		
13. Student demonstrated professionalism throughout procedure and accepted constructive feedback with a problem-solving attitude.		
14. Recognize the importance of local, state and federal legislation and regulations in the practice setting.		
Procedure documentation:	**Score:**	**10 = excellent (all correct)** **8 = good** **7 = fair** **0 = failed**

Student Name (Print)   Instructor's Name (Print & Sign)   Date

PROCEDURE COMPETENCY CHECKLIST
CHARTING
ALL MODULES

Terminal Performance Objectives

Given evaluation criteria, a file folder and preprinted forms, student will assemble a medical record, organize some sample reports, interview patients and document subjective data on a preprinted form.

Minimum Practice Requirements (As directed)

Using the list of common charting abbreviations from the student handbook and sample documentation provided on Procedure Competency Checklists, student will interview patients and record subjective data (chief complaint) for every procedure performed on classmates using pre-assembled charts and preprinted forms.

Evaluation Criteria	Satisfactory	Unsatisfactory
1. Student showed knowledge of proper organization of the medical record.		
2. Student used correct preprinted forms when documenting procedures.		
3. Student correctly interviewed patient and documented a chief complaint.		
4. Student used proper charting abbreviations when documenting procedures.		
5. Student demonstrated knowledge of subjective data versus objective data.		
6. Student's penmanship was legible.		
7. Area cleaned once exercises were finished.		
8. Student demonstrated professionalism throughout procedure and accepted constructive feedback with a problem-solving attitude.		
9. HIPAA Privacy Guidelines followed		
10. Demonstrate awareness of the consequences of not working within the legal scope of practice.		
11. Recognize the importance of local, state and federal legislation and regulations in the practice setting.		
Comments:	**Score:**	**10 = excellent (all correct)** **8 = good (-1)** **7 = fair (-2)** **0 = failed (-3)**

PROCEDURE COMPETENCY CHECKLISTS AND ASSIGNMENTS

Student Name (Print)	Instructor's Name (Print & Sign)	Date

PROCEDURE COMPETENCY CHECKLIST
ELECTROCARDIOGRAM

Terminal Performance Objectives

Given evaluation criteria, procedure sheet, a classmate, and correct supplies, students will be able, using correct technique, to a diagnostic quality resting 12 lead EKG in 15 minutes to checkoff standards.

Minimum Practice Requirements (5)

Read the skill development sheet on electrocardiogram; then complete minimum practice requirements. Document each MPR using appropriate charting formula.

Sample Documentation: 4/8/XX 10:00 am 12 Lead EKG (your signature)

Evaluation Criteria	Satisfactory	Unsatisfactory
1. Hands washed.		
2. Appropriate communication conducted with patient.		
3. Patient chart checked for signed orders and required tests.		
4. Supplies selected and prepared appropriately.		
5. Electrodes placed in correct positions.		
6. EKG machine controls set properly.		
7. Standardization appears in appropriate location on strip.		
8. EKG strip is diagnostic quality.		
9. Documentation completed correctly.		
10. Equipment cleaned and stored appropriately.		
11. EKG strip properly mounted.		
12. OSHA guidelines followed.		
13. Student demonstrated professionalism throughout procedure and accepted constructive feedback with a problem-solving attitude.		
Procedure documentation:	**Score:**	**10 = excellent** **8 = good** **7 = fair** **0 = failed**

Student Name (Print)   Instructor's Name (Print & Sign)   Date

PROCEDURE COMPETENCY CHECKLIST
PEAK FLOW METER

Terminal Performance Objectives   Given evaluation criteria, skill sheet, class mate, and the correct supplies, student will be able to obtain an accurate PFT and document in the patient's chart.

Minimum Practice Requirements (5)   Read the procedure on Peak Flow Meter and complete minimum practice requirements. Document each using appropriate charting format.

Sample Documentation: 4/8/XX 10:00am Peak Flow Meter, (your signature).

Evaluation Criteria	Satisfactory	Unsatisfactory
1. Hands washed.		
2. Appropriate communication conducted with patient.		
3. Supplies correctly selected.		
4. Patient was standing.		
5. Indicator was set at zero.		
6. Patient was instructed to inhale deeply and mouthpiece placed into patient's mouth.		
7. Insured that a tight seal was present.		
8. Instructed patient to blow hard and fast into mouthpiece.		
9. Patient was instructed to repeat this process twice.		
10. OSHA guidelines followed.		
11. Procedure correctly documented.		
Procedure documentation:	Score:	10 = excellent 8 = good 7 = fair 0 = failed

Student Name (Print)   Instructor's Name (Print & Sign)   Date

PROCEDURE COMPETENCY CHECKLIST
ASEPTIC HAND WASHING

Terminal Performance Objectives

Given evaluation criteria, and procedure sheet in text, student will perform aseptic hand washing without error.

Minimum Practice Requirements (3)

Read the skill development sheet on aseptic hand washing; then complete minimum practice requirements. Document each MPR.

Materials:

Liquid soap, nailbrush or orange cuticle stick, hot running water, paper towels, waste container.

Evaluation Criteria	Satisfactory	Unsatisfactory
1. Student removed all jewelry (except wedding bands).		
2. Student turned water on using clean, dry paper towel and discarded paper towel.		
3. Student adjusted running water to correct lukewarm temperature with clean, dry paper towel and discarded paper towel.		
4. Student applied soap to hands and worked into lather by moving it over palms, sides, and backs of both hands for 2 minutes using circular motion and friction.		
5. Student kept hands pointed downward during entire procedure.		
6. Student used hand brush and/or cuticle stick to clean under fingernails and thoroughly scrubbed wedding band if present.		
7. Student rinsed hands under running water with fingers pointing down.		
8. Student dried hands with clean, dry paper towel and discarded it.		
9. Using a clean, dry paper towel, the student turned faucet off.		
10. Student demonstrated professionalism throughout procedure and accepted constructive feedback with a problem-solving attitude.		
Comments:	**Score:**	10 = excellent 8 = good 7 = fair 0 = failed

Student Name (Print)   **Instructor's Name (Print & Sign)**   **Date**

PROCEDURE COMPETENCY CHECKLIST
PROFESSIONALISM STANDARDS
ALL MODULES

Terminal Performance Objectives

Given evaluation criteria, student will meet the minimum standards of professionalism and will demonstrate a basic understanding of how to conduct themselves as expected on the job.

Evaluation Criteria	Satisfactory	Unsatisfactory
1. Student projected a positive attitude.		
2. Student used professional language.		
3. Student exhibited good manners toward instructor and classmates.		
4. Student's uniform was complete at all times.		
5. Student was clean, neat and properly groomed.		
6. Student only wore appropriate jewelry.		
7. Student took initiative and made good use of class time.		
8. Student came to class prepared and completed assignments on time every day.		
9. Student was present when class began and was present the entire class time.		
10. Student was cooperative with instructors and classmates.		
11. Student worked in harmony with group members and interacted well with classmates.		
Comments:	**Score:**	**10 = excellent (all correct)** **8 = good (-1)** **7 = fair (-2)** **0 = failed (-3)**

| Student Name (Print) | Instructor's Name (Print & Sign) | Date |

PROCEDURE COMPETENCY CHECKLIST
PHYSICIANS' DESK REFERENCE (PDR)
ALL MODULES

Terminal Performance Objectives

Given evaluation criteria, procedure sheet, drug list and PDR, student will be able to utilize the Physicians' Desk Reference to identify one indication for use, one contraindication for use, one dosage administration and side effects for each listed drug.

Minimum Practice Requirements (as directed)

Read the procedure on the Physicians' Desk Reference; then complete the exercises. Give completed exercises to your instructor for final evaluation.

Evaluation Criteria	Satisfactory	Unsatisfactory
1. Student demonstrated an ability to identify indications for assigned medications from the PDR.		
2. Student demonstrated an ability to identify contraindications for assigned medications from the PDR.		
3. Student demonstrated an ability to identify dosage and administration of assigned medications from the PDR.		
4. Student demonstrated an ability to identify side effects of assigned medications from the PDR.		
5. Student demonstrated an ability to write a prescription based on instructions given by a physician.		
6. Student's penmanship was legible.		
7. Area cleaned once exercises were finished.		
8. Student demonstrated professionalism throughout procedure and accepted constructive feedback with a problem-solving attitude.		
Comments:	**Score:**	**10 = excellent (all correct)** **8 = good (-1)** **7 = fair (-2)** **0 = failed (-3)**

Student Name (Print)   Instructor's Name (Print & Sign)   Date

PROCEDURE COMPETENCY CHECKLIST
CODING EXERCISES
ALL MODULES

Terminal Performance Objectives

Given evaluation criteria, procedure sheet, CPT/ICD-9-CM codebooks, coding exercises and a pen, student will be able to correctly code the exercises presented.

Minimum Practice Requirements (2)

Read the procedure on CPT and ICD-9-CM codes; then complete the exercises presented. Turn the completed exercises in to your instructor for evaluation.

Evaluation Criteria	Satisfactory	Unsatisfactory
1. Student equipped coding area with appropriate items.		
2. Student demonstrated an understanding of CPT insurance coding system.		
3. Student demonstrated an understanding of ICD-9-CM insurance coding system.		
4. Student demonstrated practical application of CPT coding.		
5. Student demonstrated practical application of ICD-9-CM coding.		
6. Student completed the exercises correctly.		
7. Student's penmanship was legible.		
8. Area cleaned once exercises were finished.		
9. Student demonstrated professionalism throughout procedure and accepted constructive feedback with a problem-solving attitude.		
Comments:	**Score:**	**10 = excellent (all correct)** **8 = good (-1)** **7 = fair (-2)** **0 = failed (-3)**

| Student Name (Print) | Instructor's Name (Print & Sign) | Date |

PROCEDURE COMPETENCY CHECKLIST
VITAL SIGNS I
TEMPERATURE, PULSE AND RESPIRATION
ALL MODULES

Terminal Performance Objectives

Given evaluation criteria, procedure sheet, a classmate, thermometer and watch with second hand, student will be able to accurately measure and document temperature, pulse and respiration within 5 minutes.

Minimum Practice Requirements (5)

Read the procedure on vital signs and complete minimum practice requirements. Document each MPR using appropriate charting format.

Sample Documentation: 4/8/XX   10:00 am, T/O 98.0   P 72   R 24 SOB. (Your Signature)

Evaluation Criteria	Satisfactory	Unsatisfactory
1. Hands washed.		
2. Appropriate communication conducted with patient.		
3. Patient positioned correctly.		
4. Thermometer disinfected and inserted correctly.		
5. Procedures timed correctly		
6. Temperature reading obtained within 2 degrees accuracy.		
7. Pulse obtained within 2 beats accuracy.		
8. Respiration obtained within 2 breaths accuracy.		
9. Equipment cleaned and stored appropriately		
10. Documentation completed correctly.		
11. OSHA guidelines followed.		
12. Student demonstrated professionalism throughout procedure and accepted constructive feedback with a problem-solving attitude.		
Procedure documentation:	**Score:**	**10 = excellent (all correct)** **8 = good** **7 = fail** **0 = failed**

Student Name (Print)   Instructor's Name (Print & Sign)   Date

PROCEDURE COMPETENCY CHECKLIST
VITAL SIGNS II
BLOOD PRESSURE
ALL MODULES

Terminal Performance Objectives   Given evaluation criteria, procedure sheet, a classmate, stethoscope and sphygmomanometer, students will be able to accurately measure and document blood pressure within 5 minutes.

Minimum Practice Requirements (5)   Read the procedure on vital signs and complete minimum practice requirements. Document each MPR using appropriate charting format.

Sample Documentation: 4/8/XX   10:00 am, 130/100/96 R, MEDS: HydroDIURIL 50 mg qd, Lopressor 50 mg bid. (Your Signature)

Evaluation Criteria	Satisfactory	Unsatisfactory
1. Hands washed.		
2. Appropriate communication conducted with patient.		
3. Patient positioned correctly.		
4. Supplies selected and prepared appropriately.		
5. Palpated BP obtained and utilized accurately.		
6. Stethoscope placed and held correctly.		
7. Cuff inflated and deflated correctly.		
8. BP reading obtained within 2 mm Hg accuracy.		
9. Equipment cleaned and stored appropriately.		
10. Documentation completed correctly.		
11. OSHA guidelines followed.		
12. Student demonstrated professionalism throughout procedure and accepted constructive feedback with a problem-solving attitude.		
Procedure documentation:	**Score:**	**10 = excellent (all correct)** **8 = good (-1)** **7 = fair (-2)** **0 = failed (-3)**

Student Name (Print)   Instructor's Name (Print & Sign)   Date

PROCEDURE COMPETENCY CHECKLIST
VENIPUNCTURE

Terminal Performance Objectives

Given evaluation criteria, procedure sheet, a classmate, and correct supplies, students will be able, using correct aseptic technique, to perform a venipuncture using vacutainer, butterfly or syringe technique within 5 minutes.

Minimum Practice Requirements (4)

Read the procedure on venipuncture and complete minimum practice requirements. Document each MPR using appropriate charting format.

Sample Documentation: 4/8/XX 10:00 am, Venipuncture for FBS R basilic vein, pt NPO 12 hr, no adverse reactions. (Your Signature)

Evaluation Criteria	Satisfactory	Unsatisfactory
1. Hands washed.		
2. Appropriate communication conducted with patient.		
3. Patient chart checked for signed orders and required tests.		
4. Supplies selected and prepared appropriately.		
5. Site chosen, disinfected, and tourniquet applied correctly.		
6. Needle stabilized throughout procedure.		
7. Tubes drawn in correct order.		
8. Tourniquet, tube, needle removed in stated order.		
9. Pressure/elevation applied.		
10. Tubes labeled and mixed appropriately.		
11. Patient observed for adverse reactions.		
12. Documentation completed correctly.		
13. OSHA guidelines followed.		
14. Student demonstrated professionalism throughout procedure and accepted constructive feedback with a problem-solving attitude.		
Procedure documentation:	**Score:**	**10 = excellent (all correct)** **8 = good** **7 = fair** **0 = failed**

Student Name (Print)   Instructor's Name (Print & Sign)   Date

PROCEDURE COMPETENCY CHECKLIST
INTRADERMAL INJECTION

Terminal Performance Objectives

Given evaluation criteria, procedure sheet, a classmate, and correct supplies, students will be able, using correct aseptic technique, to administer an intradermal injection within 5 minutes.

Minimum Practice Requirements (3)

Read the procedure on syringe preparation and practice intradermal injections, and complete minimum practice requirements. Document each MPR using appropriate charting format.

Sample Documentation: 4/8/XX 10:00 am, TB, 0.1 cc ID R ant forearm, wheal card given, request CB 48-72 hr, no erythema observed. (Your Signature)

Evaluation Criteria	Satisfactory	Unsatisfactory
1. Hands washed.		
2. Appropriate communication conducted with patient, including allergy verification.		
3. Patient chart checked for signed orders.		
4. Supplies selected and prepared appropriately.		
5. Medication label checked 3 times.		
6. Site chosen, prepared correctly.		
7. Injection delivered at correct angle.		
8. Adequate wheal obtained.		
9. Needle stabilized and removed at correct angle.		
10. Patient observed for adverse reactions.		
11. Documentation completed correctly.		
12. OSHA guidelines followed.		
13. Student demonstrated professionalism throughout procedure and accepted constructive feedback with a problem-solving attitude.		
Procedure documentation:	**Score:**	**10 = excellent (all correct)** **8 = good** **7 = fair** **0 = failed**

Student Name (Print)	Instructor's Name (Print & Sign)	Date

PROCEDURE COMPETENCY CHECKLIST
SUBCUTANEOUS INJECTION
ALL MODULES

Terminal Performance Objectives	Given evaluation criteria, procedure sheet, a classmate, and correct supplies, students will be able, using correct aseptic technique, to administer a subcutaneous injection within 5 minutes.
Minimum Practice Requirements (3)	Read the procedure on syringe preparation and subcutaneous injections, and complete minimum practice requirements. Document each MPR using appropriate charting format.

Sample Documentation: 4/8/XX   10:00 am, MMR 0.5 cc SC R vastus, Patient Information Sheet (VIS) given. (Your Signature)

Evaluation Criteria	Satisfactory	Unsatisfactory
1. Hands washed.		
2. Appropriate communication conducted with patient, including allergy verification.		
3. Patient chart checked for signed orders.		
4. Supplies selected and area prepared appropriately.		
5. Medication label checked 3 times.		
6. Site chosen, prepared correctly.		
7. Injection delivered at correct angle.		
8. Injection aspirated.		
9. Needle stabilized and removed at correct angle.		
10. Patient observed for adverse reactions.		
11. Documentation completed correctly.		
12. OSHA guidelines followed.		
13. Student demonstrated professionalism throughout procedure and accepted constructive feedback with a problem-solving attitude.		
Procedure documentation:	**Score:**	**10 = excellent (all correct)** **8 = good (-1)** **7 = fair (-2)** **0 = failed (-3)**

Student Name (Print)   Instructor's Name (Print & Sign)   Date

PROCEDURE COMPETENCY CHECKLIST
INTRAMUSCULAR INJECTION (DELTOID)
ALL MODULES

Terminal Performance Objectives   Given evaluation criteria, procedure sheet, a classmate, and correct supplies, students will be able, using correct aseptic technique, to administer an intramuscular injection within 5 minutes.

Minimum Practice Requirements (3)   Read the procedure on syringe preparation and intramuscular injections, and complete minimum practice requirements. Document each MPR using appropriate charting format.

Sample Documentation: 4/8/XX   10:00 am, Vit.B_{12} 1.0 cc/1000 mcg IM, R delt, pt observed for 20 min before release. (Your Signature)

Evaluation Criteria	Satisfactory	Unsatisfactory
1. Hands washed.		
2. Appropriate communication conducted with patient, including allergy verification.		
3. Patient chart checked for signed orders.		
4. Supplies selected and area prepared appropriately.		
5. Medication label checked 3 times.		
6. Site chosen, prepared correctly.		
7. Injection delivered at correct angle.		
8. Injection aspirated.		
9. Needle stabilized and removed at correct angle.		
10. Patient observed for adverse reactions.		
11. Documentation completed correctly.		
12. OSHA guidelines followed.		
13. Student demonstrated professionalism throughout procedure and accepted constructive feedback with a problem-solving attitude.		
Procedure documentation:	**Score:**	**10 = excellent (all correct)** **8 = good (-1)** **7 = fair (-2)** **0 = failed (-3)**

Student Name (Print)   Instructor's Name (Print & Sign)   Date

PROCEDURE COMPETENCY CHECKLIST
INTRAMUSCULAR INJECTION (GLUTEAL)
ALL MODULES

Terminal Performance Objectives

Given evaluation criteria, procedure sheet, a classmate, and correct supplies, students will be able, using correct aseptic technique, to administer an intramuscular injection within 5 minutes.

Minimum Practice Requirements (3)

Read the procedure on syringe preparation and intramuscular injections, and complete minimum practice requirements. Document each MPR using appropriate charting format.

Sample Documentation: 4/8/XX   10:00 am, Ampicillin 1.0 cc/250 mg IM R glute, pt observed for 20 min before release. (Your Signature)

Evaluation Criteria	Satisfactory	Unsatisfactory
1. Hands washed.		
2. Appropriate communication conducted with patient, including allergy verification.		
3. Patient chart checked for signed orders.		
4. Supplies selected and area prepared appropriately.		
5. Medication label checked 3 times.		
6. Site chosen, prepared correctly.		
7. Injection delivered at correct angle.		
8. Injection aspirated.		
9. Needle stabilized and removed at correct angle.		
10. Patient observed for adverse reactions.		
11. Documentation completed correctly.		
12. OSHA guidelines followed.		
13. Student demonstrated professionalism throughout procedure and accepted constructive feedback with a problem-solving attitude.		
Procedure documentation:	**Score:**	**10 = excellent (all correct)** **8 = good (-1)** **7 = fair (-2)** **0 = failed (-3)**

Student Name (Print)   Instructor's Name (Print & Sign)   Date

PROCEDURE COMPETENCY CHECKLIST
INTRAMUSCULAR INJECTION (Z-TRACK)
ALL MODULES

Terminal Performance Objectives

Given evaluation criteria, procedure sheet, a classmate, and correct supplies, students will be able, using correct aseptic technique, to administer an intramuscular injection within 5 minutes.

Minimum Practice Requirements (As directed)

Read the procedure on syringe preparation and Z-Track intramuscular injections, and complete minimum practice requirements. Document each MPR using appropriate charting format.

4/8/xx 10:00 am, Depo-Estradiol 5 mg Z R glute, pt observed for 20 min before release. (Your Signature)

Evaluation Criteria	Satisfactory	Unsatisfactory
1. Hands washed.		
2. Appropriate communication conducted with patient, including allergy verification.		
3. Patient chart checked for signed orders.		
4. Supplies selected and area prepared appropriately.		
5. Medication label checked 3 times.		
6. Site chosen, prepared correctly.		
7. Injection delivered at correct angle and tension maintained.		
8. Injection aspirated.		
9. Needle stabilized and removed at correct angle.		
10. Patient observed for adverse reactions.		
11. Documentation completed correctly.		
12. OSHA guidelines followed.		
13. Student demonstrated professionalism throughout procedure and accepted constructive feedback with a problem-solving attitude.		
Procedure documentation:	**Score:**	**10 = excellent (all correct)** **8 = good (-1)** **7 = fair (-2)** **0 = failed (-3)**

Student Name (Print)   Instructor's Name (Print & Sign)   Date

PROCEDURE COMPETENCY CHECKLIST
CHARTING
ALL MODULES

Terminal Performance Objectives

Given evaluation criteria, a file folder and preprinted forms, student will assemble a medical record, organize some sample reports, interview patients and document subjective data on a preprinted form.

Minimum Practice Requirements (As directed)

Using the list of common charting abbreviations from the student handbook and sample documentation provided on Procedure Competency Checklists, student will interview patients and record subjective data (chief complaint) for every procedure performed on classmates using pre-assembled charts and preprinted forms.

Evaluation Criteria	Satisfactory	Unsatisfactory
1. Student showed knowledge of proper organization of the medical record.		
2. Student used correct preprinted forms when documenting procedures.		
3. Student correctly interviewed patient and documented a chief complaint.		
4. Student used proper charting abbreviations when documenting procedures.		
5. Student demonstrated knowledge of subjective data versus objective data.		
6. Student's penmanship was legible.		
7. Area cleaned once exercises were finished.		
8. Student demonstrated professionalism throughout procedure and accepted constructive feedback with a problem-solving attitude.		
9. HIPAA Privacy Guidelines followed		
Comments:	Score:	10 = excellent (all correct) 8 = good (-1) 7 = fair (-2) 0 = failed (-3)

Appendix C

REFERENCE TO COMMON ALLERGIES, INFECTIONS, DISORDERS, PROCEDURES, AND TESTS

TABLE 1   Common Types of Allergies

Allergy	Description
Allergic rhinitis	Inflammation of the nasal mucosa which results in nasal congestion, rhinorrhea (runny nose), sneezing and itching of the nose. Seasonal allergic rhinitis, such as seen in hay fever, occurs only during certain seasons of the year. Children suffering from this type of allergy may rub their nose in an upward movement, called the "allergic salute."
Asthma	A condition seen most frequently in early childhood in which wheezing, coughing, and dyspnea are the major symptoms. Asthmatic attacks may be caused by allergens inhaled from the air, food, and drugs. The patient's airway is affected by a constriction of the bronchial passages. Treatment is medication and control of the causative factors.
Contact dermatitis	Inflammation and irritation of the skin due to contact with an irritating substance, such as soap, perfume, cosmetics, plastic, dyes, and plants such as poison ivy. Symptoms include itching, redness, and skin lesions with blistering and oozing. Treatment consists of topical and systemic medications and removal of the causative item.
Eczema	A superficial dermatitis accompanied by papules, vesicles, and crusting. This condition can be acute or chronic.
Urticaria	A skin eruption of pale reddish wheals (circular elevations of the skin) with severe itching. It is usually associated with a food allergy, stress, or drug reactions. Also called hives.

TABLE 2   Common Skin Lesions

Type of Lesion	Description
Cyst	A fluid-filled sac or pouch under the skin.
Fissure	Crack-like lesion or groove in the skin.
Macule	Small, flat discolored area that is flush with the skin surface. An example would be a freckle and the flat rash of roseola.
Nodule	Solid, raised group of cells.
Papule	Small, solid, circular raised spot on the surface of the skin.
Polyp	Small tumor with a pedicle or stem attachment. They are commonly found in vascular organs such as the nose, uterus, and rectum.
Pustule	Raised spot on the skin containing pus.
Vesicle	Small, fluid-filled raised spot on the skin; blister.
Wheal	Small, round, raised area on the skin that may be accompanied by itching.

TABLE 3   Common Skin Infections

Infection	Description
Boil	Acute inflammation of the subcutaneous layer of skin, or hair follicle. Also called a furuncle. Treatment consists of the application of moist heat until the boil comes to a "head" or softens. An incision and drainage (I&D) may be performed to allow the purulent material to drain. Antibiotics may be prescribed.
Carbuncle	Inflammation and infection of the skin and hair follicle that may result from several untreated boils. They are most commonly found on the neck, upper back, or head. Treatment is similar to that for a single boil. Systemic antibiotics may be prescribed. A gauze bandage is applied when drainage is present.
Furuncle	Staphylococcal skin abscess with redness, pain and swelling. Also called a boil.
Herpes simplex	Infectious disease caused by the herpes simplex virus 1 and characterized by thin vesicles that tend to recur in the same area such as the lips or conjunctiva. Treatment consists of the drug acyclovir either locally or orally.
Herpes zoster	A painful, infectious viral disease which attacks the nerve endings. It is also called shingles and is caused by the same virus as chickenpox. Treatment consists of analgesics to relieve pain, and antiviral medications, such as acyclovir. In severe cases a nerve block may be necessary to relieve pain.
Impetigo	A highly contagious inflammatory skin disease with pustules that become crusted and rupture. Treatment consists of thorough cleansing using separate towels and wash cloths for the patient. These should be washed daily. Topical medications may be prescribed.
Scabies	Contagious skin disease caused by an egg-laying mite that causes intense itching. The lesions appear as small, red papules and vesicles between the fingers, toes, genitalia, and beneath the breasts. Treatment consists of a methrin cream from the neck down. All clothing and bedding need careful laundering.
Sebaceous cyst	Cyst filled with sebum (oil) from a sebaceous gland. This can grow to a large size and may need to be excised.

(continued)

TABLE 3   *(continued)*

Infection	Description
Tinea	A fungal skin disease resulting in itching, scaling lesions. Tinea pedis is also called athlete's foot. Diagnosis of tinea is made with the use of a Wood's light which are ultraviolet rays used to detect fluorescent materials in the skin and hair of patients with tinea. Topical treatment consists of fungicidal agents, such as griseofulvin.
Verruca	A benign neoplasm (tumor), which has a rough surface that is removed by chemicals and /or laser therapy, and is caused by a virus. Also called warts.

TABLE 4   Neoplasms

Benign (non-cancerous) Neoplasms	Description
Dermatofibroma	A fibrous tumor of the skin. It is painless, round, firm, red, and generally found on the extremities.
Hemangioma	Benign tumor of dilated vessels.
Keloid	The formation of a scar after an injury or surgery, which results in a raised, thickened, red area.
Keratosis	Overgrowth and thickening of cells in the epithelium located in the epidermis of the skin.
Leukoplakia	A change in the mucous membrane that results in thick, white patches on the mucous membrane of the tongue and cheek. It is considered precancerous and is associated with smoking.
Lipoma	Fatty tumor that generally does not **metastasize** (spread).
Nevus	A pigmented (colored) congenital skin blemish. It is usually benign but may become cancerous. Also called a birthmark or mole.

Malignant (cancerous) Neoplasms	Description
Basal cell carcinoma	An epithelial tumor of the basal cell layer of the epidermis. A frequent type of skin cancer that rarely metastasizes.
Kaposi's sarcoma	A form of skin cancer frequently seen in acquired immune deficiency syndrome (AIDS) patients. It consists of brownish-purple papules that spread from the skin and metastasize to internal organs.
Malignant melanoma	A dangerous form of skin cancer caused by an overgrowth of melanin in the skin. It may metastasize.
Squamous cell carcinoma	Epidermal cancer that may go into deeper tissue but does not generally metastasize.

TABLE 5   Diagnostic Procedures and Tests Relating to the Integumentary System

Procedure/Test	Description
Adipectomy	Surgical removal of fat.
Biopsy	Removal of a piece of tissue by syringe and needle, knife, punch, or brush to examine under a microscope as an aid in diagnosis.
Cauterization	The destruction of tissue with a caustic chemical, electric current, freezing, or hot iron.
Chemobrasion	Abrasion of the skin using chemicals. Also called a chemical peel.
Cryosurgery	The use of extreme cold to freeze and destroy tissue.
Curettage	The removal of superficial skin lesions with a curette or scraper.
Debridement	The removal of foreign material or dead tissue from a wound.
Dermabrasion	Abrasion or rubbing using wire brushes or sandpaper.
Dermatoplasty	The transplantation of skin. Also called skin grafting. May be used to treat large birthmarks (hemangiomas) and burns.
Electrocautery	To destroy tissue with an electric current.
Exfoliative cytology	Scraping cells from tissue and then examining them under a microscope.
Frozen section	Taking a thin piece of tissue from a frozen specimen for rapid examination under a microscope. This is often performed during a surgical procedure to detect the presence of cancer in a diseased organ.
Fungal scrapings (FS)	Scrapings taken with a curette or scraper of tissue from lesions are placed on a growth medium and examined under a microscope to identify fungal growth.
Incision and drainage (I & D)	Making an incision to create an opening for the drainage of material such as pus.
Laser therapy	Removal of skin lesions and birthmarks using a laser that emits intense heat and power at close range. The laser converts frequencies of light into one small beam.
Lipectomy	The surgical removal of fat.
Marsupialization	Creating a pouch to promote drainage by surgically opening a closed area, such as a cyst.
Needle biopsy	Using a sterile needle to remove tissue for examination under a microscope.
Plication	Taking tucks surgically in a structure to shorten it.
Rhytidectomy	Surgical removal of excess skin to eliminate wrinkles. Commonly referred to as a face lift.
Skin grafts	The transfer of skin from a normal area to cover another site. Used to treat burn victims and after some surgical procedures.
Sweat test	Test performed on sweat to see the level of chloride. There is an increase in skin chloride in some diseases, such as cystic fibrosis.

TABLE 6   Disorders of the Cardiovascular System

Disorder	Description
Anemia	A reduction in the number of circulating red blood cells per cubic millimeter of blood. It is not a disease but a symptom of disease.
Aneurysm	An abnormal dilation of a blood vessel, usually an artery, due to a congenital weakness or defect in the wall of the vessel.
Angina pectoris	Condition in which there is severe pain with a sensation of constriction around the heart. It is caused by a deficiency of oxygen to the heart muscle.
Angioma	Tumor, usually benign, consisting of blood vessels.
Angiospasm	Spasm or contraction of blood vessels.
Aortic aneurysm	Localized, abnormal dilation of the aorta, causing pressure on the trachea, esophagus, veins, or nerves. This is due to a weakness in the wall of the blood vessel.
Aortic insufficiency	A failure of the aortic valve to close completely which results in leaking and inefficient heart action.
Aortic stenosis	Condition caused by a narrowing of the aorta.
Arrhythmia	An irregularity in the heartbeat or action.
Arterial embolism	Blood clot moving within an artery. This can occur as a result of arteriosclerosis.
Arteriosclerosis	Thickening, hardening, and loss of elasticity of the walls of arteries.
Atherosclerosis	This is the most common form of arteriosclerosis. It is caused by the formation of yellowish plaques of cholesterol building up on the inner walls of the arteries.
Bradycardia	An abnormally slow heart rate (under 60 beats per minute).
Congenital heart disease	Heart defects that are present at birth, such as patent ductus arteriosus, in which the opening between the pulmonary artery and the aorta fails to close at birth. This condition requires surgery.
Congestive heart failure	Pathological condition of the heart in which there is a reduced outflow of blood from the left side of the heart. This results in weakness, breathlessness, and edema.
Coronary artery disease	A narrowing of the coronary arteries that is sufficient enough to prevent adequate blood supply to the myocardium.
Coronary thrombosis	Blood clot in a coronary vessel of the heart causing the vessel to close completely or partially.
Embolus	Obstruction of a blood vessel by a blood clot that moves from another area.
Endocarditis	Inflammation of the membrane lining the heart. May be due to microorganisms or to an abnormal immunological response.
Fibrillation	Abnormal quivering or contractions of heart fibers. When this occurs within the fibers of the ventricle of the heart, arrest and death can occur. Emergency equipment to defibrillate, or convert the heart to a normal beat, will be necessary.
Hypertensive heart disease	Heart disease as a result of persistently high blood pressure which damages the blood vessels and ultimately the heart.
Hypotension	A decrease in blood pressure. This can occur in shock, infection, anemia, cancer, or as death approaches.
Infarct	Area of tissue within an organ or part that undergoes necrosis (death) following the cessation of the blood supply.
Ischemia	A localized and temporary deficiency of blood supply due to an obstruction to the circulation.
Mitral stenosis	Narrowing of the opening (orifice) of the mitral valve which causes an obstruction in the flow of blood from the atrium to the ventricle on the left side of the heart.
Mitral valve prolapse (MVP)	Common and serious condition in which the cusp of the mitral valve drops back (prolapses) into the left atrium during systole.
Murmur	A soft blowing or rasping sound heard upon auscultation of the heart.
Myocardial infarction	Condition caused by the partial or complete occlusion or closing of one or more of the coronary arteries. Symptoms include a squeezing pain or heavy pressure in the middle of the chest. A delay in treatment could result in death. This is also referred to as MI or heart attack.
Myocarditis	An inflammation of the myocardial lining of the heart resulting in extremely weak and rapid beat, and irregular pulse.
Patent ductus arteriosus	Congenital presence of a connection between the pulmonary artery and the aorta that remains after birth. This condition is normal in the fetus.
Pericarditis	Inflammatory process or disease of the pericardium.
Phlebitis	Inflammation of a vein.
Reynaud's phenomenon	Intermittent attacks of pallor or cyanosis of the fingers and toes associated with the cold or emotional distress. There may also be numbness, pain, and burning during the attacks. It may be caused by decreased circulation due to smoking.
Rheumatic heart disease	Valvular heart disease as a result of having had rheumatic fever.
Tetralogy of Fallot	Combination of four symptoms (tetralogy), resulting in pulmonary stenosis, a septal defect, abnormal blood supply to the aorta, and the hypertrophy of the right ventricle. A congenital defect that is present at birth and needs immediate surgery to correct.
Thrombophlebitis	Inflammation and clotting of blood within a vein.
Thrombus	A blood clot.
Varicose veins	Swollen and distended veins, usually in the legs, resulting from pressure, such as occurs during a pregnancy.

TABLE 7 Diagnostic Procedures and Tests Relating to the Cardiovascular System

Procedure/Test	Description
Aneurysmectomy	The surgical removal of the sac of an aneurysm, which is an abnormal dilatation of a blood vessel.
Angiography	X-rays taken after the injection of an opaque material into a blood vessel. Can be performed on the aorta as an aortic angiogram, on the heart as an angiocardiogram, and on the brain as a cerebral angiogram.
Angioplasty	A surgical procedure of altering the structure of a vessel by dilating the vessel using a balloon inside the vessel.
Arterial blood gases	Measurement of the amount of oxygen (O_2), carbon dioxide (CO_2), and nitrogen in the blood. Also gives a pH reading of the blood. Blood gases are performed in emergency situations and provide valuable evaluation of cardiac failure, hemorrhage, and kidney failure.
Artery graft	A piece of blood vessel that is transplanted from a part of the body to the aorta to repair a defect.
Artificial pacemaker	Electrical device that substitutes for the natural pacemaker of the heart. It controls the beating of the heart by a series of rhythmic electrical impulses. An external pacemaker has the electrodes on the outside of the body. An internal pacemaker will have the electrodes surgically implanted within the chest wall.
Cardiac catheterization	Passage of a thin tube (catheter) through an arm vein and the blood vessels leading into the heart. It is done to detect abnormalities, to collect cardiac blood samples, and to determine the pressure within the cardiac area.
Cardiac enzymes	Complex proteins that are capable of inducing chemical changes within the body. Cardiac enzymes are taken by blood sample to determine the amount of heart disease or damage.
Cardiac magnetic resonance imaging (MRI)	A noninvasive procedure in which images of the heart and blood vessels are captured for examination to determine effects.
Cardiolysis	A surgical procedure to separate adhesions which involves a resection of the ribs and sternum over the pericardium.
Cardiorrhaphy	Surgical suturing of the heart.
Cardioversion	Converting a cardiac arrhythmia (irregular heart action) to a normal sinus rhythm using a cardioverter to give countershocks to the heart.
Commissurotomy	Surgical incision to change the size of an opening. For example in mitral commissurotomy, a stenosis or narrowing is corrected by cutting away at the adhesions around the mitral opening (orifice).
Coronary artery bypass surgery	Open-heart surgery in which a shunt is created to permit blood to travel around the constriction in coronary blood vessel(s).
Doppler ultrasonography	Measurement of sound-wave echoes as they bounce off tissues and organs to produce an image. Can assist in determining heart and blood vessel damage. Also called echocardiogram.
Electrocardiogram	Record of the electrical activity of the heart. Useful in the diagnosis of abnormal cardiac rhythm and heart muscle (myocardium) damage. This procedure is explained fully in Chapter 29.
Electrolytes	Measurement of blood sodium (Na), potassium (K), and chlorides (Cl).
Embolectomy	Surgical removal of an embolus or clot from a blood vessel.
Heart transplantation	Replacement of a diseased or malfunctioning heart with a donor's heart.
Holter monitor	Portable ECG monitor worn by the patient for a period of a few hours to a few days to assess the heart and pulse activity as the person goes through the activities of daily living. Used to assess a patient who experiences chest pain and unusual heart activity during exercise and normal activities when a cardiogram is inconclusive.
Lipoproteins	Measurement of blood to determine serum cholesterol and triglycerides.
Open-heart surgery	Surgery that involves the heart, coronary arteries, or the heart valves. The heart is actually entered by the surgeon.
Percutaneous balloon valvuloplasty	Insertion through the skin of a balloon catheter across a narrowed or stenotic heart valve. When the balloon is inflated, the narrowing or constriction is decreased.
Percutaneous transluminal coronary angioplasty (PTCA)	Method for treating localized coronary artery narrowing. A balloon catheter is inserted through the skin into the coronary artery and inflated to dilate the narrow blood vessel.
Phleborrhaphy	Suturing of a vein.
Prothrombin time	Measurement of the time it takes for a sample of blood to coagulate.
Stress testing	Method for evaluating cardiovascular fitness. The patient is placed on a treadmill or bicycle and then subjected to steadily increasing levels of work. An EKG and oxygen levels are taken while the patient exercises. The test is stopped if abnormalities occur on the EKG.
Treadmill test	Also called a stress test.
Valve replacement	Surgical procedure to excise a diseased heart valve and replace with an artificial valve.
Venography	X-ray of the veins by tracing the venous flow. Also called phlebography.

TABLE 8   Disorders of the Endocrine System

Disorder	Description
Acidosis	Excessive acidity of bodily fluids due to the accumulation of acids, as in diabetic acidosis.
Acromegaly	Chronic disease of middle-aged persons which results in an elongation and enlargement of the bones of the head and extremities. There can also be mood changes.
Addison's disease	A disease resulting from a deficiency in adrenocortical hormones. There may be an increased pigmentation of the skin, generalized weakness, and weight loss.
Adenoma	A neoplasm or tumor of a gland.
Cretinism	Congenital condition due to a lack of thyroid, which may result in arrested physical and mental development.
Cushing's syndrome	Set of symptoms which result from hypersecretion of the adrenal cortex. This may be the result of a tumor of the adrenal glands. The syndrome may present symptoms of weakness, edema, excess hair growth, skin discoloration, and osteoporosis.
Diabetes insipidus (DI)	Disorder caused by the inadequate secretion of the antidiuretic hormone ADH by the posterior lobe of the pituitary gland. There may be polyuria and polydipsia.
Diabetes mellitus (DM)	Chronic disorder of carbohydrate metabolism which results in hyperglycemia and glycosuria. Type I diabetes mellitus (IDDM) involves insulin dependency, which requires that the patient take daily injections of insulin. Type II (NIDDM) patients may not be insulin dependent.
Diabetic retinopathy	Secondary complication of diabetes mellitus (DM) which affects the blood vessels of the retina, resulting in visual changes and even blindness.
Dwarfism	Condition of being abnormally small. It may be the result of a hereditary condition or an endocrine dysfunction.
Gigantism	Excessive development of long bones of the body due to overproduction of the growth hormone by the pituitary gland.
Goiter	Enlargement of the thyroid gland.
Graves' disease	Disease that results from an over activity of the thyroid gland and can result in a crisis situation. Also called hyperthyroidism.
Hashimoto's disease	A chronic form of thyroiditis.
Hirsutism	Condition of having an excessive amount of hair on the body. This term is used to describe females who have the adult male pattern of hair growth. Can be the result of a hormonal imbalance.
Hypercalcemia	Condition of having an excessive amount of calcium in the blood.
Hyperglycemia	Having an excessive amount of glucose (sugar) in the blood.
Hyperkalemia	Condition of having an excessive amount of potassium in the blood.
Hyperthyroidism	Condition that results from over activity of the thyroid gland. Also called Graves' disease.
Hypothyroidism	Result of a deficiency in secretion by the thyroid gland. This results in a lowered basal metabolism rate with obesity, dry skin, slow pulse, low blood pressure, sluggishness, and goiter. Treatment is replacement with synthetic thyroid hormone.
Ketoacidosis	Acidosis due to an excess of ketone bodies (waste products) which can result in death for the diabetic patient if not reversed.
Myasthenia gravis	Condition in which there is great muscular weakness and progressive fatigue. There may be difficulty in chewing and swallowing and drooping eyelids. If a thymoma is causing the problem, it can be treated with removal of the thymus gland.
Myxedema	Condition resulting from a hypofunction of the thyroid gland. Symptoms can include anemia, slow speech, enlarged tongue and facial features, edematous skin, drowsiness, and mental apathy.
Thyrotoxicosis	Condition that results from overproduction of the thyroid gland. Symptoms include a rapid heart action, tremors, enlarged thyroid gland, exophthalmos, and weight loss.
von Rechlinghausen's disease	Excessive production of parathyroid hormone, which results in degeneration of the bones.

TABLE 9   Procedures and Tests Relating to the Endocrine System

Procedure/Test	Description
Basal metabolic rate (BMR)	Somewhat outdated test to measure the energy used when the body is in a state of rest.
Blood serum test	Blood test to measure the level of substances such as calcium, electrolytes, testosterone, insulin, and glucose. Used to assist in determining the function of various endocrine glands.
Fasting blood sugar	Blood test to measure the amount of sugar circulating throughout the body after a 12-hour fast.
Glucose tolerance test (GTT)	Test to determine the blood sugar level. A measured dose of glucose is given to a patient either orally or intravenously. Blood samples are then drawn at certain intervals to determine the ability of the patient to utilize glucose. Used for diabetic patients to determine their insulin response to glucose.
Parathyroidectomy	Excision of one or more of the parathyroid glands. This is performed to halt the progress of hyperparathyroidism.
Protein bound iodine (PBI) test	Blood test to measure the concentration of thyroxin (T4) circulating in the bloodstream. The iodine becomes bound to the protein in the blood and can be measured. This test is useful in establishing thyroid function.
Radioactive iodine uptake (RAIU) test	Test in which radioactive iodine is taken orally (PO) or intravenously (IV) and the amount that is eventually taken into the thyroid gland (the uptake) is measured to assist in determining thyroid function.
Radioimmunoassay (RIA) test	Test used to measure the levels of hormones in the plasma of the blood.
Serum glucose test	Blood test performed to assist in determining insulin levels and useful for adjusting medication dosage.
Thymectomy	Surgical removal of the thymus gland.
Thyroid echogram	Ultrasound examination of the thyroid which can assist in distinguishing a thyroid nodule from a cyst.
Thyroidectomy	Surgical removal of the thyroid gland. The patient is then placed on replacement hormone (thyroid) therapy.

(continued)

TABLE 9   (continued)

Procedure/Test	Description
Thyroid function tests	Blood tests used to measure the levels of T3, T4, and TSH in the bloodstream to assist in determining thyroid function.
Thyroparathyroidectomy	Surgical removal (excision) of the thyroid and parathyroid glands.
Thyroid scan	Test in which a radioactive element is administered which localizes in the thyroid gland. The gland can then be visualized with a scanning device to detect pathology such as tumors.
Total calcium	Blood test to measure the total amount of calcium to assist in detecting parathyroid and bone disorders.
Two-hour postprandial glucose tolerance test	Blood test to assist in evaluating glucose metabolism. The patient eats a high-carbohydrate diet and fasts overnight before the test. A blood sample is then taken two hours after a meal.

TABLE 10   Disorders and Pathology of the Digestive System

Disorder/Pathology	Description
Anorexia	Loss of appetite that can accompany other conditions such as a gastrointestinal (GI) upset.
Ascites	Collection or accumulation of fluid in the peritoneal cavity.
Bulimia	Eating disorder that is characterized by recurrent binge eating and then purging of the food with laxatives and vomiting.
Cholecystitis	Inflammation of the gallbladder.
Cholelithiasis	Formation or presence of stones or calculi in the gallbladder or common bile duct.
Cirrhosis	Chronic disease of the liver.
Cleft lip	Congenital condition in which the upper lip fails to come together. This is often seen along with cleft palate and is corrected with surgery.
Cleft palate	Congenital condition in which the roof of the mouth has a split or fissure. It is corrected with surgery.
Constipation	Experiencing difficulty in defecation or infrequent defecation.
Crohn's disease	Form of chronic inflammatory bowel disease affecting the ileum and/or colon. Also called regional ileitis.
Diverticulitis	Inflammation of a diverticulum or sac in the intestinal tract, especially in the colon.
Diarrhea	Passing of frequent, watery bowel movements. Usually accompanies gastrointestinal (GI) disorders.
Dyspepsia	Indigestion.
Emesis	Vomiting usually with some force.
Enteritis	Inflammation of only the small intestine.
Esophageal stricture	Narrowing of the esophagus which makes the flow of foods and fluids difficult.
Fissure	Cracklike split in the rectum or anal canal or roof of mouth.
Fistula	Abnormal tubelike passage from one body cavity to another.
Gastritis	Inflammation of the stomach which can result in pain, tenderness, nausea, and vomiting.
Gastroenteritis	Inflammation of the stomach and small intestine.
Halitosis	Bad or offensive breath, which is often a sign of disease.
Hepatitis	Inflammation of the liver.
Ileitis	Inflammation of the ileum of the small intestine.
Inflammatory bowel syndrome	Ulceration of the mucous membranes of the colon of unknown origin. Also known as ulcerative colitis.
Inguinal hernia	Hernia or outpouching of intestines into the inguinal region of the body. May require surgical correction.
Intussusception	Result of the intestine slipping or telescoping into another section of intestine just below it. More common in children.
Irritable bowel syndrome	Disturbance in the functions of the intestine from unknown causes. Symptoms generally include abdominal discomfort and an alteration in bowel activity.
Malabsorption syndrome	Inadequate absorption of nutrients from the intestinal tract. May be caused by a variety of diseases and disorders, such as infections and pancreatic deficiency.
Peptic ulcer	Ulcer occurring in the lower portion of the esophagus, stomach, and duodenum thought to be caused by the acid of gastric juices. Some peptic ulcers are now successfully treated with antibiotics.
Pilonidal cyst	Cyst in the sacrococcygeal region due to tissue being trapped below the skin.
Polyphagia	To eat excessively.
Polyps	Small tumors that contain a pedicle or footlike attachment in the mucous membranes of the large intestine (colon).
Reflux esophagitis	Acid from the stomach backs up into the esophagus causing inflammation and pain. Also called GERD (gastroesophageal reflux disease).
Regurgitation	Return of fluids and solids from the stomach into the mouth. Similar to emesis but without the force.
Ulcerative colitis	Ulceration of the mucous membranes of the colon of unknown source. Also known as inflammatory bowel disease.
Volvulus	Condition in which the bowel twists upon itself and causes an obstruction. Painful and requires immediate surgery.

TABLE 11 Procedures and Tests Relating to the Digestive System

Procedure/Test	Description
Abdominal ultrasonography	Using ultrasound equipment for producing sound waves to create an image of the abdominal organs.
Air contrast barium enema	Using both barium and air to visualize the colon on x-ray.
Anastomosis	Creating a passageway or opening between two organs or vessels.
Appendectomy	Surgical removal of the appendix.
Barium enema (Lower GI)	Radiographic examination of the small intestine, large intestine, or colon in which an enema containing barium is administered to the patient while the x-ray pictures are taken.
Barium swallow (Upper GI)	A barium mixture swallowed while x-ray pictures are taken of the esophagus, stomach, and duodenum used to visualize the upper gastrointestinal tract. Also called esophagram.
Colectomy	Surgical removal of the entire colon.
Cholecystectomy	Surgical excision of the gallbladder. Removal of the gallbladder through the laparoscope is a newer procedure with fewer complications than the more invasive abdominal surgery. The laparoscope requires a small incision into the abdominal cavity.
Cholecystogram	Dye given orally to the patient is absorbed and enters the gallbladder. An x-ray is then taken.
Choledocholithotomy	Removal of a gallstone through an incision into the bile duct.
Choledocholithotripsy	Crushing of a gallstone in the common bile duct. Commonly called lithotripsy.
Colonoscopy	A flexible fiberscope passed through the anus, rectum, and colon is used to examine the upper portion of the colon. Polyps and small growths can be removed during the procedure.
Colostomy	Surgical creation of an opening of some portion of the colon through the abdominal wall to the outside surface.
Diverticulectomy	Surgical removal of a diverticulum.
Endoscopic retrograde cholangiopancreatography (ERCP)	Using an endoscope to x-ray the bile and pancreatic ducts.
Esophagoscopy	The esophagus is visualized by passing an instrument down the esophagus. A tissue sample for biopsy may be taken.
Esophagram (barium swallow)	As barium is swallowed the solution is observed traveling from the mouth into the stomach over a television monitor.
Esophagogastrostomy	Surgical creation of an opening between the esophagus and the stomach. Also called Upper GI.
Esophagostomy	Surgical creation of an opening into the esophagus.
Exploratory laparotomy	Abdominal operation for the purpose of examining the abdominal organs and tissues for signs of disease or other abnormalities.
Fistulectomy	Excision of a fistula.
Gastrectomy	Surgical removal of a part of or whole stomach.
Gastrointestinal endoscopy	A flexible instrument or scope is passed either through the mouth or anus to facilitate visualization of the gastrointestinal (GI) tract.
Glossectomy	Complete or partial removal of the tongue.
Hemorrhoidectomy	Surgical excision of hemorrhoids from the anorectal area.
Hepatic lobectomy	Surgical removal of a lobe of the liver.
Ileostomy	Surgical creation of a passage through the abdominal wall into the ileum. The fecal material (stool) drains into a bag worn on the abdomen.
Intravenous cholangiogram	A dye is administered intravenously to the patient that allows for visualization of the bile vessels.
Intravenous cholecystography	A dye is administered intravenously to the patient that allows for visualization of the gallbladder.
Jejunostomy	Surgical creation of a permanent opening into the jejunum.
Lithotripsy	Crushing of a stone located within the gallbladder.
Liver biopsy	Excision of a small piece of liver tissue for microscopic examination. This is generally used to determine if cancer is present.
Liver scan	A radioactive substance is administered to the patient by an intravenous (IV) route. This substance enters the liver cells, and this organ can then be visualized. This is used to detect tumors, abscesses, and other hepatomegaly.

TABLE 12   Disorders and Pathology of the Lymphatic System

Disorder/Pathology	Description
Acquired immune deficiency syndrome (AIDS)	A disease that involves a defect in the cell-mediated immunity system. A syndrome of opportunistic infections occur in the final stages of infection with the human immunodeficiency virus (HIV). This virus attacks T4 lymphocytes and destroys them, which reduces the person's ability to fight infection.
AIDS-related complex (ARC)	A complex of symptoms which appears in the early stages of AIDS. This is a positive test for the virus but only mild symptoms of weight loss, fatigue, skin rash, and anorexia.
Elephantiasis	Inflammation, obstruction, and destruction of the lymph vessels which results in enlarged tissues due to edema.
Epstein-Barr virus	Virus which is believed to be the cause of infectious mononucleosis.
Hodgkin's disease	Lymphatic system disease that can result in solid tumors in any lymphoid tissue.
Lymphadenitis	Inflammation of the lymph glands. Referred to as swollen glands.
Lymphangioma	A benign mass of lymphatic vessels.
Lyphoma	Malignant tumor of the lymph nodes and tissue.
Lymphosarcoma	Malignant disease of the lymphatic tissue.
Mononucleosis	Acute infectious disease with a large number of atypical lymphocytes. Caused by the Epstein-Barr virus. There may be abnormal liver function and spleen enlargement.
Multiple sclerosis	Autoimmune disorder of the central nervous system in which the myelin sheath of nerves is attacked.
Non-Hodgkin's lymphoma	Malignant, solid tumors of lymphoid tissue.
Peritonsillar abscess	Infection of the tissues between the tonsils and the pharynx. Also called quinsy sore throat.
Sarcoidoisis	Inflammatory disease of the lymph system in which lesions may appear in the liver, skin, lungs, lymph nodes, spleen, eyes, and small bones of the hands and feet.
Splenomegaly	Enlargement of the spleen.
Systemic lupus erythematosis (SLE)	A chronic autoimmune disorder of connective tissue that causes injury to the skin, joints, kidneys, mucous membranes, and nervous system.
Thymoma	Malignant tumor of the thymus gland.

TABLE 13   Procedures and Tests Relating to the Lymphatic System

Procedure/Test	Description
Bone marrow aspiration	Removing a sample of bone marrow by syringe for microscopic examination. Useful for diagnosing such diseases as leukemia. For example, a proliferation (massive increase) of white blood cells could confirm the diagnosis of leukemia.
ELISA	Enzyme immunoassay test used to test blood for an antibody to the AIDS virus. A positive test means that the person has been exposed to the virus. There may be a false-positive reading and then the Western blot test would be used to verify the results.
Lymphadenectomy	Excision of a lymph node. This is usually done to test for a malignancy.
Lymphangiogram	X-ray taken of the lymph vessels after the injection of dye into the foot. The lymph flow through the chest is traced.
Splenopexy	The artificial fixation of a movable spleen.
Tonsillectomy	The surgical removable of the tonsils. Usually the adenoids are removed at the same time. This procedure is known as a T & A.
Western Blot	The test that is used as backup to the ELISA blood test to detect the presence of the antibody to HIV (AIDS virus) in the blood.

TABLE 14   Disorders of the Musculoskeletal System

Disorder	Description
Arthritis	Inflammation of the bone joints.
Bunion	Enlargement of the joint at the base of the great toe caused by inflammation of the bursa of the great toe.
Bursitis	Inflammation of the bursa, the connective tissue surrounding a joint.
Carpal tunnel syndrome	Pain caused by compression of the nerve as it passes between the bones and tendons of the wrist.
Gout	Inflammation of the joints caused by excessive uric acid.
Kyphosis	Abnormal increase in the outward curvature of the thoracic spine. Also known as hunchback or humpback.
Lordosis	Abnormal increase in the forward curvature of the lumbar spine. Also known as swayback.
Muscular dystrophy	Inherited disease causing a progressive muscle weakness and atrophy.
Myasthenia gravis	An autoimmune disorder causing loss of muscle strength and paralysis.
Osteoarthritis	Noninflammatory type of arthritis resulting in degeneration of the bones and joints, especially those bearing weight.
Osteomalacia	Softening of the bones caused by a deficiency of phosphorus or calcium. It is thought that in children the cause is insufficient sunlight and vitamin D.
Osteomyelitis	Inflammation of the bone and bone marrow due to infection; can be difficult to treat.
Osteoporosis	Decrease in bone mass that results in a thinning and weakening of the bone with resulting fractures. The bones become more porous, especially in the spine and pelvis.

(continued)

TABLE 14   *(continued)*

Disorder	Description
Paget's disease	A fairly common metabolic disease of the bone from unknown causes. It usually attacks middle-aged and elderly people and is characterized by bone destruction and deformity.
Polymyositis	A disease causing muscle inflammation and weakness from an unknown cause.
Rheumatoid arthritis	Chronic form of arthritis with inflammation of the joints, swelling, stiffness, pain, and changes in the cartilage that can result in crippling deformities.
Rickets	Deficiency in calcium and vitamin D in early childhood which results in bone deformities, especially bowed legs.
Ruptured intervertebral disk	Herniation or outpouching of a disk between two vertebrae—also called a slipped or herniated disk.
Scoliosis	Abnormal lateral curvature of the spine.
Spinal stenosis	Narrowing of the spinal canal causing pressure on the cord and nerves.
Supernumerary bone	An extra bone, generally a finger or toe, found in newborns.
Talipes	Congenital deformity of the foot. This is also referred to as a clubfoot.
Tumors: Benign	
• Epidermoid cyst	Cysts located in the skull and phalanges of the fingers.
• Ganglion cyst	Cyst found at the end of long bones.
• Giant cell tumor	Benign tumor that appears at the epiphysis but does not interfere with joint movement. It may become malignant or return after removal.
• Osteoblastoma	A benign lesion or tumor which is generally found on the spine, where it may result in paralysis.
• Osteochondroma	Tumor composed of both cartilage and bony substance.
• Osteoid osteoma	Painful tumor usually found in the lower extremities.
Malignant	
• Ewing's sarcoma	Malignant growth found in the shaft of the long bones that spreads through the periosteum. Removal is treatment of choice, as this tumor will metastasize or spread to other organs.
• Fibrosarcoma	Tumor that contains connective tissue that occurs in bone marrow. It is found most frequently in the femur, humerus, and jaw bone.
• Myeloma	Malignant neoplasm originating in plasma cells in the bone.
Whiplash	Injury to the bones in the cervical spine as a result of a sudden movement forward and backward of the head and neck. Can occur as a result of a rear-end auto collision.

TABLE 15   Procedures and Diagnostic Tests Relating to the Musculoskeletal System

Procedure/Test	Description
Amputation	Partial or complete removal of a limb for a variety of reasons, including tumors, gangrene, intractable pain, crushing injury, or uncontrollable infection.
Anterior cruciate ligament (ACL) reconstruction	Replacing a torn ACL with a graft by means of arthroscopy.
Arthrocentesis	Removal of synovial fluid with a needle from a joint space, such as in the knee, for examination.
Arthrodesis	Surgical reconstruction of a joint.
Arthrography	Visualization of a joint by a radiographic study after injection of a contrast medium into a joint space.
Arthroplasty	Surgical reconstruction of a joint.
Arthroscopic surgery	Use of an arthroscope, a lighted instrument with camera/video capabilities, to facilitate performing surgery on a joint.
Arthrotomy	Surgically cutting into a joint.
Bone graft	Piece of bone taken from the patient that is used to take the place of a removed bone or a bony defect at another site, or to be wedged between bones for fusion of a joint.
Bone scan	Use of scanning equipment to visualize bones. It is especially useful in observing progress of treatment for osteomyelitis and cancer metastases to the bone.
Bunionectomy	Removal of the bursa at the joint of the great toe.
Carpal tunnel release	Surgical cutting of the ligament in the wrist to relieve nerve pressure caused by repetitive motion, for example typing (carpal tunnel disease).
Computerized axial tomography (CAT)	Computer-assisted x-ray used to detect tumors and fractures. Also referred to as CT-scan.
Electromyography	Study and record of the strength of muscle contractions as a result of electrical stimulation. Used in the diagnosis of muscle disorders and to distinguish nerve disorders from muscle disorders,.
Fasciectomy	Surgical removal of the fascia, which is the fibrous membrane covering and supporting muscles.
Laminectomy	Removal of the vertebral posterior arch to correct severe back problems caused by compression of the lamina.
Magnetic resonance imaging (MRI)	Medical imaging that uses radio-frequency radiation as its source of energy. It does not require the injection of contrast medium or exposure to ionizing radiation. The technique is useful for visualizing large blood vessels, the heart, brain, and soft tissues.

(continued)

TABLE 15   *Continued*

Procedure/Test	Description
Menisectomy	Removal of the knee cartilage (meniscus).
Muscle biopsy	Removal of muscle tissue for pathological examination.
Myelography	Study of the spinal column after injecting opaque contrast material.
Photon absorptiometry	Measurement of bone density using an instrument for the purpose of detecting osteoporosis.
Reduction	Correcting a fracture by realigning the bone fragments. A closed reduction of the fracture is the manipulation of the bone into alignment and the application of a cast or splint to immobilize the part during the healing process. Open reduction is the surgical incision at the site of the fracture to perform the bone re-alignment. This is necessary when there are bone fragments to be removed.
Spinal fusion	Surgical immobilization of adjacent vertebrae. This may be done for several reasons, including correction of a herniated disk.
Total hip replacement	Surgical reconstruction of a hip by implanting a prosthetic or artificial joint.

TABLE 16   Disorders and Diseases of the Nervous System

Disorder/Disease	Description
Amnesia	Loss of memory in which people forget their identity as a result of head injury or a disorder, such as epilepsy, senility, and alcoholism. This can be either temporary or permanent.
Amyotrophic lateral sclerosis (ALS)	Disease with muscular weakness and atrophy due to degeneration of motor neurons of the spinal cord. Also called Lou Gehrig's disease, after the New York Yankees' baseball player who died from the disease.
Aneurysm	Localized abnormal dilatation of a blood vessel, usually an artery; the result of a congenital defect or weakness in the wall of the vessel.
Anorexia nervosa	Loss of appetite, which generally occurs in females between the ages of 12 and 21, due to a fear of obesity. The patient believes that she is fat even when thin. Psychiatric treatment may be necessary if the patient refuses to eat, since death can occur.
Aphasia	Loss of ability to speak.
Asthenia	Lack or loss of strength, causing extreme weakness.
Astrocytoma	Tumor of the brain or spinal cord that is composed of astrocytes.
Ataxia	Lack of muscle coordination as a result of a disorder or disease.
Autism	Form of mental introversion in which the patient, usually a child, shows no interest in anything or anyone except himself or herself.
Bell's palsy	One-sided facial paralysis caused by herpes simplex virus. The person cannot control salivation, tearing of the eyes, or expression but will usually recover.
Brain tumor	Intracranial mass, either benign or malignant. A benign tumor of the brain can be fatal since it will grow and cause pressure on normal brain tissue. The most malignant form of brain tumor in children is the glioma.
Cerebral palsy	Nonprogressive paralysis resulting from a defect or trauma at the time of birth.
Cerebrovascular accident (CVA)	Hemorrhagic lesion in the brain which can result in paralysis and the inability to speak.
Chorea	Involuntary nervous disorder that results in muscular twitching of the limbs or facial muscles.
Coma	Abnormal deep sleep or stupor resulting from an illness or injury.
Concussion	Injury to the brain that results from an illness or injury.
Convulsion (seizure)	Sudden severe involuntary muscle contractions and relaxations. These have a variety of causes, such as head injury, epilepsy, fever, and toxic conditions.
Encephalitis	Inflammation of the brain due to disease factors, such as rabies, influenza, measles, or smallpox.
Embolism	Obstruction of a blood vessel by a blood clot or foreign substance, such as air and/or fat.
Epidural hematoma	Mass of blood in the space outside the dura mater of the brain and spinal cord.
Epilepsy	A recurrent disorder of the brain in which convulsive seizures and loss of consciousness occurs.
• Grand mal	Severe seizures in which loss of consciousness and muscular contractions occur.
• Petit mal	Form of epilepsy in which there is an alteration in the level of consciousness but an absence of seizures or convulsions.
• Jacksonian	A localized form of epilepsy with spasms confined to one part or one group of muscles.
Glioma	Sarcoma of neurological origin.
Hematoma	Swelling or mass of blood confined to a specific area, such as in the brain.
Herniated nucleus pulposa	Protrusion of the nucleus pulposa of the intervertebral disk into the spinal canal. This is also called a herniated disk.
Huntington's chorea	Disease of the central nervous system that results in progressive dementia with bizarre involuntary movements of parts of the body.
Hydrocephalus	Accumulation of cerebrospinal fluid within the ventricles of the brain, causing pressure on the brain and for the head to be enlarged. It is treated by creating an artificial shunt for the fluid to leave the brain.
Meningioma	Slow-growing tumor in the meninges of the brain.
Meningitis	Inflammation of the membranes of the spinal cord and brain that is caused by a microorganism.

(continued)

TABLE 16   *(continued)*

Disorder/Disease	Description
Meningocele	Congenital hernia in which the meninges, or membranes, protrude through an opening in the spinal column or brain.
Multiple sclerosis	Degenerative, demyelination, inflammatory disease of the central nervous system in which there is extreme weakness and numbness.
Narcolepsy	Chronic disorder in which there is an extreme uncontrollable desire to sleep.
Neuritis	Inflammation of a nerve or nerves, causing pain.
Neuroblastoma	Malignant metastatic hemorrhagic tumor that originates in the sympathetic nervous system, especially in the adrenal medulla. Occurs mainly in infants and children.
Palsy	Temporary or permanent loss of the ability to control movement.
Paralysis	A temporary or permanent loss of the ability to control movement.
• Paraplegia	Paralysis of the lower portion of the body and both legs.
• Hemiplegia	Paralysis of only one side of the body. This is the same as hemiparesis.
• Quadriplegia	Paralysis of all four limbs. This is the same as tetraplegia.
Parkinson's disease	Chronic progressive disorder of the nervous system with fine tremors, muscular weakness, rigidity, and a shuffling gait.
Pica	An eating disorder in which there is a craving for material that is not food, such as clay, grass, wood, dirt, paper, soap, and plaster.
Reye's syndrome	A combination of symptoms that generally occurs in children under 15 years of age one week after they have had viral infection. It begins with a rash, vomiting, and confusion and may lead to coma, seizures, or respiratory arrest.
Shingles	Eruption of vesicles on the trunk of the body along a nerve path. Can be painful and generally occurs on only one side of the body. It is caused by the herpes zoster.
Spina bifida	Congenital defect in the walls of the spinal canal in which the laminae of the vertebra do not meet or close. May cause membranes and/or the spinal cord to herniate through the opening. This condition can also result in other defects such as hydrocephalus (fluid on the brain).
Subdural hematoma	Mass of blood forming beneath the dura mater of the brain.
Syncope	Fainting.
Tic douloureaux	Painful condition in which the trigeminal nerve is affected by pressure or degeneration. The pain is of a severe stabbing nature and radiates from the jaw and along the face.
Transient ischemic attack (TIA)	Temporary interference with blood supply to the brain, causing neurological symptoms, such as dizziness, numbness, and hemiparesis. May lead eventually to a full-blown stroke (CVA).

TABLE 17   Procedures and Tests Relating to the Nervous System

Procedure/Test	Description
Babinski's sign	Reflex test developed by John Babinski, a French neurologist, to determine lesions and abnormalities in the nervous system. The Babinski reflex is present, for a positive Babinski, if the great toe extends instead of flexes when the lateral sole of the foot is stroked. The normal response to this stimulation would be a flexion, or upward movement of the toe.
Brain scan	Injection of radioactive isotopes into the circulation to determine the function and abnormality of the brain.
Carotid endarterectomy	A surgical procedure for removing an obstruction within the carotid artery. It was developed to prevent strokes but is found to be useful only in severe stenosis with TIA.
Cerebral angiogram	X-ray of the blood vessels of the brain after the injection of radiopaque dye.
Cerebrospinal fluid shunts	Surgical creation of an artificial opening to allow for the passage of fluid. Used in the treatment of hydrocephalus.
Cordectomy	Removal of part of the spinal cord.
Craniotomy	Surgical incision into the brain through the cranium.
Cryosurgery	Use of extreme cold to produce areas of destruction in the brain. Used to control bleeding and treat brain tumors.
Echoencephalogram	Recording of the ultrasonic echoes of the brain. Useful in determining abnormal patterns of shifting in the brain.
Electromyogram	Written recording of the contraction of muscles as a result of receiving electrical stimulation.
Laminectomy	Removal of a vertebral posterior arch.
Lumbar puncture	Puncture with a needle into the lumbar area (usually the fourth intervertebral space) to withdraw fluid for examination and for the injection of anesthesia.
Nerve block	A method of regional anesthetic to stop the passage of sensory stimulation along a nerve path.
Pneumoencephalography	X-ray examination of the brain following withdrawal of cerebrospinal fluid and injection of air or gas via spinal puncture.
Positron emission tomography (PET)	Use of positive radionuclides to reconstruct brain sections. Measurement can be taken of oxygen and glucose uptake, cerebral blood flow, and blood volume.
Romberg's sign	Test developed to establish neurological function in which the person is asked to close their eyes and place their feet together. This test for body balance is positive if the patient sways when the eyes are closed.
Spinal puncture	Puncture with a needle into the spinal cavity to withdraw spinal fluid for microscopic analysis. Anesthetic is also administered by this route. This is also called a spinal tap.
Sympathectomy	Excision of a portion of the sympathetic nervous system. Could include a nerve or ganglion.
Transcutaneous electrical nerve stimulation (TENS)	Application of a mild electrical stimulation to skin electrodes placed over a painful area, causing interference with the transmission of the painful stimuli. Can be used in pain management to interfere with the normal pain mechanism.
Trephination	Process of cutting out a piece of bone in the skull to gain entry into the brain to relieve pressure.
Vagotomy	Surgical incision into the vagus nerve. Medication can be administered into the nerve to prevent its function.

TABLE 18   Common Disorders of the Eye

Disorder	Description
Achromatopsia	The condition of color blindness. This is more common in males.
Astigmatism	An eye disorder in which light rays are focused unevenly on the retina, resulting in a distorted image due to the abnormal curvature of the cornea.
Blepharitis	Inflammatory condition of the eyelash follicles and glands of the eyelids which results in swelling, redness, and crusts of dried mucus on the lids. This can be the result of allergy or infection.
Blepharochalasis	In this condition, the upper eyelid increases in size due to loss of elasticity, which is followed by swelling and recurrent edema of the lids. The skin may droop over the edges of the eyes when the eyes are open.
Cataract	Diminished vision resulting from the lens of the eye becoming opaque or cloudy. Treatment is usually surgical removal of the cataract.
Chalazion	A small, hard tumor or mass, similar to a sebaceous cyst, developing on the eyelid. This may require incision and drainage (I & D).
Conjunctivitis	An inflammation of the conjunctiva which is also called pinkeye.
Diabetic retinopathy	Small hemorrhages and edema that develop as a result of diabetes mellitus. Laser surgery and vitrectomy may be necessary for treatment.
Ectropion	Refers to an enversion (outward turning) of the eyelid, exposing the conjunctiva.
Entropion	Inversion (inward turning) of the eyelid.
Esotropia	Inward turning of the eye. An example of strabismus (muscle weakness of the eye).
Exophthalmus	Abnormal protrusion of the eyeball. Can be due to hyperthyroidism.
Esotropia	Outward turning of the eye. Also an example of strabismus (muscle weakness of the eye).
Glaucoma	Increase in intraocular pressure, which, if untreated, may result in atrophy (wasting away) of the optic nerve and blindness. Glaucoma is treated with medication and surgery. There is an increased risk of developing glaucoma in persons over 60 years of age, in people of African ancestry, after sustaining a serious eye injury, and in anyone with a family history of diabetes or glaucoma. Figure 22-8 [ID23-19] illustrates a glaucoma test.
Hemianopia	Loss of vision in half of the visual field. A stroke patient may suffer from this condition.
Hordeolum	Refers to a sty which is a small purulent inflammatory infection of a sebaceous gland of the eye. This is treated with hot compresses and, if necessary, surgical incision.
Hyperopia	With this condition a person can see things in the distance but has trouble reading material at close vision. It is also known as farsightedness.
Keratitis	Inflammation of the cornea.
Macular degeneration	Degeneration or deterioration of the macular area of the retina of the eye. It may be treated with laser surgery to destroy the blood vessels beneath the macula.
Myopia	With this condition a person can see things close up but distance vision is blurred. It is also known as nearsightedness.
Nystagmus	Jerky-appearing involuntary eye movement.
Presbyopia	Visual change due to aging, resulting in difficulty in focusing for near vision (such as reading).
Retinal detachment	A disorder that occurs when the two layers of the retina become separated or detached. The treatment is surgery.
Retinitis pigmentosa	Progressive disease of the eye which results in the retina becoming hard (sclerosed), pigmented, and atrophying (wasting away). There is no known cure for this condition.
Strabismus	An eye muscle weakness resulting in the eyes looking in different directions at the same time. (The eyes may be divergent or convergent). May be corrected with glasses, and/or surgery. Also called lazy eye, crossed eyes, or squint.
Trachoma	A chronic infectious disease of the conjunctiva and cornea caused by bacteria. This occurs more commonly in people living in hot, dry climates. Untreated, it may lead to blindness when the scarring invades the cornea. Trachoma can be treated with antibiotics.

TABLE 19   Procedures and Diagnostic Tests Relating to the Eye

Procedure/Test	Description
Fluorescein angiography	The process of injecting a dye (fluorescein) to observe the movement of blood for detecting lesions in the macular area of the retina. This is used to determine if there is a detachment of the retina.
Gonioscopy	Use of an instrument called a gonioscope to examine the anterior chamber of the eye to determine ocular motility and rotation.
Keratometry	Measurement of the cornea using an instrument called a keratometer.
Laser Surgery	Surgical procedure performed with a laser handpiece that transfers light into intense, small beams capable of destroying or fixing tissue in place.
Slit lamp microscope	The instrument used in ophthalmology for examining the posterior surface of the cornea.
Tonometry	Measurement of the intraocular pressure of the eye using a tonometer to check for the condition of glaucoma. After a topical anesthetic is applied, the physician places the tonometer lightly upon the eyeball and a pressure measurement is taken. An air-puff tonometer similarly records the cornea's resistance to pressure, but uses more expensive equipment. This is generally part of a normal eye examination for adults.
Visual acuity	Measurements of the sharpness of a patient's vision. Usually a Snellen chart is used for this test and the patient identifies letters from a distance of 20 feet.
Vitrectomy	A surgical procedure for replacing the contents of the vitreous chamber of the eye.

TABLE 20   Common Disorders of the Ear

Disorder	Description
Acoustic neuroma	Benign tumor of the eighth cranial nerve sheath which can cause symptoms from pressure being exerted on tissues.
Anacusis	Total loss of hearing. Also called deafness.
Cerumen block	Ear wax causing a blockage in the external canal of the ear.
Conductive hearing loss	Loss of hearing as a result of the blocking of sound transmission in the middle ear or outer ear.
Meniere's disease	An abnormal condition within the labyrinth of the inner ear that can lead to a progressive hearing loss. The symptoms are dizziness or vertigo, hearing loss, and tinnitus (ringing in the ears).
Otitis media	Commonly referred to as a middle ear infection. This is seen frequently in children and is often preceded by an upper respiratory infection.
Otosclerosis	Progressive hearing loss caused by immobility of the stapes bone.
Presbycusis	Loss of hearing that can accompany the aging process.

TABLE 21   Procedures and Diagnostic Tests Relating to the Ear

Procedure/Test	Description
Audiogram	A chart that shows the faintest sounds a patient can hear during audiometry testing.
Audiometric test	A test of hearing ability by determining the lowest and highest intensity and frequencies that a person can distinguish. The patient may sit in a soundproof booth and receive sounds through earphones as the technician decreases and changes the volume or tones.
Falling test	A test used to observe balance and equilibrium. The patient is observed on one foot, then with one foot in front of the other, and then walking forward with eyes open. The same test is conducted with the patient's eyes closed. Swaying and falling with the eyes closed can indicate an ear and equilibrium malfunction.
Mastoid antrotomy	Surgical opening made in the cavity within the mastoid process to alleviate pressure from infection and allow for drainage.
Mastoid x-ray	X-ray taken of the mastoid bone to determine the presence of an infection, which can be an extension of a middle ear infection.
Myringoplasty	Surgical reconstruction of the eardrum.
Myringotomy	Surgical puncture of the eardrum with removal of fluid and pus from the middle ear, to eliminate a persistent ear infection and excessive pressure on the tympanic membrane. A tube is placed in the tympanic membrane to allow for drainage of the middle ear cavity.
Otoplasty	Corrective surgery to change the size of the external ear or pinna. The surgery can either enlarge or decrease the size of the pinna.
Otoscopy	The use of a lighted instrument (otoscope) to examine the external auditory canal and the middle ear.
Rinne and Weber tuning-fork tests	The physician holds a tuning fork, an instrument that produces a constant pitch when it is struck, against or near the bones on the side of the head. These tests assess both nerve and bone conduction of sound.
Sensorineural hearing loss	A type of hearing loss in which the sound is conducted normally through the external and middle ear but there is a defect in the inner ear or with the auditory nerve (eighth cranial nerve), resulting in the inability to hear.
Stapedectomy	Removal of the stapes bone to treat otosclerosis (hardening of the bone). A prosthesis or artificial stapes is implanted.
Tympanometry	Measurement of the movement of the tympanic membrane. Can indicate the presence of pressure in the middle ear.
Tympanoplasty	Another term for the surgical reconstruction of the eardrum. Also called myringoplasty.

TABLE 22   Common Disorders and Pathology of the Reproductive System

Disorder/Pathology	Description
Abruptio placenta	An emergency condition in which the placenta tears away from the uterine wall before the 20th week of pregnancy. This requires immediate delivery of the baby.
Amenorrhea	An absence of menstruation, which can be the result of many factors, including pregnancy, menopause, and dieting.
Breech presentation	Position of the fetus within the uterus in which the buttocks or feet are presented first for delivery rather than the head.
Carcinoma in situ	Malignant tumor that has not extended beyond the original site.
Cervical cancer	A malignant growth in the cervix of the uterus. This is an especially difficult type of cancer to treat, and causes 5 percent of the cancer deaths in women. PAP tests have helped to detect early cervical cancer.
Cervical polyps	Fibrous or mucous tumor or growth found in the cervix of the uterus. These are removed surgically if there is a danger that they will become malignant.
Cervicitis	Inflammation of the cervix of the uterus.
Choriocarcinoma	A rare type of cancer of the uterus which may occur following a normal pregnancy or abortion.
Condyloma	A wartlike growth on the external genitalia. *(continued)*

TABLE 22   *(continued)*

Disorder/Pathology	Description
Cystocele	Hernia or outpouching of the bladder that protrudes into the vagina. This may cause urinary frequency and urgency.
Dysmenorrhea	Painful cramping that is associated with menstruation.
Eclampsia	Convulsive seizures and coma occurring between the 20th week of pregnancy and the first week of postpartum.
Ectopic	A fetus that becomes abnormally implanted outside the uterine cavity. This is a condition requiring immediate surgery.
Endometrial cancer	Cancer of the endometrial lining of the uterus.
Fibroid tumor	Benign tumor or growth that contains fiberlike tissue. Uterine fibroid tumors are the most common tumors in women.
Mastitis	Inflammation of the breast, which is common during lactation but can occur at any age.
Menorrhagia	Excessive bleeding during the menstrual period. Can be either in the total number of days or the amount of blood or both.
Ovarian carcinoma	Cancer of the ovary.
Ovarian cyst	Sac that develops within the ovary.
Pelvic inflammatory disease (PID)	Any inflammation of the female reproductive organs, generally bacterial in nature.
Placenta previa	When the placenta has become attached to the lower portion of the uterus and, in turn, blocks the birth canal.
Preeclampsia	Toxemia of pregnancy which if untreated can result in true eclampsia. Symptoms include hypertension, headaches, albumin in the urine, and edema.
Premature birth	Delivery in which the infant (neonate) is born before the thirty-seventh week of gestation (pregnancy).
Premenstrual syndrome (PMS)	Symptoms that develop just prior to the onset of a menstrual period, which can include irritability, headache, tender breasts, and anxiety.
Prolapsed uterus	A fallen uterus that can cause the cervix to protrude through the vaginal opening. It is generally caused by weakened muscles from vaginal delivery or as a result of pelvic tumors pressing down.
Rh factor	A condition developing in the baby when the mother's blood type is Rh-negative and the father's is Rh-positive. The baby's red blood cells can be destroyed as a result of this condition. Treatment is early diagnosis and blood transfusion.
Salpingitis	Inflammation of the fallopian tube or tubes.
Spontaneous abortion	Loss of a fetus without any artificial aid. Also called a miscarriage.
Stillbirth	Birth in which the fetus dies before or at the time of delivery.
Toxic shock syndrome	Rare and sometimes fatal staphylococcus infection that generally occurs in menstruating women.
Tubal pregnancy	Implantation of a fetus within the fallopian tube instead of the uterus. This requires immediate surgery.
Vaginitis	Inflammation of the vagina, generally caused by a microorganism.

TABLE 23   Procedures and Diagnostic Tests Relating to the Female Reproductive System

Procedure/Test	Description
Abortion	The termination of a pregnancy before the fetus reaches a viable point in development.
Amniocentesis	Puncturing of the amniotic sac using a needle and syringe for the purpose of withdrawing amniotic fluid for testing. Can assist in determining fetal maturity, development, and genetic disorders.
Cauterization	The destruction of tissue using an electric current, a caustic product, a hot iron, or freezing.
Cervical biopsy	Taking a sample of tissue from the cervix to test for the presence of cancer cells.
Cesarean section (C-section)	Surgical delivery of a baby through an incision into the abdominal and uterine walls.
Colposcopy	Visual examination of the cervix and vagina.
Conization	Surgical removal of a core of cervical tissue or a partial removal of the cervix.
Cryosurgery	Exposing tissues to extreme cold in order to destroy tissues. This procedure is used in treating malignant tumors, to control pain and bleeding.
Culdoscopy	Examination of the female pelvic cavity using an endoscope.
Dilation and curettage (D&C)	Surgical procedure in which the opening of the cervix is dilated and the uterus is scraped or suctioned of its lining or tissue. A D & C is performed after a spontaneous abortion and to stop excessive bleeding from other causes.
Doppler ultrasound	Using an instrument placed externally over the uterus to detect the presence of fibroid tumors to outline the shape of the fetus.
Endometrial biopsy	Taking a sample of tissue from the lining of the uterus to test for abnormalities.
Episiotomy	Surgical incision of the perineum to facilitate the delivery process. Can prevent an irregular tearing of tissue during birth.
Fetal monitoring	Using electronic equipment placed on the mother's abdomen to monitor the baby's heart rate and strength of uterine contractions during labor.
Hymenectomy	Surgical removal of the hymen.
Hysterectomy	Surgical removal of the uterus.
Hysterosalpingography	Taking an x-ray after injecting radiopaque material into the uterus and oviducts.
Hysteroscopy	Inspection of the uterus using a special endoscope instrument.
Intrauterine device (IUD)	A device inserted into the uterus by a physician for the purpose of contraception.

(continued)

TABLE 23   *(continued)*

Procedure/Test	Description
Kegel exercises	Exercises named after A.H. Kegel, an American gynecologist, who developed them to strengthen female pelvic muscles. The exercises are useful in treating incontinence and as an aid in childbirth.
Laparoscopy	Examination of the peritoneal cavity using an instrument called a laparoscope. The instrument is passed through a small incision made by the surgeon into the peritoneal cavity.
Laparotomy	Making a surgical opening into the abdomen.
Oophorectomy	Surgical removal of an ovary.
Panhysterectomy	Excision of the entire uterus, including the cervix.
Panhysterosalpingo-oophorectomy	Surgical removal of the entire uterus, cervix, ovaries, and fallopian tubes. Also called a total hysterectomy.
PAP (Papanicolaou) smear	Test for the early detection of cancer of the cervix named after the developer of the test, George Papanicolaou, a Greek physician. A scraping of cells is removed from the cervix for examination under a microscope.
Pelvic examination	The physical examination of the vagina and adjacent organs performed by a physician by placing the fingers of one hand into the vagina. A visual examination is performed using a speculum.
Pelvimetry	Measurement of the pelvis to assist in determining if the birth canal will allow the passage of the fetus for a vaginal delivery.
Pelvic ultrasonography	The use of ultrasound waves to produce an image or photograph of organ or fetus.
Pregnancy test	A chemical test on urine that can determine pregnancy during the first few weeks. This can be performed in the physician's office or with an at-home test.
Salpingo-oophorectomy	Surgical removal of the fallopian tube and ovary.
Tubal ligation	Surgical tying off of the fallopian tube to prevent conception from taking place. This results in the sterilization of the female.

TABLE 24   Disorders of the Male Reproductive System

Disorder	Description
Anorchism	A congenital absence of one or both testes.
Aspermia	The lack of, or failure to, eject sperm.
Azoospermia	Absence of sperm in the semen.
Balanitis	Inflammation of the skin covering the glans penis.
Benign prostatic hypertrophy	Enlargement of the prostate gland commonly seen in males over 50.
Carcinoma of the testes	Cancer of one or both testes.
Cryptorchidism	Failure of the testes to descend into the scrotal sac before birth. Generally, the testes will descend permanently before the boy is one year old. A surgical procedure called an orchidopecy may be required to bring the testes down into the scrotum permanently and secure them permanently. Failure of the testes to descend could result in sterility in the male.
Epididymitis	Inflammation of the epididymis which causes pain and swelling in the inguinal area.
Epispadias	Congenital opening of the male urethra on the dorsal surface of the penis.
Hydrocele	Accumulation of fluid within the testes.
Hypospadias	Congenital opening of the male urethra on the underside of the penis.
Impotent	Inability to copulate due to inability to maintain an erection or to achieve orgasm.
Perineum	In the male, the external region between the scrotum and the anus.
Phimosis	Narrowing of the foreskin over the glans penis which results in difficulty with hygiene. The condition can lead to infection or difficulty with urination. The condition is treated with circumcision, the surgical removal of the foreskin.
Prostate cancer	A slow-growing cancer that affects a large number of males after 50. The PSA (prostate-specific antigen) test is used to assist in early detection of this disease.
Prostatic hyperplasia	Abnormal cell growth within the prostate.
Prostatitis	An inflamed condition of the prostate gland which may be the result of infection.
Varicocele	Enlargement of the veins of the spermatic cord which commonly occurs on the left side of adolescent males. This seldom needs treatment.

TABLE 25   Procedures and Diagnostic Tests Relating to the Male Reproductive System

Procedure/Test	Description
Castration	Excision of the testicles in the male or the ovaries in the female.
Cauterization	Destruction of tissue with an electric current, a caustic agent, hot iron, or by freezing.
Circumcision	Surgical removal of the end of the prepuce or foreskin of the penis. Generally performed on the newborn male at the request of the parents. The primary reason is for ease of hygiene. Circumcision is also a ritual practiced in some religions.
Orchidopexy	Surgical fixation to move undescended testes into the scrotum, and attaching them to prevent retraction.
Prostatectomy	Surgical removal of the prostate gland.
Sterilization	Process of rendering a male or female sterile or unable to conceive children.
Transurethral resection of the prostate (TUR)	Surgical removal of the prostate gland by inserting a device through the urethra and removing prostate tissue.
Vasectomy	Removal of a segment or all of the vas deferens to prevent sperm from leaving the male body. Used for contraception purposes. A bilateral vasectomy would render the male sterile.
Semen analysis	This procedure is used when performing a fertility workup to determine if the male is able to produce sperm. Sperm is collected by the patient after abstaining from sexual intercourse for a period of three to five days. Also used to determine if a vasectomy has been successful. After a period of six weeks, no further sperm should be present in a sample from the patient.

TABLE 26   Sexually Transmitted Diseases

Disease	Description
Acquired immune deficiency syndrome (AIDS)	The final stage of infection from the human immunodeficiency virus (HIV). At present there is no cure.
Candidiasis	A yeastlike infection of the skin and mucous membranes which can result in white plaques on the tongue and vagina.
Chancroid	Highly infectious nonsyphilitic ulcer.
Chlamydial infection	Parasitic microorganism causing genital infections in males and females. Can lead to pelvic inflammatory disease (PID) in females and eventual infertility.
Genital herpes	Growths and elevations of warts on the genitalia of both males and females which can lead to cancer of the cervix in females. These painful vesicles on the skin and mucosa erupt periodically and can be transmitted through the placenta or at birth.
Genital warts	Growths and elevations of warts on the genitalia of both males and females which can lead to cancer of the cervix in females. There is currently no cure.
Gonorrhea	Sexually transmitted inflammation of the mucous membranes of either sex. Can be passed on to an infant during the birth process.
Hepatitis	Infectious, inflammatory disease of the liver. Hepatitis B and C types are spread by contact with blood and bodily fluids of an infected person.
Syphilis	Infectious, chronic, venereal disease that can involve any organ. May exist for years without symptoms.
Trichomoniasis	Genitourinary infection that is usually without symptoms (asymptomatic) in both males and females. In women the disease can produce itching and/or burning, a foul-smelling discharge, and results in vaginitis.

TABLE 27   Genetic Disorders

Disorder	Description
Alopecia	Baldness in particular patterns, especially on the head.
Cooley's anemia	A rare form of anemia or a reduction of red blood cells which is found in some people of Mediterranean origin.
Cystic fibrosis	A disorder of the exocrine glands which causes these glands to produce abnormally thick secretions of mucus. The disease affects many organs, including the pancreas and the respiratory system. One reliable diagnostic test in children is the sweat test, which will show elevated sodium and potassium levels. There is presently no known cure for the disease, which can shorten the life span.
Down syndrome	A disorder which produces moderate-to-severe mental retardation and multiple defects. The physical characteristics of a child with this disorder are a sloping forehead, flat nose or absent bridge to the nose, low-set eyes, and a general dwarfed physical growth. The disorder occurs more commonly when the mother is over 40. Also called Trisomy 21.
Duchene muscular dystrophy	A muscular disorder in which there is progressive wasting away of various muscles, including leg, pelvic, and shoulder muscles. Children with this disorder have difficulty climbing stairs and running. They may eventually be confined to a wheelchair. Other complications relating to the heart and respiratory system can be present. It is caused by a recessive gene and is more common in males. This disorder often results in a shortened life-span.

(continued)

TABLE 27 *(continued)*

Disorder	Description
Hemophilia	A bleeding disorder in which there is a deficiency in one of the factors necessary for blood to clot. There is an abnormal tendency to bleed, and victims of this disorder may require frequent blood transfusions. The female (mother) carries this recessive gene and it is passed on to males. Therefore, it is found almost exclusively in boys.
Huntington's chorea	A rare condition characterized by bizarre involuntary movements called chorea. The patient may have progressive mental and physical disturbances, which generally begin around 40.
Retinitis pigmentosa	Chronic progressive disease that begins in early childhood and is characterized by degeneration of the retina. This can lead to blindness by middle age.
Sickle cell anemia	Severe, chronic, incurable disorder that results in anemia and causes joint pain, chronic weakness, and infections. Occurs more commonly in people of Mediterranean and African heritage. The blood cell in this disease is sickle shaped.
Spina bifida	A congenital disorder that results in a defect in the walls of the spinal column, causing the membranes of the spinal cord to push through to the outside. It may be associated with other defects, such as hydrocephalus, which is an enlarged head as a result of the accumulation of fluid on the brain.
Tay-Sachs disease	A disorder caused by a deficiency of an enzyme, which can result in mental and physical retardation and blindness. It is transferred by a recessive trait and is most commonly found in families of Eastern European Jewish decent. Death generally occurs before the age of 4.

TABLE 28   Respiratory Disorders and Pathology

Disorder	Description
Asthma	Disease caused by various conditions, such as allergens, and resulting in constriction of the bronchial airways and labored respirations. It can cause violent spasms of the bronchi (bronchospasms) but is not generally life-threatening. Medication can be very effective.
Atelectasis	A condition in which the lung tissue collapses, which prevents the respiratory exchange of oxygen and carbon dioxide. It can be caused by a variety of conditions, including pressure upon the lung from a tumor or other object.
Bronchiectasis	An abnormal stretching of the bronchi which results from a dilation of a bronchus or the bronchi that can be the result of an infection. The major symptom is a large amount of purulent (pus-filled) sputum. Rales (bubbling chest sounds) and hemoptysis (spitting up blood) may be present. This can be irreversible and may result in destruction of the bronchial walls.
Bronchitis	Inflammation of the mucous membranes of the bronchial tubes which results in a typical barking cough, fever, and **malaise** or discomfort.
Bronchogenic carcinoma	Malignant lung tumor that originates in the bronchi. It is usually associated with a history of cigarette smoking.
Chronic obstructive pulmonary disease (COPD)	Progressive, chronic, and usually irreversible condition in which the lungs have a diminished capacity for inspiration (inhalation) and expiration (exhalation). The patient may have difficulty breathing upon exertion (dyspnea) and a cough. Also called chronic obstructive lung disease.
Croup	An acute respiratory condition found in infants and children which is characterized by a barking type of cough or stridor.
Emphysema	Pulmonary condition that can occur as a result of long-term heavy smoking. Air pollution also worsens this disease. The patient may not be able to breath except in a sitting or standing position.
Empyema	Pus within the plural space, usually the result of infection.
Epistaxis	Nosebleed.
Histoplasmosis	A pulmonary disease from dust in the droppings of pigeons and chickens.
Hyaline membrane disease	Condition seen in premature infants whose lungs have not had time to develop properly. The lungs are not able to expand fully and a membrane (hyaline membrane) actually forms which causes extreme difficulty in breathing and may result in death. It is also known as infant respiratory distress syndrome (IRDS).
Laryngitis	Inflammation of the larynx (voicebox) causing difficulty in speaking.
Legionnaires' disease	Severe, often fatal disease characterized by pneumonia and gastrointestinal symptoms. It is caused by a gram-negative bacillus and named after people who came down with it at an American Legion Convention in 1976.
Paroxysmal nocturnal dyspnea	Attacks of shortness of breath (SOB) which occur only at night and awaken the patient.
Pertussis	Commonly called whooping cough, due to the "whoop" sound made when coughing. It is an infectious disease which children receive immunization against as part of their DPT shots.
Pleural effusion	The abnormal presence of fluid or gas in the pleural cavity. Physicians can detect the presence of fluid by tapping the chest (percussion) or listening with a stethoscope (auscultation).
Pleurisy	Inflammation of the pleura surrounding the lungs. The patient will experience pain upon inspiration due to friction caused by a rubbing of the pleural lining.
Pneumonia	Inflammatory condition of the lung which can be caused by bacterial and viral infections, diseases, and chemicals.
Pneumoconiosis	A condition that occurs as a result of inhaling environmental particles that become toxic. Can be the result of inhaling coal dust (anthracosis), or asbestos (asbestosis).
Pneumonomycosis	A disease of the lungs caused by a fungus.
Pneumothorax	Collection of air or gas in the pleural cavity which may result in collapse of the lung.
Pulmonary edema	Condition in which lung tissue retains an excessive amount of fluid. This results in labored breathing.

(continued)

TABLE 28 *(continued)*

Disorder	Description
Pulmonary embolism	Blood clot or air bubble that moves to the pulmonary artery or one of its branches.
Respiratory distress syndrome (RDS)	Impairment of the respiratory function in premature infants due to immaturity.
Silicosis	A form of respiratory disease resulting from the inhalation of silica (quartz) dust. It is considered an occupational disease.
Sudden infant death syndrome (SIDS)	Unexpected and unexplained death of an apparently well infant.
Tracheostenosis	A narrowing and stenosis of the lumen or opening into the trachea.
Tuberculosis	An infectious disease caused by the tubercle bacillus, Mycobacterium tuberculosis. It most commonly affects the respiratory system and causes inflammation and calcification of the system. Tuberculosis is again on the uprise and is seen in many patients who have an impaired immune system, such as in AIDS.

TABLE 29 Procedures and Tests Relating to the Respiratory System

Procedure/Test	Description
Arterial blood gases	Testing for the gases present in the blood. This test is generally used to assist in determining the levels of oxygen (O_2) and carbon dioxide (CO_2) in the blood.
Bronchography	X-ray of the lung after a radiopaque substance has been inserted into the trachea or bronchial tube.
Bronchoplasty	The surgical repair of a bronchial defect.
Bronchoscopy	Using an instrument, the bronchoscope, to visualize the bronchi. During this procedure, tissue can be obtained for biopsy and foreign bodies can be removed.
Bronchotomy	A surgical incision of a bronchus, larynx, or trachea.
Cardiopulmonary resuscitation (CPR)	Emergency treatment provided by persons trained in CPR given to patients when their respirations and heart stop. CPR provides oxygen to the brain, heart, and other vital organs until medical treatment can restore a normal heart and pulmonary function. See an illustration of adult and infant CPR in Chapter 35.
Chest x-ray	Taking a radiographic picture of the lungs and heart from the back and front of the patient.
Endotracheal intubation	Placing a tube through the mouth to create an airway.
Heimlich maneuver	A technique for removing a foreign body from the trachea or pharynx by exerting diaphragmatic pressure.
Hyperbaric oxygen therapy	The use of oxygen under greater than normal pressure to treat cases of smoke inhalation, carbon monoxide poisoning, and other conditions. In some cases, the patient is placed in a hyperbaric oxygen chamber for this treatment.
Intermittent positive pressure breathing (IPPB)	A method for assisting the breathing of patients with a mask that is connected to a machine that produces an increased pressure.
Laryngectomy	The surgical removal of the larynx. This procedure is most frequently performed for excision of cancer.
Laryngoplasty	Surgical repair of the larynx.
Laryngoscopy	Examination of the interior of the larynx with a lighted instrument.
Lobectomy	Surgical removal of a lobe of the lung. Often the treatment of choice for lung cancer.
Pneumonectomy	The surgical removal of lung tissue.
Postural drainage	Drainage of secretions from the bronchi by placing the patient in a position that uses gravity to promote drainage. It is used for the treatment of cystic fibrosis, bronchiectasis, and before lobectomy surgery. May be combined with clapping and vibrating maneuvers to dislodge secretions.
Pulmonary angiography	Injecting dye into a blood vessel for the purpose of taking an x-ray of the arteries and veins of the lungs.
Pulmonary function test (PFT)	Breathing equipment used to determine respiratory function and measure lung volumes and gas exchange. Also called spirometry.
Rhinoplasty	Plastic surgery of the nose performed for cosmetic reasons and to facilitate breathing.
Sinus x-ray	An x-ray view of the sinus cavities from the front of the head.
Spirometry	Using a device to measure the breathing capacity of the lungs.
Sputum culture and sensitivity (CS)	Testing sputum by placing it on a culture medium and observing any bacterial growth. The specimen is then tested to determine antibiotic effectiveness.
Sputum cytology	Testing for malignant cells in sputum.
Throat culture	Removing a small sample of tissue or material from the pharynx and placing it upon a culture medium to determine bacterial growth.
Thoracentesis	The surgical puncture of the chest wall for the removal of fluids.
Thoracostomy	An insertion of a tube into the chest for the purpose of draining off fluid or air.
Tracheotomy	Surgical incision into the trachea to provide an airway. This is generally performed as an emergency procedure to provide oxygen.
Tuberculin skin tests (TB test)	Applying a chemical agent (Tine or Mantoux tests) under the surface of the skin to determine if the patient has been exposed to tuberculosis.

TABLE 30   Disorders and Diseases of the Urinary System

Disorder/Disease	Description
Anuria	No urine formed by the kidneys and a complete lack of urine excretion.
Bladder neck obstruction	Blockage of the bladder outlet.
Dysuria	Abnormal secretion of large amounts of urine.
Enuresis	Involuntary discharge of urine after the age by which bladder control should have been established. This usually occurs by the age of 5. Also called bed-wetting at night.
Glomerulonephritis	Inflammation of the kidney (primarily of the glomerulus). Since the glomerular membrane is inflamed, it becomes more permeable and this results in protein (proteinuria) and blood (hematuria) in the urine.
Hematuria	A condition of blood in the urine. This is a symptom of disease process.
Hypospadius	A congenital opening of the male urethra on the underside of the penis.
Interstitial cystitis	Disease of an unknown cause in which there is inflammation and irritation of the bladder. It is most commonly seen in middle-aged women.
Lithotomy	Surgical incision to remove kidney stones.
Meatotomy	A surgical enlargement of the urinary opening (meatus).
Nocturia	Excessive urination during the night. This may or may not be abnormal.
Pyelitis	Inflammation of the renal pelvis.
Pyelonephritis	Inflammation of the renal pelvis and the kidney. This is one of the most common types of kidney disease. It may be the result of a lower urinary tract infection that moved up to the kidney via the ureters. There may be large quantities of white blood cells and bacteria in the urine. Hematuria may also be present. This condition can occur whenever there is an untreated or persistent case of cystitis.
Pyuria	Presence of pus in the urine.
Renal colic	Pain caused by a kidney stone. This type of pain can be excruciating and generally requires medical treatment.

TABLE 31   Procedures and Tests Relating to the Urinary System

Procedure/Test	Description
Catheterization	The insertion of a sterile tube through the urethra and into the urinary bladder for the purpose of withdrawing urine. This procedure is used to obtain a sterile urine specimen and also to relieve distension when the patient is unable to void on their own. See Chapter 26 for procedure.
Cystography	The process of instilling a contrast material or dye into the bladder by catheter to visualize the urinary bladder.
Cystoscopy	Visual examination of the urinary bladder using an instrument called a cystoscope. The patient may receive a general anesthetic for this procedure.
Dialysis	The artificial filtration of waste material from the blood. It is used when the kidneys fail to function.
Excretory urography	Injection of dye into the bloodstream followed by taking an x-ray to trace the action of the kidney as it excretes the dye.
Hemodialysis	Use of an artificial kidney that filters the blood of a person to remove waste products. Use of this technique in patients who have defective kidneys is lifesaving.
Intravenous pyelogram (IVP)	An x-ray examination of the kidneys, ureters, and bladder by injecting a radiopaque dye into the circulatory system and tracing its route as it is excreted.
Lithotripsy	Destroying or crushing kidney stones in the bladder or urethra with a device called a lithotriptor.
Peritoneal dialysis	The removal of toxic waste substances from the body by placing warm chemically balanced solutions into the peritoneal cavity. This is used in treating renal failure and in certain types of poisonings.
Renal transplant	Surgical placement of a donor kidney.
Urinalysis	A laboratory test that consists of the physical, chemical, and microscopic examination of urine.
Urography	The use of a contrast medium to provide an x-ray of the urinary tract.

INDEX